*Third Edition*

# Psychosocial Aspects of Health Care

**Meredith E. Drench, PT, PhD**
*Director*
*Adaptive Health Associates, Inc.*
*East Greenwich, RI*
*Adjunct Faculty*
*Department of Physical Therapy*
*Northeastern University, Boston, MA*

**Ann Cassidy Noonan, PT, EdD**
*Associate Professor*
*Physical Therapy Program Director*
*Brooks College of Health*
*Department of Clinical and Applied Movement Sciences*
*University of North Florida, Jacksonville, FL*

**Nancy Sharby, PT, DPT, MS**
*Associate Clinical Professor*
*Department of Physical Therapy*
*Northeastern University, Boston, MA*

**Susan H. Ventura, PT, MEd, PhD**
*Associate Clinical Professor*
*Department of Physical Therapy*
*Northeastern University, Boston, MA*

**Pearson**
Boston   Columbus   Indianapolis   New York   San Francisco   Upper Saddle River
Amsterdam   Cape Town   Dubai   London   Madrid   Milan   Munich   Paris   Montreal   Toronto
Delhi   Mexico City   Sao Paulo   Sydney   Hong Kong   Seoul   Singapore   Taipei   Tokyo

**Publisher:** Julie Levin Alexander
**Publisher's Assistant:** Regina Bruno
**Editor-in-Chief:** Mark Cohen
**Executive Editor:** John Goucher
**Development Editor:** Melissa Kerian
**Editorial Assistant:** Rosalie Hawley
**Marketing Manager:** Katrin Beacom
**Marketing Specialist:** Michael Sirinides
**Marketing Assistant:** Crystal Gonzalez
**Production Liaison:** Frances Russello
**Full Service Production and Composition:** Nitin Agarwal/Aptara®, Inc.
**Art Director:** Jayne Conte
**Cover Image:** Javarman/Shutterstock
**Cover Designer:** Bruce Kenselaar
**Printing and Binding:** Edwards Brothers
**Cover Printing:** Lehigh Phoenix

The names contained in the journal entries found in this book are fictitious. Any connection to real people is unintended.

Notice: The authors and the publisher of this volume have taken care that the information and technical recommendations contained herein are based on research and expert consultation, and are accurate and compatible with the standards generally accepted at the time of publication. Nevertheless, as new information becomes available, changes in clinical and technical practices become necessary. The reader is advised to carefully consult manufacturers' instructions and information material for all supplies and equipment before use, and to consult with a healthcare professional as necessary. This advice is especially important when using new supplies or equipment for clinical purposes. The authors and publisher disclaim all responsibility for any liability, loss, injury, or damage incurred as a consequence, directly or indirectly, of the use and application of any of the contents of this volume.

**Library of Congress Cataloging-in-Publication Data**
Psychosocial aspects of health care / Meredith E. Drench . . . [et al.].—3rd ed.
    p. cm.
   Includes bibliographical references and index.
   ISBN-13: 978-0-13-139218-2 (alk. paper)
   ISBN-10: 0-13-139218-2 (alk. paper)
   1. Clinical health psychology.   2. Medical personnel and patient.   3. Social medicine.
I. Drench, Meredith E.
   R726.7.P7953 2012
   610.69'6—dc22

                                                   2010037232

10 9 8 7 6 5 4 3 2 1

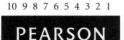

www.pearsonhighered.com

ISBN 10:    0-13-139218-2
ISBN 13: 978-0-13-139218-2

## Dedication

*To our clients, for teaching us the art of healing and reinforcing the need to integrate psychosocial concerns into our therapeutic interventions*

*To our colleagues, for their collaboration, mutual teaching, and learning*

*To our families, for supporting, loving, and sharing us with this project*

*To our students, that they may understand that a key ingredient for clinical competence and professional excellence is based on compassion and understanding*

# CONTENTS

# PART IV  Transitions Across the Lifespan 221

# PREFACE

*Psychosocial Aspects of Health Care* addresses a variety of integrated psychosocial topics, involving clients, families, and other caregivers affected by pathology, impairment, functional limitation, or disability. This book is intended for students in the health care professions, such as nurses, physical and occupational therapists, speech-language pathologists, physicians and physician assistants, respiratory therapists, social workers, and students in medical laboratory sciences. The text may also serve as a reference for those already practicing in their respective disciplines.

As a textbook, *Psychosocial Aspects of Health Care* could fit well into various levels of the curriculum, incorporated into basic, intermediate, and advanced courses. It is appropriate wherever a course specifically addresses or includes psychosocial aspects of illness and disability, such as courses in social psychology of disability and rehabilitation, chronic illness, and rehabilitation psychology. This textbook would also be useful in courses that include issues in communication, family relationships, client–professional relationships, characteristics of illness and disability, adaptation to impairment and disability, manifestations of client behavior, grieving and adjusting to loss, sources of stress and support, and attitudinal and cultural differences. In addition, the text will also assist clinicians in identifying possible cases of abuse or neglect across the life span, making recommendations to appropriate referral sources, and caring for adult survivors of child sexual abuse.

We had three compelling reasons to write such a text. The primary purpose was to help readers understand that a key ingredient for clinical competence and professional excellence is the human factor. Second, we strongly believe in the need for clinicians to understand psychosocial aspects of health care so that they may best help patients/clients optimize their therapeutic outcomes. This foundation area is often overlooked or devalued in favor of the "hard-core" components of health care. Last, as educators with collectively over 100 years of experience with clients and students, we are concerned with the reported and perceived lack of students' interest in textbooks, level of readership, and appreciation of the importance of this subject in their treatment armamentarium. We believe that the style and approach of this book will hold readers' attention and enhance their understanding of the material.

The book is divided into five parts, each subdivided into chapters. Relevant clinical examples are interspersed throughout each chapter, punctuating topic points. Student journal entries introduce and are entwined throughout every chapter, reinforcing the subject and identifying biases and "too-quick" conclusions. The description and reflection of realistic clinical situations add to the fabric of the discussion, creating a real-life case study, an actual client problem.

Part I, "Knowing Self/Knowing Others," addresses the foundations of health care, including client–professional relationships, health care ethics, and models of care; components of recognizing your own attitudes, beliefs, and values as a health provider; multicultural perspectives of therapeutic care; and spirituality in health care and the connections of the mind, body, and spirit. Part II, "Making Connections," explores communication and the client interview, as well as motivation, adherence, and collaborative treatment planning. Part III, "Loss/Grief, Coping, and Family," delves into understanding loss, grief, and adjustment as related to disease, disability, and death, as well as discerning family needs, roles, and responsibilities. Part IV, "Transitions Across the Life Span," presents issues of disability, chronic conditions, and sexuality. Finally, Part V, "Conditions That Challenge Care," considers psychiatric disorders, self-destructive behaviors, and abuse and neglect.

Because readers of this text come from many health care disciplines, each with its own jargon, we have had to make editorial decisions for the sake of consistency. We have used *client* to name those with whom we work. *Caregiver* refers to personal caregivers and may be family, friends, or others with caregiving responsibilities. Variations of *health care professionals* and *health care providers* represent the readership, those who have chosen to make a career of providing care. Examples of clients and caregivers reflect both the diversity and life-span issues inherent in today's health care environment. Similarly, the health professions and the students in the journal entries also depict our changing world.

Reflective Questions and Case Studies with topical questions, both popular features of earlier editions, conclude each chapter of the text. Based on our own experience and the feedback of other faculty and students who have used this text in learning about psychosocial aspects of health care, these will continue to allow individual musings, classroom discussion, small-group exercises, and student assignments.

This third edition includes updated information and references, where applicable, a change in sequencing and renaming of some of the chapters and parts, an integration of some topics with others, and an expansion and addition of some areas. There is also the introduction of both an online Instructors' Manual and a Student Workbook at www.myhealthprofessionskit.com. Additional Readings, suggested to engage readers in further personal accounts, histories, and insights, have been updated and included in the new complementary online teaching tools rather than at the end of each part as they were in the first and second editions. Readers will develop self-awareness as they learn more about the psychosocial issues of health care.

# ACKNOWLEDGMENTS

A work of this nature is not created in a vacuum. We express our thanks and gratitude to all those who have helped us in our journey toward the publication of this book. Throughout our lives, many have nurtured us, taught us how to nurture others, and provided lessons in the costs and rewards of caregiving.

Special thanks to our families and friends, who supported us throughout this project. They have forgiven our absences from social events and family meals, as well as late hours spent at the computer, rather than in front of the fire.

We also thank the many educators who have facilitated our development, including George Goldin, Ruthie Hall, Ruth Purtilo, Shirley Stockmeyer, Fran Tappan, and Marie Winston. They helped shape our ability to provide skilled and compassionate care that is based on a strong moral and ethical foundation.

We are grateful for the review and critique of selected material by David Borrelli, MD, Psychiatrist, Massachusetts General Hospital, for his time, wisdom, and clarification of the psychiatric concepts. We appreciate the insights of the people at the Manic Depressive-Depressive Association, McLean Hospital Chapter, whose struggles and successes of living with mental illness remind us of the resilience of the human spirit.

We also acknowledge the members of our professional communities, who challenge and guide us. Northeastern University and the University of North Florida, in particular, facilitated this endeavor by providing a climate conducive to intellectual pursuits. Special thanks to our graduate assistants for the hours spent "in the stacks."

Finally, we recognize Mark Cohen, Editor-in-Chief, and Melissa Kerian, development editor, at Pearson Health Science, for their belief in this project and its valuable contribution to health care.

# REVIEWERS

## Reviewers of the Third Edition

Denise Abrams, PT, DPT, MA
*Broome Community College*
*Binghamton, New York*

Linda M. Barnes, MSED, OT/L
*Pennsylvania College of Technology*
*Williamsport, Pennsylvania*

Linda Biggers, PT, MHS, CLT
*University of Indianapolis*
*Indianapolis, Indiana*

Kathy Dieruf, PT, PhD, NCS
*University of New Mexico*
*Albuquerque, New Mexico*

Cindy Kief, ND, COTA/L, CAPS, ROH
*Cincinnati State College Technical*
*and Community College*
*Cincinnati, Ohio*

Claudia Miller, OTD, OTR/L
*Cincinnati State College Technical and*
*Community College*
*Cincinnati, Ohio*

Leslie Russek, PT, DPT, PhD, OCS
*Clarkson University*
*Potsdam, New York*

Ann Vendrely, PT, DPT, EdD
*Governors State University*
*University Park, Illinois*

## Reviewers of Previous Editions

Denise Abrams, PT, DPT, MA
*Broome Community College*
*Binghamton, New York*

Debbie Amini, EdD, OTR/L, CHT
*Cape Fear Community College*
*Wilmington, North Carolina*

Sherry Borcherding, MA, OTR/L
*University of Missouri*
*Columbia, Missouri*

Donna Calvert, PhD, PT
*Rockhurst University*
*Kansas City, Missouri*

Larry Chinnock, PT, EdD, MBA
*Loma Linda University*
*Loma Linda, California*

Kimberly K. Cleary, PhD, PT
*Idaho State University*
*Pocatello, Idaho*

Peggy DeCelle Newman, PT, MHR
*Oklahoma City Community College*
*Oklahoma City, Oklahoma*

Elaine Eckel, PT, MA
*Fayetteville Technical Community*
*College*
*Fayetteville, North Carolina*

Joan E. Edelstein, MA, PT, FISPO
*Columbia University*
*New York, New York*

Yolanda Griffiths, OTD, OTR/L, FAOTA
*Creighton University Medical Center*
*Omaha, Nebraska*

Christine Helfrich, PhD, OTR/L, FAOTA
*University of Illinois at Chicago*
*Chicago, Illinois*

Cathy Hinton, PhD, PT
*Belmont University*
*Nashville, Tennessee*

Debbie Ingram, PT, EdD
*University of Tennessee at Chattanooga*
*Chattanooga, Tennessee*

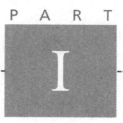

# Knowing Self/ Knowing Others

# 1

# Foundations

I still can't get over the conversation I had with my client Paula today. Apparently, the orthopedic surgeon came by to discuss her surgery. What impressed her most was the amount of time that he spent with her. He perched himself on the edge of her bed, asked her about her concerns, and then actually listened and responded to them! First, she shared her fears about anesthesia and that the surgery might make things worse. She had expected him to be interested in that much. But then he asked her about her home life, what her duties would be upon discharge, and how she planned to deal with the fact that she would have to remain on bedrest for several days after the surgery. She felt that he really cared about her answers. He also took the time to draw a picture for her so that she would clearly understand just what would happen in the operating room. He assured her that everyone who touched her would be as gentle as possible. As if to prove his point, he gently touched her arm. Once she was fully comfortable with the explanation, he continued to chat for a few minutes longer, even getting her to laugh at a joke or two. Only then did he ask her to sign a consent form. She felt like she was this doctor's only patient. I wonder how he knew the best approach to dispel Paula's fears.

—*From the journal of Antonella Molinari, nursing student*

The approach taken by the physician described above to prepare his patient for surgery amazed the nursing student who witnessed her client's encounter. She wondered how the surgeon knew how to address her client's fears so effectively. Some psychosocial skills come naturally to health professionals, but many are not intuitive and must be taught. Students often inaccurately assume that the knowledge about how to perform sensitive and effective client interactions is merely common sense. This could not be further from the truth. Much of what we know to guide our clinical decisions relies on research used to standardize care. Evidence from multiple disciplines, including biology, physiology, pharmacology, psychology, sociology, medical anthropology, and ethics, informs clinical practice (Shepard, 2007).

Just as each health care provider is a unique person with individual talents, skills, strengths, and weaknesses, so too is each client. Common sense may tell us that the best course of care is to treat every client the same, but research tells us otherwise. It is important to account for unique cultural beliefs and values, as well as personal experiences that determine what style of interaction is most effective for good clinical outcomes. What we say and do matters, as does how we say and do it. In this chapter, we lay the foundation for the best practices that can be used to establish relationships with clients, make ethical decisions to guide clinical practice, and create inviting environments of care that foster comfort and support.

## CLIENT–PROFESSIONAL RELATIONSHIPS

Health care providers must remember that it is always the providers' responsibility to establish and maintain effective relationships with their clients. We cannot expect clients to change their beliefs or values to be congruent with ours or to put aside their personal pain or discouragement when they are in distress. Think about who you might consider to be a "good" client. Is it the person who is quiet, pleasant, grateful, and adherent? How would you feel about working with people who have different beliefs or those who challenge our sense of authority? What about clients who are "unmotivated" or nonadherent or those who are depressed or "needy?" Do we consider it part of our responsibility to address issues of substance abuse or domestic violence? It is, in fact, our professional obligation to identify and address all of our clients' needs and use evidence-based knowledge to develop individualized treatment plans that respond to psychosocial, as well as physical, concerns. It is the only way we will be able to achieve optimal outcomes. Attention to the concepts summarized below will help early career practitioners establish and hone their interaction skills.

### Boundaries

A good relationship between a client and a health care provider depends on effective communication, mutual respect, and shared trust. Clients have a relatively dependent and vulnerable role in the relationship, and it is important for them to communicate their needs to providers as honestly and effectively as possible.

Emotional boundaries are complex and difficult. Compassion is essential, and this requires emotional involvement but only to a certain point. The clinician must maintain enough emotional distance to preserve professional judgment and objectivity. It is important to avoid establishing friendships or romantic relationships with clients, which is in conflict with maintaining the professional distance required in the health care relationship.

Clinicians must also be careful about disclosing personal information to clients. Although we want to invite clients into warm and engaging professional relationships, an essential concept to remember is that the relationship is always for the benefit of the client, never the provider. The differences between personal and professional relationships are significant. Personal relationships are mutual in nature and serve the needs of all participants equally. The parties engage in a reciprocal give-and-take relationship, with each expecting to give and receive support and attention. Unlike family or friends, however, clients pay money to spend time with health care providers. They are entitled to receive health care services, empathy, and compassion but should never feel the need to return the same. Developing and honoring professional boundaries works to ensure that clients' interests remain central in the health care relationship. Before making decisions or taking any action, ask yourself, "What are the client's needs?" and "How will this help him (or her)?"

The health professional is responsible for establishing and maintaining financial, emotional, and physical boundaries (Jacobson, 2002). Financial expectations should be clearly defined. If an insurance company is to be billed, the client must agree to this in advance. If the client is to provide a copayment at the time of the visit, this should be made clear, too. At times, clients wish to express their gratitude by giving health care providers small gifts. Many employers have formal policies about employees accepting gifts, and these policies must be observed. It is generally felt to be ethical to accept small gifts, such as a batch of home-baked cookies, a box of candy, or flowers, but some gifts are clearly inappropriate. These include money, gifts of a personal nature, such as clothing or jewelry, and expensive gifts, such as theater tickets. It is helpful to let clients know at the beginning of the relationship what these boundaries are. Some clinics post discreet signs or include this with other relevant information in brochures that are distributed to clients. This can help prevent embarrassment or hurt feelings.

Touch is another important element in the healing relationship. Because touch is also associated with personal relationships, it is critical that the touch we use in health care not be confused with personal touch. As highlighted in Chapter 3, comforting touch and other physical boundaries are culturally sensitive. It is important to acknowledge and respect the client's personal space and enter into this only with permission. This can be accomplished by providing the client with advanced warning, such as, "I would like to look in your ears" or "May I take a look at that shoulder now?"

## Preservation of Dignity

I began my rotation in the cardiac care unit at the hospital today and was appalled by what I saw. An older woman came in to have a stress echocardiogram. The client never had this experience before and was noticeably anxious. She waited in the room wearing only a thin johnny. Soon the male technician came in and began setting her up by exposing her chest and putting her in the correct position. The client was quite alarmed and said, "Who are you?" He seemed surprised that she asked and stated, "Oh, I'm Jack!" "No," she said, "What is your job? What do you do here?" Somehow Jack didn't think it was important for him to explain his role or even provide his name.

—*From the journal of Meredith Spencer, nursing student*

A client's dignity is threatened in the presence of illness or impairment because the client's self-image of the past may be inconsistent with the present (Chochinov, 2004). The threat to dignity may be the primary source of the client's anxiety about the medical visit. By doing everything possible to eliminate this threat, the provider can minimize the client's anxiety. This can be as simple as observing common courtesies, such as knocking before entering a treatment or examination room, introducing yourself appropriately, and demonstrating warmth and concern. It is also helpful to apologize to clients if they are inconvenienced by unavoidable delays or offended by something we have said or done. In addition, even when providers are personally offended or flustered, composure needs to be maintained, putting their own needs aside in favor of clients' needs (White, 1999). The role of health care providers is to serve clients. This means that goals must be client centered. Providers have a responsibility to carefully plan treatments, think critically about choices, and review any information about which they feel uncertain. An important goal of client interactions is to achieve mutual respect.

Medical examinations involve taking a history, asking about personal and social circumstances, and inquiring about spiritual beliefs and values. When collecting this information, it is important to honor the client's right to privacy and do whatever possible to help preserve his or her dignity. Be certain that what is being asked is needed to establish or clarify treatment goals rather than as a means to get to know the client on a personal basis. Clients generally seek a feeling of security in the health care relationship, which can be established only if there is mutual trust and respect, and the client's dignity is preserved. They deserve to feel that they are genuinely respected, which providers can demonstrate by utilizing effective communication skills, such as active listening, appropriate education, and answering questions with thoughtful answers.

## Trust, Respect, and Compassion

Although we cannot always cure clients (eliminate health concerns), we can always facilitate healing (making or restoring a sense of wholeness). No matter how sophisticated the technology of health care becomes, healing relies on three simple human elements: compassion, touch, and conversation (Sulmasy, 1997). The physician described in the journal entry at the beginning of this chapter displayed each of these important elements. In doing so, he invited the patient to enter into a trusting relationship. Just because the invitation is extended, though, does not ensure that the client will accept it. Trust does not come easily in today's health care environment. By definition, trust involves risk and uncertainty, which can create anxiety (Sulmasy, 1997). Some people will do almost anything to avoid the latter.

Consider the case of Rob Jones, a 42-year-old lawyer who sought medical care for frequent headaches. He had avoided seeing a doctor, assuming his headaches were stress related and that nothing could be done. However, he became frightened when his cousin had a stroke and died. Although his doctor had little reason to believe that Rob was at risk for a stroke, Rob demanded a magnetic resonance imaging (MRI) test to avoid the anxiety of uncertainty. He even went so far as to threaten his doctor with a malpractice suit if he did not order the test. Because of his own need to avoid risk, the physician ordered the test.

There are many barriers to developing a trusting health care relationship. One that is all too common occurs when clients feel rushed during medical encounters. The ability to understand and absorb information can be seriously hampered by this, especially when coupled with the stress that clients report feeling when they discuss matters of failing health.

Specialization of care creates another barrier (Amalberti, Auroy, Berwick, & Barach, 2005). Specialists work within their own "silos," and little infrastructure exists to facilitate integration of information across specialties. As a result, clients are left to sort out information, some of which may be conflicting. Clients may feel overwhelmed, confused, and discouraged. At times, the burden of care may seem greater than the potential benefits (D'Incà et al., 2008).

The involvement of third-party payers is another barrier to developing trust. Trust between clients and health care professionals can be affected by clients' knowledge that other people will view their medical records. As a result, they may be reluctant to share certain information, such as drug or alcohol problems, psychiatric symptoms, abuse, sexual dysfunction, or incontinence.

Growing commercialism in medicine is another source of mistrust. Commercial advertising of medications, for-profit ownership of hospitals, and other commercial aspects of health care are common, and this has contributed to a perception of decreased professionalism and an increased focus on profits. Providers are always obligated to place clients' interests above their own. This includes avoiding conflicts of interest, such as owning stock in drug companies, health maintenance organizations, and medical equipment companies. Providers are frequently called on to advocate for their clients, particularly when third-party payers have denied health care benefits. In the best interest of clients, providers should remain free from conflicts of interest to ensure availability to act as advocates whenever and wherever required.

Health care, as a commercial enterprise, relegates clients to the role of consumers, who are empowered by lawsuits when they believe they have not obtained the outcomes for which they have paid (Stelfox, 2005). This threatens the ability of health providers to trust clients. As clients and practitioners get to know one another, a sense of security, trust, and respect either grows or diminishes. An effective practitioner does whatever he or she is able to do to establish relationships based on the virtues of client-centered care, but success is not always possible. Clinics can be understaffed, and people may come from many cultures, speaking different languages. Whenever a provider does not feel compassion for a particular client or believes that he or she cannot trust a client, that provider has a responsibility to refer the client elsewhere for care.

Consider the case of Renate Justin, a Jewish physician, who reported on a client experience that was influenced by prejudice and strong emotional overtones. A patient was referred to her because they both spoke German. Unaware that her new physician was Jewish, the patient spoke freely during her initial visit, revealing that she was involved in the Nazi party and had been assigned to supervise Jewish slave labor during World War II. Her story was riddled with slanderous remarks about the Jewish slaves under her watch. Dr. Justin was able to contain her emotional response in the presence of the patient. After serious personal deliberation and soul-searching, she decided that, although she felt capable of providing basic medical care to this patient, she also had a duty to let the patient know that she was Jewish. She experienced significant relief when the patient opted to change providers (Justin, 2000).

Dr. Justin believed that she could feel compassion for her patient because of her medical illness but doubted that she could establish trust and respect for the patient. In spite of this, she believed that it would be possible to treat the patient (Justin, 2000). Health care professionals have a duty to put the client's needs first and examine potential conflicts from the client's point of view.

The Hippocratic oath (Figure 1–1), long accepted as the "fundamental expression of medical ethics," extends to all health care professionals who work to bring about benefit to the client (Bulger & Barbato, 2000, p. S7). There have been many modifications to this original oath. In fact, physicians now have a choice about which oath they take, but many of the ideals expressed in the Hippocratic oath still apply today. These include making the commitment to remain competent through continuing education, caring for clients in a way that always seeks what is best for clients, respecting and keeping clients' personal information confidential, and avoiding any behavior that takes advantage of the clients' dependence and vulnerability. Because of a significant increase in diagnostic and treatment options, we now also have the obligation to provide care in a way that reflects responsible utilization of services in the interest of all clients and the health care system (Minogue, 2000).

"I will look upon him who shall have taught me this art even as one of my parents. I will share my substance with him, and will supply his necessities, if he be in need. I will regard his offspring even as my own brethren, and I will teach them this art, if they would learn it, without fee or covenant. I will impart this art by precept, by lecture, and by every mode of teaching, not only to my own sons but to sons of him who has taught me, and to disciples bound by covenant and oath, according to the law of medicine. The regimen I adopt shall be for the benefit of my patients according to my ability and judgment, and not for their hurt or for any wrong. I will give no deadly drug to any, though it be asked of me, nor will I counsel such, and especially will I not aid a woman to procure abortion. Whatsoever house I enter, there will I go for the benefit of the sick, refraining from all wrongdoing or corruption, and especially from an act of seduction of male or female, of bond or free. Whatsoever things I see or hear concerning the life of men, in my attendance upon the sick or even apart therefrom, which ought not to be noised abroad, I will keep silence thereon, counting such things to be as sacred secrets.

**FIGURE 1–1**   The Original Hippocratic Oath   (*Source:* Bulger & Barbato, 2000, p. S6.)

## HEALTH CARE ETHICS

Providers' responsibilities to both clients and the health care system are often divergent, causing daily ethical dilemmas in health care. A *dilemma* is a conflict that requires careful consideration of all possible solutions to identify the one that balances the interests of all involved. The guidelines for solving health care dilemmas lie in the legal and ethical parameters defined specifically for each health care profession. The first determination is always to ensure that the proposed solutions are legal. If not, they are immediately ruled out. If they are legal, ethical principles are then applied to ensure that the interests of all parties are observed.

Ethics complement legal guidelines, which stem from federal, state, and local laws, as well as case law. Federal legislation governs the "big picture," known as the health care system, guiding the practices of insurance companies, health maintenance organizations, and government subsidies, including Medicare. Each state then governs the activities of its own hospitals, Medicaid programs, and the medical professionals who practice within its borders. Professional practice acts, established within each state, outline the guidelines that medical practitioners must agree to follow to become and remain licensed. Case law provides an historical collection of legal decisions that help to interpret medical questions brought before the courts.

Ethics are a set of moral principles that serve as a guiding philosophy for behavior. They help to ensure that health providers make the best possible decisions that honor the rights of clients. Most professional practice acts adopt the related professions' code of ethics within their legal guidelines. However, health care ethics can also be examined by using professionally neutral frameworks that provide a common basic language across disciplines.

Beauchamp and Childress (2001) introduced an approach that relies on four basic ethical principles: autonomy, beneficence, nonmaleficence, and justice. Others endorse this model (Adedeji, Sokol, Palser, & McKneally, 2009; Breier-Mackie, 2008). It provides a simple means to examine all possible solutions to an ethical dilemma, with respect to these four ethical principles, in order to identify the one best solution. It is important to acknowledge that this model of ethical decision making reflects health care practices and systems typical of Western cultures. Clinicians engaged in the care of clients who are from other cultures may need to modify their approach to meet the individualized needs of clients, as discussed in Chapter 3.

In a case described in the previous section, Rob insisted on having a MRI to rule out the risk of a stroke. The physician might have chosen another route if he had used this approach to solving his dilemma. In the interest of *autonomy*, clients have the right to request any diagnostic or treatment option that they believe might be helpful. Rob felt that the MRI was needed to rule out the possibility of stroke and to reduce his stress. *Beneficence* requires health care practitioners to do whatever is in the best interest of their clients. Because the MRI would probably reduce the client's stress and rule out certain differential diagnoses, it could be considered to be in Rob's best interest. *Nonmaleficence* requires the provider to do no harm. The known risks of MRI are minimal and, therefore, probably not an issue. *Justice*, however, was not upheld in this case. Justice requires that resources be distributed responsibly. The physician in this case did not honor this ethical principle. By choosing lower cost diagnostics, prior to proceeding with a more expensive test, he may have been able to honor all four ethical principles.

## Autonomy

Autonomy, or self-determination, calls for a client–provider relationship based on trust, respect, truthfulness, information sharing, and confidentiality. The right to informed consent is rooted in this principle. Most clients exercise their right to autonomy by requesting full disclosure of their medical condition and options for treatment. However, others may prefer to leave the decision making to family members or the provider. Whatever option is preferred by the client is the appropriate one for that particular client.

The legal doctrine of informed consent stems from autonomy and the right to self-determination; that is, adults who are of sound mind have the right to make their own decisions about medical care. Although verbal consent may have been enough in the early days of this mandate, written consent is required for legal protection today and must be kept with clients' records. Several issues must be addressed in the process: (1) Clients must be informed in a language that they can understand (lay terms and in their primary language), (2) all risks and benefits must be outlined, (3) any and all reasonable alternatives must be discussed, and (4) clients must sign a statement that indicates their understanding and acceptance of the treatment. This right can be waived in certain situations. For example, consent can be assumed if a client is brought into an emergency department in an unconscious state. Treatment can also be administered without parental consent in some cases, particularly if a legal mandate supports the decision. One of the best illustrations of this occurs when a parent refuses lifesaving treatment for a minor child based on religious beliefs. A court can order a health care facility to provide the treatment necessary to save that child's life (Yale-New Haven Hospital & Yale University School of Medicine, 2000).

Clients faced with death have a heightened need and legal right to self-determination. Any ethical dilemmas in end-of-life care must be based on clients' own beliefs and values. When clients are dying, the role of health care providers is to support clients, offer palliative care for the relief of suffering, enhance autonomy and self-control, and assist the clients in achieving spiritual comfort (Carney & Meier, 2000). Health care providers must exercise caution when acting as advocates to clients near the end of life. There is a fine line between advocacy and paternalism when clients are this vulnerable (Zomorodi & Foley, 2009).

The availability of experimental therapies, life-sustaining technologies, and active life-ending options (euthanasia) has complicated end-of-life decisions. If experimental therapies seem appropriate, health care providers need to provide clients with the information and documentation regarding known risks and possible benefits that will allow clients to make an informed decision about treatment. Regarding termination of life-sustaining treatment, health care providers are obligated to comply with client wishes, even if this hastens death (Carr & Moorman, 2009).

Technological mechanisms, developed in the interest of organ transplantation, are capable of indefinitely sustaining the function of many body systems. This has complicated the legal definition of death and caused dilemmas for families and health care practitioners alike (Shabanzadeh, Sadr, Ghafari, Nozari, & Toushih, 2009). Advance directives and legislative efforts to define "legal death" are intended to clarify the issues involved, but uncertainty over the withdrawal of life-sustaining treatment still occurs. Many hospitals today employ clinical ethicists to review cases marked by ethical uncertainty to help in making "right and good decisions in individual cases" (Siegler, 2000, p. S19). The emotional toll on family members and health care providers involved in such cases can be overwhelming.

Advance directives allow competent adults to express their wishes regarding life-sustaining treatment should they become unable to make such decisions later. These directives seek to realize the basic values of human dignity, respect for self-determination, and the right to refuse treatment. Common directives include the living will and the medical durable power of attorney. The living will provides an opportunity to outline specific wishes regarding life-sustaining measures. The medical durable power of attorney names a successor to make these decisions, if the client becomes unable to do so (Rubin, Strull, Fialkow, Weiss, & Lo, 1994).

Although advance directives may protect a client's right to self-determination, any ambiguity in the language may complicate decisions made on behalf of the client. Consider Caitlin, an infant who was born with anencephaly (literally "without a brain"), rendering her prognosis for survival limited. Her parents directed the hospital staff to provide only palliative treatment. Over the weekend, Caitlin developed an apparently painful ear infection. This presented a clinical dilemma. The staff agonized over the decision to order antibiotics, wondering whether this would violate the parents' wishes. Ultimately, they administered the medication, and the parents were grateful that the staff chose to provide this comfort measure.

Physicians involved in critical care are often faced with moral dilemmas regarding resuscitation and withdrawal of treatment (Smith & O'Neill, 2008). This is particularly true in the absence or ambiguity of advance directives. If the decision is made to provide life-sustaining treatment, such as mechanical ventilation, the family and health care team may later be faced with the dilemma of whether to continue or discontinue use in the absence of improvement.

Euthanasia is an especially controversial topic. Whereas some people believe that it is simply a matter of clients exercising their right to autonomy by hastening death and "dying with dignity," others consider it to be an act of suicide and believe it is morally and legally wrong. Euthanasia could be viewed as the ultimate example of avoiding risk and uncertainty. Clients who are near death seek relief of symptoms that could include pain, depression, fear, and anxiety, especially if they expect their condition will only worsen. Most people would not voluntarily choose to experience pain and adversity, but numerous personal accounts support the idea that adversity can be a positive experience, even at the end of life (Bauby, 1997; Coughlin, 1993; Galli, 2000).

If euthanasia becomes a legal right, how long will it take to become an obligation in the interest of justice and cost containment? Will people who are elderly or catastrophically disabled feel obligated to make this choice to avoid being a burden on their families? We will see in the next section that under the principles of beneficence and nonmaleficence, every person deserves to feel loved, welcomed, and protected. Each is entitled to end-of-life care, not expedient elimination.

To date, few states in the United States recognize physician-assisted suicide as a legal option. However, the Assisted Suicide Consensus Panel of the Finding Common Ground Project, at the University of Pennsylvania Center for Bioethics, reported that more states are likely to permit euthanasia unless negative issues arise (Tulsky, Ciampa, & Rosen, 2000). Physicians are not ethically bound to provide this intervention if it is in direct contrast to their own beliefs and values. However, there is always an ethical obligation to provide information in a value-neutral manner. If client and provider beliefs are incongruent, the client should be referred elsewhere. The provider's ethical obligation to avoid either emotional or physical abandonment, when values are conflicting, is of utmost importance (Tulsky et al., 2000).

## Beneficence and Nonmaleficence

A career in health care is a form of humanitarianism. Its purpose is to help clients, guided by the virtues of benevolence and concern. The motivation for most people who choose to become health care professionals is the simple desire to help others. However, scientific and technological advances sometimes cloud our vision. What is "helpful" may not always be immediately obvious.

The ethical principle of beneficence guides providers to "do good" or "provide benefit," while nonmaleficence means to "do no harm." These two principles should be considered simultaneously because there is always a risk of harm when doing something to help a client (Beauchamp & Childress, 2001). When harm is unavoidable, everything possible should be done to minimize it. The benefit(s) must clearly outweigh the risk(s) of harm. Consider the benefits and potential risks involved in immunization. The potential benefit, immunization against infectious disease, probably outweighs the risk of pain from the injection and possible side effects, such as mild flu-like symptoms.

To honor beneficence and nonmaleficence, we must also honor autonomy, because clients' perceptions of benefit will vary. Consider Joan and Marie. Both required a radical mastectomy for breast cancer. In Joan's opinion, the potential benefit of eliminating cancer overwhelmingly outweighed the harm of disfigurement. Conversely, Marie felt that benefit would outweigh harm only if she could receive reconstructive surgery at the same time as the mastectomy.

## Justice

Justice is the ethical obligation to be fair. Three types of justice are involved in health care. *Rights-based justice* applies to the obligation providers have to respect client rights. As mentioned above, these rights stem from legal, as well as ethical, principles. *Legal justice* requires providers to honor morally acceptable laws. This means that licensed clinicians must observe all legal guidelines for practice, with the exception of laws that entitle clients to services that are morally objectionable to the provider. The most obvious examples are abortion and euthanasia. The law protects clinicians who refuse to provide services that are in conflict with their own personal values, as long as they refer their clients to someone else who may be able to provide them with the services requested.

*Distributive justice* refers to the distribution of scarce resources. No nation can afford to provide *all* health care options to *all* citizens, so a fair and equitable formula for distribution is needed (Cassell, 2000). This means that society has a responsibility to provide care for the poor, less educated, and those racial or ethnic minorities who may bear disproportional burdens of morbidity and mortality (Orsi, Margellos-Anast, & Whitman, 2010). Although medical professionals and politicians agree on this concept in health care, a solution has yet to be identified within the complex American health care system. The health care reform legislation recently signed in March 2010 by President Obama provides a beginning, but significant change will be necessary during the coming years.

## CREATING INVITING ENVIRONMENTS OF CARE

I started my new clinical rotation in primary care today, and I'm not sure how I will make it through this one. It seems like all I'm expected to do is dispense prescriptions for medication or refer my patients to specialists! The office schedules patients every ten minutes, and I barely have enough time to hear the patient's primary complaint before I have to make a diagnosis and decide what to do. The tools at my disposal include a prescription pad and a computer that I can use to order diagnostic tests, make referrals, and record the highlights about what little information I've been able to collect. I wanted to work in primary care so that I could really get to know my patients and help them discover the best ways to stay healthy, but I can see that's not going to happen here.

—*From the journal of Jesse Perrault, physician assistant student*

Scholars have established conceptual models to guide the processes of establishing client–provider relationships and informing clinical decision making (i.e., the biomedical model), as well as those that also improve the psychosocial sensitivity of health care delivery systems (i.e., the biopsychosocial model and the integrative models of health care delivery).

### The Biomedical Model

The scenario above, described by the physician assistant student, is likely familiar to anyone who has sought help from a conventional health care provider in the United States. Based on the biomedical model of health care, conventional medical practices like the one described in this journal entry seek expeditious evidence-based resolutions to presenting symptoms. To its credit, the biomedical model is characterized by remarkable scientific and technological advances that have made it possible to cure or control many diseases. Unfortunately, another distinguishing characteristic is the primacy of pharmaceutical interventions and surgery over integrative approaches to wellness and health promotion that have been shown to improve other aspects of clients' health. Medical ethicist W. A. Rogers (2004) pointed out that, because of the way in which research is commissioned and designed, the biomedical model fails to account for social, cultural, and other factors that influence health. Evidence is rarely gathered from persons whose health is affected by poverty, ethnicity, age, gender, and disability. As a result, some health care interventions may not be relevant to people who bear the greatest burden of illness (Rogers, 2004).

In contrast to the controlled trials used to generate biomedical evidence to demonstrate the efficacy and safety of interventions, social scientists study interactions between clients and providers for the purpose of establishing models of care that are sensitive to all aspects of clients' health experiences. Psychosocial evidence is typically gathered in the form of qualitative research. Although it is more subtle than the quantitative approach used in "hard science," it is equally important in the development of interventions that improve client care. Gathered evidence is typically "reduced" and placed into the context of a model so it can be tested to determine if it offers a valid, reliable, and usable tool across practice environments. If the model holds up under the scrutiny of repeated testing, it eventually becomes a theory that can be utilized to guide clinical practice (Finfgeld-Connett, 2008; Morse, 2004).

## The Biopsychosocial Model

Beginning with the 1970s, social scientists and clinicians have made significant contributions to health care. Most notably, Dr. George Engel (1977) introduced the concept of the biopsychosocial model, which extended the biomedical approach to health care by including three important additions: (1) the client's subjective experience of illness, (2) a comprehensive model of causation incorporating client-specific psychosocial factors, and (3) relationship-centered care, which empowers the client to assume an active role in his or her own health. An examination of Engel's biopsychosocial model "25 years later" noted that his most enduring contribution was to "broaden the scope of the clinician's gaze" and "[transform] the way illness, suffering, and healing are viewed" (Borrell-Carrio, Suchman, & Epstein, 2004, p. 576).

The principles of the biopsychosocial model are included in many health care education programs today. Presented as a model that guides clinicians to move beyond the primacy of the biomedical model, it encourages clinicians to address all aspects of clients' health experiences by fully engaging clients in a collaborative model of care. This approach teaches health providers to facilitate client recognition of personal resources that they can access to take charge of their health and healing. As trust builds in the relationship, it is more likely that providers will discover client attitudes, beliefs, and practices that help reinforce health and those that do not. This approach creates the opportunity for building health care partnerships in which clients can access the expertise of health professionals to augment their own efforts to maintain or improve their health.

Unfortunately, the biopsychosocial model does not consistently receive support in clinical health care environments, so as students move into the clinical components of their education programs, they may lose focus on the principles of care embedded in the biopsychosocial model. The most commonly cited barrier to implementing the biopsychosocial model stems from the perceived amount of time needed to conduct in-depth discussions. Some clinicians believe that the need to more fully engage clients will lead to extended time for which they will not be adequately reimbursed. This perception is often reinforced by reimbursement systems that pay more for procedures and tests than for listening and collaborating. This type of reimbursement system can increase the risk that health care providers will order unnecessary diagnostic tests, referrals, and other services, which drive up health care costs and decrease client satisfaction without improving outcomes (Lin & Dudley, 2009). Despite the presumption that client-centered care is time consuming and complex, this is not the case. With client-centered care, time is reallocated from provider-driven questions to client-driven concerns that are more effectively and efficiently addressed by the provider (Edwards, Jones, Carr, Braunack-Mayer, & Jensen, 2004; Lin & Dudley, 2009; Platt & Platt, 2003).

Another barrier to realizing the goals of the biopsychosocial model relates to health providers whose primary area of practice is associated with the physical aspects of health. They may naturally feel better equipped to deal with the physical aspects of presenting symptoms and uncomfortable exploring clients' emotional symptoms. For example, one study documented that physical therapists asked clients questions regarding their feelings, expectations, and perceptions only 19 percent of the time (Tripicchio, Bykerk, Wegner, & Wegner, 2009). Another study focusing on geriatric rehabilitation found that physical therapists rarely discussed goals with their clients or considered any aspect of function outside the realm of biomechanical or neurological function (Wallin, Talvitie, Cattan, & Karppi, 2008). In physical therapy, this discomfort with psychosocial issues has led many therapists to "believe that anything that is not physical is not our therapy" (Shepard, 2007, p. 1547).

Even though occupational therapists are educated to address psychiatric as well as physical diagnoses, they demonstrate similar clinical behaviors to those of physical therapists. Many have a preference for interviewing skills that are problem focused rather than client centered (Franits, 2005). A potential explanation beyond the discomfort of dealing with the psychosocial-emotional aspects of health relates to the authority of the therapist working in a clinical culture that assumes clients are seeking the opinions of "experts" and will automatically choose to work toward goals established by expert therapists (Tripicchio et al., 2009). Workplace cultures in which professionals are viewed this way tend to undermine the client–provider collaboration that is central to the biopsychosocial model. Depending on how it plays out in the clinical setting, a power differential can emerge between clients and providers (Franits, 2005). Clinicians are perceived as the "experts"— those who know the right answers and have no need for additional information from the client. In this culture, clients who make an attempt to engage in collaborative treatment planning by challenging health professionals' opinions may be deemed "difficult" (Greenfield, Anderson, Cox, & Tanner, 2008; Stacey, Henderson, MacArthur, & Dohan, 2009).

Although progress toward implementing the biopsychosocial model has been made since its introduction by Engel in 1977, the evidence presented here suggests that we still have a long way to go before the principles of the biopsychosocial model will be fully embraced. Ultimately, the goal is to empower clients with the knowledge and skills they need to take charge of their own health. This requires an approach in which clients feel confident that health providers are their partners in health management and safe enough to provide honest accounts of their fears, hopes, histories, resources, and preferences. Recognizing that there may be features beyond Engel's formulation of the biopsychosocial model that could facilitate progress, other models of care have emerged.

## Emerging Models

The Institute of Medicine (IOM) hosted a health care summit in 2009 with the goals of facilitating more rapid development of alternative health care models and generating themes associated with the successes enjoyed by recently established centers of integrative health care. Eleven themes emerged from the summit, which are discussed in detail in the final report (IOM, 2009). They are also outlined here in Table 1–1. The first six themes are already included within the

| Table 1–1   Themes That Emerged from the 2009 Summit on Integrative Health Care | |
|---|---|
| **Existing Themes** | 1. Include all established health determinants (e.g., physical, psychological, socioeconomic). |
| | 2. Strive for person- and relationship-centered care. |
| | 3. Prevent or minimize the effects of disease. |
| | 4. Establish a team-based approach with the client as the central team member. |
| | 5. Elevate the importance of client and family insights. |
| | 6. Provide supportive follow-up. |
| **New Themes** | 7. Optimize health and healing by aligning health care services across the life span. |
| | 8. Integrate personal, predictive, preventive, and participatory care across the life span. |
| | 9. Integrate conventional and complementary practices as per evidence of need and benefits. |
| | 10. Facilitate seamless integration of care across caregivers and institutions. |
| | 11. Contribute evidence of success to the literature, education, and health care policies. |

biopsychosocial model. However, the last five themes (7 through 11) present new ideas. Themes 7 and 8 are associated with integrating care across the life span from the perspectives of both the health care system and personal management. These goals will help eliminate unnecessary repetition of storytelling, diagnostic testing, and other health care activities that waste time and money and cause frustration for clients.

Theme 9 calls for the integration of conventional and complementary practices, based on the needs of clients and the existing sources of evidence that support the practices being considered. The following journal entry illustrates many of the characteristics and benefits associated with an integrative model of health care, designed to promote healing, even when a cure for an illness may not be possible (Cohen, Wheeler, & Scott, 2001).

I love this clinical education experience! Today my supervisor and I had the honor of leading a yoga session for people who are here being treated for cancer. Before I came to the Center for Integrative Medicine, I never would have believed I would enjoy working with people who have a cancer diagnosis, but it's nothing like I expected. Even though they are receiving very toxic chemotherapies, I've seen few side effects. My clients claim that the combination of exercise, meditation, and acupuncture make it possible for them to receive the treatments they need to cure their cancers while maintaining relatively good health. They all seem so hopeful!

—*From the journal of Marcus Lowe, physical therapist student*

Theme 10 calls for seamless integration of health care across caregivers and institutions, a very worthy goal that promises to improve client satisfaction by reducing the stressors that occur when clients try to manage multiple caregivers on their own. Finally, theme 11 calls for researchers and clinicians to contribute evidence to the literature, education, and health care policy. As we have seen in the more than three decades since Engel (1977) introduced the concept of the biopsychosocial model, progress toward positive change can be extremely slow, but carefully gathered evidence, which is quickly translated into clinical practice, can help facilitate the changes needed.

An important goal of integrative models of health care is to empower clients to take responsibility for their own health. Integrative models of care offer all of the traditional aspects of Western health care plus a new mandate to help clients develop individualized interventions that enable them to adopt behaviors needed to improve health and well-being. Health care programs structured around this framework acknowledge that "health is a personal matter, as is the way each of us chooses to integrate concerns about health into our lives" (IOM, 2009, p. ix).

Studies designed to explore the benefits of integrative health care have discovered that mutual benefits exist for both clients and health professionals. Clients report high levels of satisfaction with their care, while providers express greater levels of job satisfaction, decreased signs of burnout, and a personal sense of fulfillment that is often associated with altruism and being part of a caring community. In short, health providers believe they are making meaningful contributions to their clients' lives, and this has been confirmed by their clients (Cohen et al., 2001; Graber & Johnson, 2001; Malloch, 2000; VandeCreek & Burton, 2001). It will be exciting to watch the progress of integrative models of care as the supporting evidence continues to grow.

The emergence of integrative models of health care delivery offers hope for improvements in health care that move even further beyond the biopsychosocial model of care. Unfortunately, availability is currently limited to centers that can afford to make the change from more conventional approaches. Further expansion will depend on health care financing, a topic that is beyond the scope of this text. It is important for health care professionals to advocate for the changes needed to bring about more supportive environments of care, as indicated by the evidence, and to make such services available to all potential clients.

While it is helpful for clinicians to be aware of the health care models that guide health care policies, they also need models of clinical reasoning that guide day-to-day interactions with clients. Standardized guidelines can help clinicians remain mindful about the importance of interacting with clients in a manner that is client centered and capable of eliciting information not just about symptoms, but also about feelings, beliefs, experiences, and goals.

## Clinical Reasoning

It is safe to say that virtually all health care providers are now expected to conform to the standards of evidence-based practice (EBP), which mandate that we rely on data rather than assumptions to make decisions about the treatments we provide for our clients. Placing significant emphasis on the evidence derived from the basic and social sciences is important, but it is insufficient to provide all of the information needed to make informed decisions. EBP requires that we integrate high-quality research evidence with clinical expertise and client values (Sackett, Straus, Richardson, Rosenberg, & Haynes, 2000).

Clinical experience is an important source of information that helps us make judgments about how research findings can inform individualized treatment decisions that are based on clients' unique symptoms, comorbidities, and responses to past interventions. In addition, we also have to consider acceptable standards of practice, ethical guidelines, and, most importantly, what clients feel is best for them. To provide optimal care, it is important to include the goals, expectations, beliefs, and values that clients bring to health care encounters and incorporate them into the clinical decision-making process (Edwards et al., 2004; Sackett et al., 2000). Diagnostic tests and measures provide important information, but ". . . spoken language is the most powerful diagnostic and therapeutic tool in medicine" (Platt et al., 2001, p. 1079). As we will see, the interplay of these factors in all aspects of client care will provide much of the evidence we need to make good clinical decisions.

Edwards and colleagues (2004) provide an excellent conceptual model for clinical reasoning that is consistent with the biopsychosocial model. Described as a dialectical reasoning model, it explains the process clinicians use to make sense of two fundamentally different processes of reasoning when using a biopsychosocial model of care. On the one hand, clinicians use *objective, rational diagnostic reasoning* to establish diagnoses, utilize evidence, select tests and measures, and guide other procedural aspects of care. On the other, they utilize *interactive, narrative reasoning* to obtain and understand clients' beliefs and values, cultures, experiences of illness or disability, and the meanings they attribute to their circumstances. The interplay between these two approaches is fluid and expressed through clinical reasoning strategies comprised of procedures, interactions, teaching, collaborating, predicting, and ethical decision making. Table 1–2 provides descriptions of the clinical reasoning strategies that the authors observed in clinical practice.

The process of clinical reasoning is continuous and dynamic, requiring rapid interpretation and integration of both objective, rational diagnostic reasoning and interactive, narrative reasoning to formulate health provider actions The remaining chapters of this text are devoted to deeper exploration of factors that influence clinical care and our ability to practice within the framework of the biopsychosocial model of care.

| Table 1–2 | Clinical Reasoning Strategies |
| --- | --- |
| **Clinical Reasoning Strategy** | **Description** |
| Reasoning about procedures | Strategies used to select and carry out treatment procedures |
| Interactive reasoning | Strategies used to establish and manage client–provider relationships |
| Collaborative reasoning | Strategies used to establish client–provider collaboration for the interpretation of exam findings, development of goals and priorities, and implementation/progression of interventions |
| Reasoning related to teaching | Strategies used to establish teaching methods and content and to conduct assessments to ensure clients understand what we teach |
| Predictive reasoning | Strategies used to envision future scenarios, including choices clients may make and the implications of those choices |
| Ethical reasoning | Strategies used to articulate ethical and practical dilemmas that affect interventions and desired goals and the actions needed to resolve them |

*Source:* Edwards et al. (2004).

## Summary

This chapter discussed the importance of balancing biomedical and psychosocial aspects of health care in order to address all factors that influence the health and well-being of our clients. We also addressed the different approaches used to gather the biomedical and psychosocial evidence needed to support clinical decision making and reviewed changes that have occurred in models of health care delivery. The movement away from a strictly bio-medical model to the biopsychosocial model has improved client satisfaction and enhanced the experiences of health care providers, who enjoy the benefits of altruism and being part of a caring community. The movement toward fully integrative models of health care was explored, and we presented guidelines set forth by experts who are practicing integrative health care, which can be used to facilitate further development in this direction.

## Reflective Questions

1. Consider the journal entry at the beginning of this chapter. What makes this encounter seem so remarkable?
2. Think about a health care provider with whom you have a good relationship.
   a. What makes the relationship a good one?
   b. What does he or she do that demonstrates compassion?
   c. What does he or she do to earn your trust and respect?
   d. How does he or she encourage effective communication?
3. Boundaries are relative to the situation. Consider the following:
   • receiving a gift
   • disclosing personal information
   • making physical contact.
   a. Contrast the boundaries that exist for each of these situations with respect to a personal relationship and a professional relationship.
   b. Explain what circumstances would help you decide whether a boundary has been crossed in a professional relationship.

4. At times, clients cross the boundaries we have established. Without embarrassing the client, how could you reestablish boundaries in the following situations:
   a. A client asks you on a date.
   b. A client gives you an expensive gift.
   c. A client makes an offensive remark.
   d. A client asks you a personal question.
   e. A client touches you inappropriately.

5. Your client's insurance company will only pay for treatment as long as progress is being documented. You believe that your client has reached a plateau but know that his or her condition will deteriorate if treatment is withdrawn. Consider the ethical principles of autonomy, beneficence, nonmaleficence, and justice.
   a. What would you do?
   b. What factors contributed to your decision?

## Case Study

Beverly is a 60-year-old woman with diagnoses of multiple sclerosis and chronic back pain. She is well known to the other therapists in your clinic. When the referral to treat her arrives in the office, it is met with moans and groans along with stories about how "impossible" it is to meet this client's expectations. After all, she has two chronic conditions. She can't expect to be cured! As a new therapist, you have been assigned to pick up her case. You are sensitive to the needs of people with multiple sclerosis because your mother has the same diagnosis, including a long history of chronic pain. You are actually excited about the challenge of developing an effective plan of care for Beverly.

1. Describe the differences in the care Beverly could expect to receive under each of the following models: (a) the biomedical model, (b) the biopsychosocial model, and (c) an emerging model (with special attention to themes 7 through 11; see Table 1–1).

2. Having just been trained in the most appropriate professional behaviors, you are appalled by the response of the other therapists in your clinic to this referral. Will you mention your reaction to anyone? Why or why not?

3. One of your colleagues mentioned that Beverly's conditions cannot be cured. Discuss how your plan of care will be designed to promote healing. What does this mean to you? How will you determine what it means to Beverly?

4. Your familiarity with multiple sclerosis and chronic pain from your mother's experiences will help to inform your approach to Beverly's care. In what ways will you use this to your advantage? What, if anything, will you share about your own experiences with Beverly? What principles will guide you?

## References

Adedeji, S., Sokol, D., Palser, T., & McKneally, M. (2009). Ethics of surgical complications. *World Journal of Surgery, 33*(4), 732–737.

Amalberti, R., Auroy, Y., Berwick, D., & Barach, P. (2005). Five system barriers to achieving ultrasafe health care. *Annals of Internal Medicine, 142*(9), 756–764.

Bauby, J. D. (1997). *The diving bell and the butterfly.* New York, NY: Vintage.

Beauchamp, T. L., & Childress, J. F. (2001). Principles of biomedical ethics (5th ed.). New York, NY: Oxford University Press.

Borrell-Carrio, F., Suchman, A. L., & Epstein, R. M. (2004). The biopsychosocial model 25 years later: Principles, practice and scientific inquiry. *Annals of Family Medicine, 2*(6), 576–582.

Breier-Mackie, S. (2008). What's your contribution to the clinical ethics process? *Nursing Management, 39*(2), 35–43.

Bulger, R. J., & Barbato, A. L. (2000). On the Hippocratic sources of Western medical practice. *Hastings Center Report, 30*(4), S4–S7.

Carney, M. T., & Meier, D. E. (2000). Palliative care and end-of-life issues. *Anesthesiology Clinics of North America, 18*(1), 183–209.

Carr, D., & Moorman, S. (2009). End-of-life treatment preferences among older adults: An assessment of psychosocial influences. *Sociological Forum, 24*(4), 754–778.

Cassell, E. J. (2000). The principles of the Belmont Report revisited: How have respect for persons, beneficence and justice been applied to clinical medicine? *Hastings Center Report, 30*(4), 12–21.

Chochinov, H. M. (2004). Dignity in the eye of the beholder. *Journal of Clinical Oncology, 22*(7), 1336–1340.

Cohen, C. B., Wheeler, S. E., & Scott, D. A. (2001). Walking a fine line: Physicians inquiries into patients' religious and spiritual beliefs. *Hastings Center Report, 31*(5), 29–39.

Coughlin, R. (1993). *Grieving: A love story.* New York, NY: Random House.

D'Incà, R., Bertomoro, P., Mazzocco, K., Vettorato, G., Rumiati, R., & Sturniolo, G. C. (2008). Risk factors for non-adherence to medication in IBD patients. *Alimentary Pharmacology & Therapeutics, 27*(2), 166–172.

Edwards, I., Jones, M., Carr, J., Braunack-Mayer, A., & Jensen, G. (2004). Clinical reasoning strategies in physical therapy. *Physical Therapy, 84*(4), 312–330.

Engel, G. L. (1977). The need for a new medical model: A challenge for biomedicine. *Science, 196,* 129–136.

Finfgeld-Connett, D. (2008). Qualitative convergence of three nursing concepts: Art of nursing, presence and caring. *Journal of Advanced Nursing, 63*(5), 527–534.

Franits, L. E. (2005). Nothing about us without us: Searching for the narrative of disability. *American Journal of Occupational Therapy, 59*(5), 577–579.

Galli, R. (2000). *Rescuing Jeffrey.* Chapel Hill, NC: Algonquin Books.

Graber, D. R., & Johnson, J. A. (2001). Spirituality and health care organizations. *Journal of Health Care Management, 46*(1), 39–50.

Greenfield, B. H., Anderson, A., Cox, B., & Tanner, M. C. (2008). The meaning of caring to seven novice physical therapists during their first year of clinical practice. *Physical Therapy, 88*(10), 1154–1166.

Institute of Medicine. (2009). *Integrative medicine and the health of the public: A summary of the February 2009 summit.* Washington, DC: National Academies Press.

Jacobson, G. A. (2002). Maintaining professional boundaries: Preparing nursing students for the challenge. *Journal of Nursing Education, 4*(6), 279–281.

Justin, R. G. (2000). Can a physician always be compassionate? *Hastings Center Report, 30*(4), 26–27.

Lin, G. A., & Dudley, R. A. (2009). Patient-centered care. *Archives of Internal Medicine, 169(17),* 1551–1553.

Malloch, K. (2000). Healing models for organizations: Description, measurement, and outcomes. *Journal of Healthcare Management, 45*(5), 332–350.

Minogue, B. (2000). The two fundamental duties of the physician. *Academic Medicine, 75*(5), 431–442.

Morse, J. M. (2004). Constructing qualitatively derived theory: Concept construction and concept typologies. *Qualitative Health Research, 14,* 1387–1395.

Orsi, J. M., Margellos-Anast, H., & Whitman, S. (2010). Black-white health disparities in the United States and Chicago: A 15-year progress analysis. *American Journal of Public Health, 100*(2), 349–356.

Platt, F. W., Gaspar, D. L., Coulehan, J. L., Fox, L., Adler, A. J., Weston, W. W., . . . Steward, M. (2001). "Tell me about yourself": The patient-centered interview. *Annals of Internal Medicine, 134*(11), 1079–1085.

Platt, F., & Platt, C. (2003). Two collaborating artists produce a work of art. *Archives of Internal Medicine, 163*(10), 1131–1132.

Rogers, W. A. (2004). Evidence based medicine and justice: A framework for looking at the impact of EBM upon vulnerable or disadvantaged groups. *Journal of Medical Ethics, 30*(2), 141–146.

Rubin, S. M., Strull, W. M., Fialkow, M. F., Weiss, S. J., & Lo, B. (1994). Increasing the completion of the durable power of attorney for health care. *Journal of the American Medical Association, 271*(3), 209–212.

Sackett, D. L., Straus, S. E., Richardson, W. S., Rosenberg W., & Haynes, R. B. (2000). *Evidence-based medicine* (2nd ed.). Edinburgh, Scotland: Churchill Livingstone.

Shabanzadeh, A., Sadr, S., Ghafari, A., Nozari, B., & Toushih, M. (2009). Organ and tissue donation knowledge among intensive care unit nurses. *Transplantation Proceedings, 41*(5), 1480–1482.

Shepard, K. F. (2007). Are you waving or drowning? *Physical Therapy, 87(11), 1543–1554.*

Siegler, M. A. (2000). Professional values in modern clinical practice. *Hastings Center Report, 30*(4), S19–S22.

Smith, C. B., & O'Neill, L. (2008). Do not resuscitate does not mean do not treat: How palliative care and other modalities can help facilitate communication about goals of care in advanced illness. *Mt. Sinai Journal of Medicine, 75*(5), 260–265.

Stacey, C. L., Henderson, S., MacArthur, K. R., & Dohan, D. (2009). Demanding patient or demanding encounter? A case study of cancer. *Social Science and Medicine, 69,* 729–737.

Stelfox, H. T. (2005). The relation of patient satisfaction with complaints against physicians and malpractice lawsuits. *American Journal of Medicine, 118*(10), 1126–1133.

Sulmasy, D. P. (1997). *The healer's calling.* Mahwah, NJ: Paulist Press.

Sulmasy, D. (2006). *The rebirth of the clinic: An introduction to spirituality in health care.* Washington, DC: Georgetown University Press.

Tripicchio, B., Bykerk, K., Wegner, C., & Wegner, J. (2009). Increasing patient participation: The effects of training physical and occupational therapists to involve geriatric patients in the concerns-clarification and goal-setting processes. *Journal of Physical Therapy Education, 23*(1), 55–61.

Tulsky, J. A., Ciampa, R., & Rosen, E. J. (2000). Responding to legal requests for physician-assisted suicide. *Annals of Internal Medicine, 132*(6), 494–499.

VandeCreek, L., & Burton, L. (Eds.). (2001). A white paper. Professional chaplaincy: Its role and importance in health care. *Journal of Pastoral Care, 55*(1), 81–97.

Wallin, M., Talvitie, U., Cattan, M., & Karppi, S. L. (2008). Physiotherapists' accounts of their clients in geriatric inpatient rehabilitation. *Scandinavian Journal of Caring Science, 22,* 543–550.

White, A. A., III. (1999). Compassionate patient care and personal survival in orthopaedics: A 35-year perspective. *Clinical Orthopaedics and Related Research, 361,* 250–260.

Yale-New Haven Hospital & Yale University School of Medicine. (2000). Patient's rights. In *Risk management handbook.* Retrieved from http://info.med.yale.edu/caim/risk/patient_rights/patient_rights_2.html

Zomorodi, M., & Foley, B. (2009). The nature of advocacy vs. paternalism in nursing: Clarifying the "thin line." *Journal of Advanced Nursing, 65*(8), 1746–1752.

# chapter 2

# Recognizing Attitudes, Beliefs, and Values

I was sitting in the conference room today, waiting for our team meeting to begin. I couldn't believe the discussion that was going on. Mrs. Garjulo had been admitted last night with a left hip fracture, due to falling out of bed. Apparently, she was well-known to the staff, with a long history of obesity, diabetes, coronary artery disease, and arthritis. She was now scheduled to undergo surgery. I couldn't believe what the staff members were saying. One of them actually said it was her own fault, and she deserved what she got.

Angie, the nutritionist, stated, "I've worked with her over and over again. I've explained the importance of a balanced diet to her, but she just doesn't listen. She always loses weight while she's in the hospital, but as soon as she's home, she's back to her old habits of eating candy, ice cream, and cookies. The pounds go right back on. I've warned her that it's affecting her health, but she doesn't seem to care."

Pam, the physical therapist, said, "I'm glad I'm rotating to the outpatient department tomorrow. I would hate to be the one to have to get her out of bed and walking. She's so big! She only fits into *one* of the wheelchairs in the hospital. Every time she's admitted, I end up wasting time trying to find it."

At that point, the charge nurse arrived, and the conference began. All day long, I kept thinking about poor Mrs. Garjulo. Imagine how she would feel if she knew what the staff thought about her. I've always been a few pounds overweight myself, but I've never thought too much of it. Now, I'm wondering if others talk about me behind my back.

—*From the journal of Donald Spencer, occupational therapy student*

Health care professionals are presumed to treat all individuals with respect and dignity. Codes of ethics provide a list of professional values and describe ethical responsibilities. It is important to recognize, however, that as one enters into therapeutic relationships, providers and clients do so having developed distinct personalities, temperaments, natural abilities, talents, values, and beliefs. Lessons learned in life shape the way individuals view the world. Developing self-awareness and an understanding of one's strengths and limitations is an important personal and professional lesson. Individuals begin to develop personal values at a very early age. Parents, extended families, society, schools, and culture all serve to mold and shape personal values. People tend to be more comfortable when they are with individuals who are similar to themselves. Although hesitant to admit it, everyone has personal biases. Individuals may be aware of some biases, but others may exist in the subconscious mind. Both overt and covert prejudices can affect interactions with clients and colleagues. When individuals become aware of their biases, they are less likely to make inappropriate or incorrect judgments about others.

This chapter discusses the importance of recognizing our own attitudes, beliefs, and values and identifying how they shape what we think and feel and how we behave. Developing awareness helps avoid stereotyping and discrimination. The significance of valuing interdisciplinary viewpoints and working together in teams is emphasized.

## UNDERSTANDING VALUES

"The less a person understands his own feelings, the more he will fall prey to them. The less a person understands the feelings, the responses, and the behaviors of others, the more likely he will interact inappropriately with them" (Gardner, 1993, p. 254). To develop a sense of self, every individual needs to develop both intrapersonal and interpersonal intelligence. Intrapersonal intelligence involves developing an understanding of one's own feelings and emotions so that you can discriminate among them and be able to purposefully use them to guide your behaviors. Interpersonal intelligence involves understanding the feelings, behaviors, and motivations of those around you. It is the ability to recognize changes in other's moods, intentions, or motivations (Gardner, 2006). By developing a sense of self, an individual is able to grow, mature, and interact intelligently and appropriately in society. To do this, health care providers need to take time to examine and understand their personal value systems.

Values are strong beliefs and attitudes about the worth of a thought, idea, object, or course of action (Purtilo & Haddad, 2007). An individual's values represent aspects of life important to personal satisfaction (Johnson, 2009). These beliefs and attitudes develop during the formative years, as parents teach children *their* values and what is important to them. Values may include religious beliefs, honesty, the importance of a good education, a strong work ethic, and/or taking care of family. Socioeconomic status and culture influence value systems. One's early beliefs are often very personal, and they have not been examined or questioned in any way. Critically thinking about values and looking at them from multiple perspectives may be uncomfortable for some individuals (Triezenberg & Davis, 2000). However, to be effective, health care practitioners need to examine, understand, and reflect on their own values and beliefs, and appreciate and respect those of their clients and colleagues (Whalley Hammell, 2009).

When people enter health professions, in addition to their own personal values, they are expected to embrace professional values. Formulated over many years, professional values express ideals that members of the organization believe are important, such as critical thinking, problem solving, professionalism, altruism, autonomy, compassion, client advocacy, and evidence-based practice (Johnson, 2009; Triezenberg & Davis, 2000). These values are reflected in professional ethics and are typically presented in the form of a code of ethics; ethical principles, such as autonomy, beneficence, justice, nonmaleficence, and equal distribution of resources, are also codified and interpreted (Kasar & Clark, 2000; Wharton, 2005).

Health care providers recognize that they may not always be able to adhere to all of these principles equally. When demand for resources is high and the supply of resources is low, decisions must be made to determine who will receive the limited assets. Priorities and decisions that achieve a balance among these principles and serve the best interest of the clients are made in conjunction with clients, families, and other health care providers. A health professional who receives incentives for containing costs in a managed care environment may experience a dilemma when weighing the costs/benefits of self-interest and organizational survival against fidelity to a client (Swisher, 2002).

At times, the values of a health professional are in conflict with those of clients or colleagues. It is the provider's responsibility to respect clients' and colleagues' values while maintaining personal values. For example, Mrs. Mahoney has been receiving treatments for cancer for several months. She calls the clinic and indicates that she has decided to terminate conventional therapy and substitute herbal treatments. The provider might believe that this will be detrimental to her health and explain why she should continue treatments. However, she insists on her new course of action. Despite disagreeing with her decision and rationale, the provider needs to respect her autonomy.

## Moral Reasoning, Self-Assessment, and Reflection

Health care professionals have a duty to act in the best interest of their clients. Yet, changes in health care environments, including managed care, productivity requirements, reimbursement by third-party payers, and advancements in technology, have exposed providers to more ethical dilemmas than ever before (Triezenberg & Davis, 2000). As professional responsibilities expand, providers must be able to function in these challenging environments and be prepared to make ethical, as well as clinical, judgments in order to balance professional and organizational obligations with client needs (Dieruf, 2004; Sisola, 2000).

To be successful, providers must first develop moral sensitivity. They must recognize the attitudes and skills needed to identify an ethical issue. Then, they must develop moral reasoning, the ability to analyze a situation and come to a moral decision. Finally, they must develop the skills to act on the decisions they made. Understanding and being sensitive to the well-being of others is at the core of moral reasoning. Effective health care professionals recognize how their actions affect the lives of their clients. Studies show that the most successful providers understand the importance of the client–provider relationship, identify their own personal beliefs and values, examine differences between their beliefs and values and those of their clients, and promote awareness of ethical issues found in practice (Andre, 1991; Kohlberg, 1984; Rest, 1994; Triezenberg & Davis, 2000).

Practitioners develop moral reasoning skills by practicing self-assessment. Through ongoing self-assessment, they identify strengths and weaknesses related to their knowledge, skills, experiences, and values; improve critical thinking skills; and develop a plan for continuing competence (Moyers, 2005; Rodts & Lamb, 2008). The use of reflection and reflective writing has been shown to be a useful tool in developing these skills (Craft, 2005). Dewey (1933) first spoke about the importance of reflective thinking. Schon (1983) later expanded on Dewey's recommendation and suggested that professionals could modify their practice and further develop ideas by thinking about what they did. Practitioners who take the time to "reflect-*on*-practice" will become aware of what they do not know and will be better prepared to "reflect-*in*-practice" when faced with similar situations in the future (Musolino & Mostrom, 2005). Schon (1983) further recommended that "reflection in and on action" should be integral parts of professional education to assist students as they move toward professional practice. Students develop these skills by thinking about what they did in clinical situations, maintaining reflective journals, documenting their thoughts and feelings related to events that took place in the clinic, and receiving feedback from classroom and clinical faculty (Craft, 2005).

## ATTITUDES, STIGMA, AND PREJUDICE IN HEALTH CARE DELIVERY

Attitudes are favorable or unfavorable emotions or sentiments toward individuals or groups that strongly predict behaviors. Although we may believe that we are unbiased and treat all individuals fairly, hidden or covert biases may emerge. People within a particular group tend to share common values, habits, and customs, which they may not share with those from outside the group (Bizumic, Duckitt, Popadic, Dru, & Krauss, 2009; Capell, Dean, & Veenstra, 2008). As a result, individuals often feel more comfortable with people who they perceive as similar to themselves. Ethnocentrism was first defined by Sumner (1906) as the tendency to favor *in-groups* and disparage members of the *out-groups*. As a result, many groups/cultures feel or believe they are superior to others and reject or exploit those from other groups/cultures (Bizumic et al., 2009).

Research shows that when asked to attribute positive or negative qualities, distribute resources, or indicate liking for several different groups, individuals, in general, favor those who are similar to themselves (Brauer, 2001). Favoritism for like individuals is so embedded in people's value systems that pronouns such as "us" are more favorably valued than those such as "them." Social behavior often operates in an unconscious manner, and people may not realize that past experiences affect future judgments. This supports the findings that people who adamantly disavow prejudice have been shown to discriminate against others. The ethnocentrism of health care providers may lead to stigma and prejudice in health care delivery, impair one's ability to provide culturally appropriate care, and contribute to inadequate treatment and even misdiagnosis (Capell et al., 2008).

Stigma and prejudice are complex concepts, often related to interactions between nonmarginalized and marginalized groups. Research in this area stems from the seminal works of Goffman (1963) and Allport (1954). Prejudice is defined as having a poor attitude toward an individual simply because he or she belongs to a group to which negative qualities have been assigned, resulting in erroneous assumptions. Stereotyping can lead to avoidance and lack of respect for those who are stigmatized. Studies show that health care professionals may unconsciously stigmatize and discriminate against individuals or groups who have certain diagnoses or come from different cultures (Balsa, McGuire, & Meredith, 2005; Crisp, Gelder, Rix, Meltzer, & Rowlands, 2000). The population in the United States is becoming increasingly diverse, and health care providers need to be aware of the factors that effect how clients understand and manage their illnesses, in order to provide effective, culturally sensitive interventions (Ekelman, Dal Bello-Hass, Bazyk, & Bazyk, 2003; Suarez-Balcazar et al., 2009).

In its 2002 report "Unequal Treatment," the Institute of Medicine defined racial disparity as differences in treatment provided to individuals from dissimilar racial or ethnic groups, not justified by the underlying health conditions or clients' treatment choices. The report suggests that this may occur due to unconscious bias or prejudice, being uncertain about a diagnosis, and/or recognizing that members of some minority groups are more prone to certain diseases than others. These biases may be so subtle that most providers are not even aware of them. In addition, race or ethnicity might be associated with poor client–provider communication and interfere with one's ability to understand and respond appropriately to clients' health needs (Balsa & McGuire, 2001; McGuire et al., 2008). It is a significant concern that, despite the fact that health disparities were identified 20 years ago, little progress has been made in reducing these inequalities; they continue to have a very real and negative effect on the lives of individuals who are members of minority groups.

One goal of the United States' *Healthy People 2010* (U.S. Department of Health and Human Services [DHHS], 2002) was to eliminate health disparities. Unfortunately, that goal has not yet been achieved. Prejudice, stigma, and discrimination are thought to be significant contributors to the existing disparities in the health care system. Recognizing personal bias, understanding differences, and avoiding stigmatization and discrimination are important components of providing effective health care. Developing awareness of biases can help reduce stereotyping and discrimination and increase appreciation for diversity and respect for all clients and colleagues. Sumsion and Smith (2000) reported that therapists and clients from different ethnic backgrounds frequently had differing goals. This was cited as the major barrier to providing client-centered care. Including case study examples, such as those featuring interactions between health care providers and members of minorities, in academic and continuing education programs was shown to be the most effective method for resolving this problem. While we have made some progress, reducing health care disparities continues to be a goal of *Healthy People 2020* (DHHS, 2009).

As a result of advances in health care research, risk factors for many illnesses and conditions have been identified. Some are within a person's control, such as cigarette smoking, substance abuse, obesity, sedentary lifestyle, multiple sex partners, and failure to wear seat belts (Gunderman, 2000). Consequently, some health care providers "blame" clients for their illnesses or conditions because they failed to take responsibility for their personal well-being. Do providers treat clients who abuse alcohol and need liver transplants the same way they treat those who never drank? Do they treat clients with lung cancer who never smoked the same way they treat those who smoked two packs of cigarettes a day? These are important questions for health providers to ask themselves as they strive to increase self-awareness. Other factors need to be considered; socioeconomic, cultural, educational, and geographical influences all affect behavior. Yet, providers may lose patience and blame those who overreact to illness or who fail to recognize they are sick and wait until it is too late to seek help. When unable to "cure" a client, it is sometimes easier to say the client "failed to respond to treatment," when in truth, the health care system may have failed the client. The role of health care professionals is not to blame but to assist clients with their illnesses or disabilities. Although it is appropriate to inform clients as to how their habits may be jeopardizing their health, "blaming the victim can inhibit care-seeking, erode hope, and undermine the therapeutic alliance between clients and health professionals" (Gunderman, 2000, p. 10). The choices one makes are influenced by the choices one has available and may be related to social determinants, including income, education, housing, neighborhood safety, and availability of healthy food and safe recreational space. According to the World Health Organization (WHO, 2010), social determinants include the conditions into which people are born and where they live, work, and age. They are shaped by power, money, and available resources; inequities in these areas are primarily responsible for inequities in health care.

## Discrimination in Health Care

Access to health care and utilization of services vary by gender, race, age, and socioeconomic status. Experiences with discrimination result in delays in clients seeking care and poor adherence to treatment recommendations (Casagrande, Gary, LaVeist, Gaskin, & Cooper, 2007; Penner et al., 2009). Although the population in the United States continues to grow increasingly diverse, Bass-Haugen (2009) noted that segregation, dissimilar treatment, and racism continued to be factors in the epidemiological gap between the majority (White) and minority groups. Studies show that the "significant underrepresentation of minorities in the health professions and in the health care industry is one reason behind the disparity" (Gonzales, Gooden, & Porter, 2000, p. 56).

Attitudinal barriers to health care include past experiences, mistrust of health care professionals and institutions, and perceptions and acts of discrimination (Casagrande et al., 2007). Studies have found that people who are Black, Hispanic, Native American, and Asian receive less adequate and less intensive health care than those who are White, and those disparities exist even when factoring in such issues as health insurance, status, age, income, gender, and education. Researchers found that members of these minority groups stated that they believed they would receive better medical care if they belonged to a different race. They further believed that providers judged them unfairly or treated them disrespectfully because of their race or their limited English skills (Johnson, Saha, Arbelaez, Beach, & Cooper, 2004). Whether or not discrimination truly occurs, clients' perceptions of racial and ethnic bias are common among minority health care users (Stepanikova & Cook, 2008). These perceptions result in lower satisfaction with care, higher rates of depression (Bird, Bogart, & Delahanty, 2004), postponing of medical tests and treatments (Van Houtven et al., 2005), and a lower likelihood of seeking and receiving preventive care (Trivedi, Zaslavsky, Schneider, & Ayanian, 2005). As a result, clients who experience discrimination or who perceive that they are being discriminated against tend to suffer (Williams & Neighbors, 2001; William, Neighbors, & Jackson, 2003).

Another form of bias is gender bias. The Society for the Advancement of Women's Health Research was founded in 1990 to bring national attention to the problem of gender bias in health care research and to promote a women's health research agenda (Greenberger, 1999). Until that time, women's health issues were largely ignored. Most medical research focused on a White male population, and findings could not be generalized to a larger, diverse population, including women (Marrocco & Stewart, 2001). Although more women are entering the field of medicine today, generations of gender inequities in health care have not yet been eliminated.

Consider the case of Mrs. Rawls, who for several months complained of pain in her jaw. The doctor suggested that she see her dentist because her dentures probably needed adjusting. One morning, she woke up with severe jaw pain and vomiting. She was admitted to the hospital through the emergency department and diagnosed with acute myocardial infarction. Because she did not present with the typical male symptoms of chest pain, her diagnosis was missed, and she almost died. Failure to distinguish the differences between men's and women's symptoms perpetuates gender bias in health care (Marrocco & Stewart, 2001; Nicolette & Jacobs, 2000). Providers must guard against dismissing women's complaints just because they do not fit into predetermined categories. The incidence of cardiovascular disease among women is now recognized as a major challenge and is the leading cause of death among women. Despite recent gains in identifying women's health issues, societal stereotyping and gender bias still exist.

Another type of bias is ageism. In spite of advancements in medical care and improved health and life expectancy, bias against older adults continues today (Reyna, Goodwin, & Ferrari, 2007; Rybczyk, Haut, Lacey, Fogg, & Nicholas, 2001).

Hattie Williams worked part time as a fashion designer, right up until her stroke weeks ago. I'm totally amazed at how sharp she is! She has a quick wit and is the "youngest" 84-year-old person I've ever met.

Yesterday, I commented on the new bathrobe she was wearing. She wrinkled her nose and said, "My daughter-in-law bought it for me. She's very sweet and means well, but this is for an old lady. It's too frumpy! I'd have picked one that is stylish."

I see her improve everyday, and she's able to do more independently. We've been discussing where she might go after discharge. Although her son wants to bring her into his home, the doctor thinks she should go to a nursing home "because she's 84 and has had a stroke." Hattie, however, wants to go to her own house. I hope they don't make this decision based on age alone.

*—From the journal of Diane Patel, social work student*

In a society that emphasizes youth and beauty, the tendency to view aging in a negative light is common. The media portrays few positive images of older people, especially older women. Some older individuals fear declining health and the potential lack of independence. Yet, many older adults maintain health and independence well into their 90s and beyond. Chronological age is not necessarily a reflection of biological age (Shortt, 2001). However, health care professionals, perhaps because of their frequent exposure to older clients who are "ill," have been shown to be particularly susceptible to ageism, and caring for people who are elderly is often an unpopular career choice (Kearney, Miller, Paul, & Smith, 2000; Reyna et al., 2007). Given the current demographics, a "declining interest in geriatrics could foreshadow a crisis in the future of long-term health care for older adults" (Reyna et al., 2007, p. 50).

Unfortunately, "a client's age is often inappropriately used as a factor in selecting treatment options" (Madan, Aliabadi-Wahle, & Beech, 2001, p. 282). Chronological age has been used as one criterion for discontinuing life support. Underrepresentation of older clients in research studies has been shown to lead to health care decisions based on assumptions, observations, past experiences, and bias rather than on evidence-based practice (Kearney et al., 2000).

Older clients are sometimes not offered the same medical treatments as younger clients (Madan et al., 2001). Although biological factors and comorbidities may limit the use of certain procedures, ageism may also influence the options offered to older clients. In one study, researchers found that when treating clients diagnosed with breast cancer, second-year medical students did not offer the same options regarding breast reconstruction to clients over age 59 as they did to those under age 31. However, they would choose the option they suggested to younger clients if they or their family members were placed in a similar situation (Madan et al., 2001). Decisions need to be made using evidence-based criteria, not the health care provider's attitudes and beliefs. Regardless of client age, all available options need to be presented to clients, and they should be included in determining which treatment option is the best one for them (Shortt, 2001).

## Other Common Biases and Their Effects on Health Care Delivery

**HIV/AIDS**   ". . . HIV stigma continues to be a significant barrier to HIV prevention and treatment efforts nearly 30 years after the start of the epidemic" (Earnshaw & Chaudoir, 2009, p. 1160). While prejudice and discrimination directed at people infected with HIV has lessened since the 1980s, the goal of eliminating this stigma and its consequences has shown only moderate success (Colbert, Kim, Sereika, & Erlen, 2010; Earnshaw & Chaudoir, 2009). Perceived discrimination could discourage individuals infected with HIV from seeking health care, following treatment protocols, or returning for follow-up visits (Schuster et al., 2005), leading to less than optimal outcomes.

As with other stigmatized conditions, self-awareness of potential bias is important. When health professionals ask clients how they became infected, clinicians need to know why they are asking. Is it out of curiosity about the client's lifestyle, or is it to enable them to provide more effective client education? Will a health provider's attitude toward a client change if the client was infected as the result of a blood transfusion rather than as the result of using a tainted needle or participating in unprotected sex (Bormann & Kelly, 1999)?

**MENTAL ILLNESS**    People with mental illness are severely stigmatized, which poses real barriers to diagnosis, treatment, and social integration. Epidemiological surveys suggest that stigmatization and discrimination of individuals with mental illness are based on lack of knowledge about the causes and treatments available for mental illness, ignorance about how to access evaluation and treatment, and expectations of prejudice against those diagnosed with mental illness. The stigma related to a diagnosis of mental illness has led to feelings of shame for clients and family members and blame from others (Thornicroft, 20008). Even among soldiers returning from battle, most do not seek mental health care because of concerns related to possible stigmatization (Hoge et al., 2004). Stigmatization against people with mental illness presents barriers to social inclusion and to appropriate access to mental health care for many individuals (Thornicroft, 2008).

A study of nursing students assigned to a rotation working with clients diagnosed with mental illness found that students entering the experience did not know what to expect. They described feelings of fear, apprehension, and worry based on the stigma associated with clients with psychiatric conditions During the rotation, students indicated how easy it was to develop assumptions about clients—without having even met them—after reading a report. Students began to understand the stigmatizing beliefs about mental illness as they grew to know the clients. They also practiced self-reflection by writing in their journals. At the end of the experience, they indicated that by working with and reflecting on experiences with clients with psychiatric conditions, they learned about themselves and the clients and let go of their previous assumptions (Webster, 2009).

Each year, although approximately 30 percent of the population worldwide is diagnosed with some form of mental illness, many do not seek help because of their fear of stigma if they are diagnosed, and their fear of shame and rejection if they disclose the conditions. Although the majority of individuals with mental disorders eventually seek services, they wait a long time before doing so. The average delays are 8 years for mood disorders and 9 years for anxiety disorders (Thornicroft, 2008). Unmet mental health care needs are greatest for individuals who are poor, elderly, members of minority ethnic groups, those with low income or who lack insurance, and individuals from rural areas (Wang et al., 2005). Evidence suggests that even when there are no financial burdens related to care, many people do not seek treatment in an attempt to avoid being labeled as "mentally ill" (Corrigan, 2004a). According to DHHS (2001), people of racial and ethnic minorities have less access to mental health services than do those who are White, are less likely to receive needed care, and more likely to receive poor quality care when treated.

**OBESITY**    In the United States, obesity has reached epidemic proportions, with 50 percent of the adult population meeting the definition of being overweight (Luber, Fischer, & Venkat, 2008). Stigmatization of obese individuals has not decreased in our society, despite its increasing prevalence (Latner & Stunkard, 2003; Ross, Shivy, & Mazzeo, 2009). Obesity bias is the tendency to negatively judge an overweight individual, considering them to be lazy, lacking in self-discipline, incompetent, and/or unclean (Puhl, Moss-Racusin, Schwartz, & Brownell, 2008; Ross et al., 2009). Weight bias leads to stereotyping of individuals. Those who feel the impact of obesity bias often develop symptoms of depression, body image distress, decreased self-esteem, and lack of self-acceptance. It has been suggested that individuals who are obese often internalize the stereotypes held against them, and they, themselves, demonstrate bias toward other individuals who are overweight (Schwartz, Vartanian, Nosek, & Brownell, 2006). Many people believe that obesity and other eating disorders are self-inflicted, perpetuating stereotypes and stigma. Little empathy exists for people who are obese (Crisp et al., 2000).

Obesity is a chronic disease affected by genetic, environmental, and behavioral factors, with no easy remedies. Although dieting may result in short-term success, most weight is later regained. Obese individuals are at risk for a number of conditions that can lead to increased mortality, including type 2 diabetes, hypertension, sleep apnea, and cardiovascular and gallbladder disease (Must et al., 1999). Overweight individuals are discriminated against in educational settings, in the workforce, and in health care environments (Puhl et al., 2008).

As health professionals, we need to understand how personal lifestyle choices may affect one's ability to relate to clients. If you are overweight, would you feel comfortable counseling a client who is obese? By avoiding the topic, we do a disservice to our clients. The role of client–provider communication is essential to decrease disparities. The health care professionals discussing Mrs. Garjulo, in the journal entry at the beginning of this chapter, seem to believe that she was undisciplined and self-indulgent. With such an attitude, would they be able to develop an honest rapport with her and provide effective treatment?

**DRUG AND ALCOHOL ADDICTIONS**   Many clinicians avoid treating clients who have drug or alcohol addictions. Although some health professionals think they lack the necessary training and support to treat clients with these problems, others prefer not to work with them. Practitioners who do care for those who use alcohol or abuse drugs describe the experience as extremely challenging (McLaughlin & Long, 1996). Clients may be perceived as out of control, self-indulgent, and having self-inflicted problems. Practitioners may fear that clients are unpredictable and dangerous, and they may expect clients to relapse. This leads to feelings of frustration, pessimism, and anger. Derogatory comments made by health professionals may contribute to clients' hiding their problems and, when internalized, result in depression, self-criticism, and possibly a return to or accelerated use of drugs or alcohol in an attempt to escape these negative feelings (Howard & Chung, 2000). However, treatment is available for substance abuse problems, and some clients do recover.

**DISABILITY**   As a result of advancements in medical care and the aging of the population, the number of individuals living with disabilities in the United States has grown and is more visible than ever before (Smart, 2008). Yet, despite the passage of the Americans with Disabilities Act in 1990, negative societal perceptions of individuals with disabilities continue to exist (Corrigan, 2004b). People with disabilities are often considered out of the ordinary, because they often do not fit commonly accepted standards of beauty, attractiveness, and being able bodied, as portrayed by the media (Seo & Chen, 2009). Our socialization, professional education, personal experiences, and health profession specialization all influence and shape our perceptions of disability.

As a result of well-intentioned fund-raising campaigns, people with disabilities may be stereotyped as having suffered great misfortunes. They may be looked on as individuals whose lives have been damaged forever. When pursuing their interests and strengths, they may be perceived as compensating for their disabilities. Yet, when they hold back from engaging in certain activities because they recognize their limitations, they may be viewed as inferior to others. People are often amazed when they see a person with a disability who is happy and leading a successful life; they do not expect this. Some believe that having a disability must be intolerable and that people with disabilities must spend their entire lives wishing they were "normal."

As a result of this stigmatization and stereotyping, people may try to hide their disabilities. A person who has limited sight may pretend to be lost. An individual diagnosed with multiple sclerosis may pretend to be clumsy. People with "hidden" disabilities, such as diabetes, high blood pressure, or other conditions not visible to the naked eye, may attempt to conceal their diagnoses. The time and energy spent "hiding" the disability can increase stress, which may affect their overall health. However, some people would prefer to hide their disabilities rather than face the pity they fear from their peers who are not disabled.

Health care professionals have a duty to promote equality and reduce prejudice and discrimination in society, especially in the health care arena. One of the most powerful strategies for reducing prejudice involves promoting interpersonal contact between members of different groups. Encouraging intergroup communication may help reduce prejudice and bias if the circumstances surrounding the contact ensure equal status for both groups, shared goals, and interdependence (Allport, 1954; Seo & Chen, 2009).

## CROSS-PROFESSIONAL VALUES AND BIASES: EFFECTS ON TEAMWORK AND CLIENT OUTCOMES

Technological advances, a focus on health promotion, changes in reimbursement policies, and a movement away from acute care to outpatient and home-based services have all affected the role of health professionals. In today's health care environment, professionals are expected to take on a leadership role, with an emphasis on delegation, education, and supervision (Mawn & Reece, 2000). In this new system, no one works alone. Teamwork has been shown to be a key component of providing services essential for safe, efficient, and effective client care (Begley, 2009; Finn, Learmonth, & Reedy, 2010; Solheim, McElmurry, & Kim, 2007). High-quality clinical outcomes require collaboration among health care professionals. Members of a team need to understand each other's roles and contributions and be clear about how they are going to work together (Martin, 2000). This is not always as easy as it might seem. Our personal beliefs, attitudes, and values, as well as our previous experiences and professional socialization, may differ from those of our colleagues. Ethnocentrism may surface, and individuals from one group of professionals may think that they are more valuable than those from another profession, leading to competition rather than collaboration (Bizumic et al., 2009; Capell et al., 2008).

The health care system is an example of a culture. Within that culture exist many subcultures, such as nurses, doctors, physical therapists, occupational therapists, speech and language pathologists, dietitians, and social workers. Professional ethnocentrism, based on the in-group and out-group model, may pose a barrier to effective communication. Members of each in-group share a specialized educational experience, culminating in a specific degree or license. Each group has an umbrella organization that affords its members greater professional identity and separateness. To work together effectively, members of each group must first acknowledge the existence of professional ethnocentrism, recognize each others' strengths, and then work together for the common goal of promoting optimal health care for all clients (Brauer, 2001).

Success in today's health care system demands a balance between quality client care and cost effectiveness. Information from all involved disciplines must be obtained, consolidated, updated, and shared. Communication is vital, and team meetings can facilitate this exchange.

Working as a team, members can achieve more than working independently; quality client care depends on it (Begley, 2009; Finn et al., 2010; Solheim et al., 2007).

For a team to be effective, three conditions need to be present. First, all members must trust one another. Second, the team needs to have a sense of group identity. Members must feel that they belong to a unique and worthwhile team. Finally, members need to believe that they can be more effective working together, rather than as individuals, and that each person on the team can perform competently. Although a team may function when one or more of these conditions are missing, it will not be as effective (Druskat & Wolff, 2001).

One building block of a team is human emotions. Individuals need to understand and be able to control their emotions, be sensitive to others, and support team members. When health care professionals accurately listen and assess each other's feelings and concerns, they are more willing to cooperate with each other, improving morale. If one team member is being disruptive, other members of the team must be willing to confront the individual. This can be accomplished in a positive way, conveying the message that his or her contributions to the group are valued. However, it must be clear that disruptive behavior will not be tolerated. Similarly, if an individual appears upset, members need to acknowledge that person's feelings and express a caring attitude. If feelings are not addressed early, disruptive behaviors can escalate and erode any sense of trust in the team.

Taking time to build team spirit and allowing members to vent frustrations help develop effectiveness. Emotionally intelligent groups make better decisions, develop creative strategies for problem solving, and are more productive. Health care professionals can foster emotional intelligence by comprehending their own personal and professional identity, attitudes, beliefs and values, as well as gaining a clear awareness of their colleagues' strengths and skills. As a by-product, quality of care improves, and everyone benefits (Campion-Smith, 2001; Gardner, 2006).

## Summary

This chapter addressed the importance of understanding personal and professional beliefs and values. The significance of identifying attitudes and recognizing how they affect behaviors was explored. We described how both overt and covert personal biases can result in stigmatization, generalization, and stereotyping of individuals who are different from "us." The need for group cohesiveness, when working in interdisciplinary teams, was explained. Optimal health care requires knowledge, experience, mutual respect, and tolerance.

## Reflective Questions

1. a. List 10 values that are personally important to you, such as faith, appearance, power, and success.
   b. Once you have completed your list, prioritize your values in order of importance to you.
   c. Discuss how your values affect your behavior.
   d. How do you feel about people whose behavior conflicts with your values?
2. Imagine you have a colleague who makes offensive comments about people.
   a. How would you feel?
   b. What would your opinion be about this person?
   c. What would you do?
3. Although we may consider ourselves fair and unbiased, it is likely that we harbor stereotypes or negative images, to varying degrees, toward some individuals or groups. Consider your feelings and beliefs carefully and honestly.
   a. Do you hold negative stereotypes about any racial or ethnic groups, older people, those with mental retardation or mental illness, people with HIV/AIDS, or others? If so, describe what they are.
   b. Biases and stereotypes can interfere with our ability to be nonjudgmental, build relationships, and work effectively with clients. What can you

do to move beyond your current beliefs, attitudes, and feelings?

4. People with disabilities often state that health care providers have lower expectations and goals for them than they themselves do. How might you respond to clients who challenge your expectations of them?

5. a. What might your response be to clients with disabilities who you consider to have unrealistic goals or expectations for their rehabilitation?

   b. How might you support clients in achieving mutually established goals?

## Case Study

As part of the service learning component of her nursing curriculum, Jackie has been assigned to volunteer in a shelter for homeless women that is located in the inner city. Having grown up in an affluent suburban neighborhood, she is very uncomfortable taking the bus into the city and is somewhat afraid of the clients. Although she is unaware of their medical status, several appear to her to have some form of mental illness, and others appear to be drug or alcohol dependent. Many do not speak English.

Jackie is expected to spend 3 hours each week assisting the nursing staff and serving the clients. Her role includes monitoring vital signs, preparing and serving meals, discussing the importance of diet and exercise and other healthy behaviors, and spending time talking with the women.

1. Discuss Jackie's possible preconceived biases and how she may have internalized these values.

2. What can Jackie do to modify her beliefs and values to reduce her biases?

3. Stigmatization is a serious obstacle for people perceived to be out of the mainstream, such as the women in this shelter. Identify how stereotypes and biases can create barriers to care.

4. What can health care providers do to eliminate barriers to care for stigmatized populations?

## References

Allport, G. W. (1954). *The nature of prejudice.* Reading, MA: Addison-Wesley.

Andre, J. (1991). Beyond moral reasoning: A wider view of the professional ethics course. *Teaching Philosophy, 14,* 359–373.

Balsa, A. L., & McGuire, T. G. (2001). Statistical discrimination in health care. *Journal of Health Economics, 20,* 881–907.

Balsa, A. I., McGuire, T. G., & Meredith, L. S. (2005). Testing for statistical discrimination in health care. *Health Services Research, 40*(1), 227–252.

Bass-Haugen, J. (2009). Health disparities: Examinations of evidence relevant for occupational therapy. *American Journal of Occupational Therapy, 63*(1), 24–35.

Begley, C. M. (2009). Developing inter-professional learning: Tactics, teamwork and talk. *Nurse Education Today, 29,* 276–283.

Bird, S. T., Bogart, L. M., & Delahanty, D. I. (2004). Health-related correlates of perceived discrimination in HIV Care. *AIDS Patient Care and STDS, 18*(1), 19–26.

Bizumic, B., Duckitt, J., Popadic, D., Dru, V., & Krauss, S. (2009). A cross-cultural investigation into a reconceptualization of ethnocentrism. *European Journal of Social Psychology, 39,* 871–899.

Bormann, J., & Kelly, A. (1999). HIV and AIDS: Are you biased? *American Journal of Nursing, 99*(9), 38–39.

Brauer, M. (2001). Intergroup perception in the social context: The effects of social status and group membership on perceived out-group homogeneity and ethnocentrism. *Journal of Experimental Social Psychology, 37,* 15–31.

Campion-Smith, C. (2001). Putting patients first will help interprofessional education. *British Medical Journal, 322*(7287), 676.

Capell, J., Dean, E., & Veenstra, G. (2008). The relationship between cultural competence and ethnocentrism of health care professionals. *Journal of Transcultural Nursing, 19*(2), 121–125.

Casagrande, S. S., Gary, T. L., LaVeist, T. A., Gaskin, D. J., & Cooper, A. (2007). Perceived discrimination and adherence to medical care in a racially integrated community. *Society of General Medicine, 22*, 389–395.

Colbert, A. M., Kim, K. H., Sereika, S. M., & Erlen, J. A. (2010). An examination of the relationships among gender, health status, social support, and HIV-related stigma. *Journal of the Association of Nurses in AIDS Care, 21*(4), 302–313.

Corrigan, P. (2004a). How stigma interferes with mental health care. *American Psychology, 59*(7), 614–625.

Corrigan, P. W. (2004b). Target-specific stigma change: A strategy for impacting mental illness stigma. *Psychiatric Rehabilitation Journal, 28*(2), 113–123

Craft, M. (2005). Reflective writing and nursing education. *Journal of Nursing Education, 44*(2), 53–57.

Crisp, A. H., Gelder, M. G., Rix, S., Meltzer, H. I. & Rowlands, O. J. (2000). Stigmatization of people with mental illnesses. *British Journal of Psychiatry, 177*, 4–7.

Dewey, J. (1933). *How we think. A restatement of the relation of critical thinking to the educative process.* Lexington, MA: D. C. Heath.

Dieruf, K. (2004). Ethical decision-making by students in physical and occupational therapy. *Journal of Allied Health, 33*(1), 24–30.

Druskat, V. U., & Wolff, S. B. (2001). Building the emotional intelligence of groups. *Harvard Business Review, 79*(3), 81–90.

Earnshaw, V. A., & Chaudoir, S. R. (2009). From conceptualizing to measuring HIV stigma: A review of HIV stigma mechanism measures. *AIDS Behaviors, 13*, 1160–1177.

Ekelman, B., Dal Bello-Hass, V. D., Bazyk, J., & Bazyk, S. (2003). Developing cultural competence in occupational therapy and physical therapy education. *Journal of Allied Health, 32*(2), 131–137.

Finn, R., Learmonth, M., & Reedy, P. (2010). Some unintended effects of teamwork in healthcare. *Social Science and Medicine, 70*(8), 1148–1154.

Gardner, H. (1993). *Frames of mind: The theory of multiple intelligences.* New York, NY: Basic Books.

Gardner, H. (2006). *Multiple intelligences. New horizons.* New York, NY: Basic Books.

Goffman, E. (1963). *Stigma.* New York, NY: Simon & Schuster.

Gonzalez, R. I., Gooden, M. B., & Porter, C. P. (2000). Eliminating racial and ethnic disparities in health care. *American Journal of Nursing, 100*(3), 56–58.

Greenberger, P. (1999). The women's health research coalition: A new advocacy network. *Journal of Women's Health and Gender-Based Medicine, 8*(4), 441–442.

Gunderman, R. (2000). Illness as failure: Blaming patients. *Hastings Center Report, 30*(4), 7–11.

Hoge, C. W., Castro, C. A., Messer, S. C., McGurk, D. Cotting, D. I., & Koffman, R. L. (2004). Combat duty in Iraq and Afghanistan, mental health problems, and barriers to care. *New England Journal of Medicine, 351*(1), 13–22.

Howard, M. O., & Chung, S. S. (2000). Nurses' attitudes toward substance misusers. I. Surveys. *Substance Use and Misuse, 35*(3), 347–365.

Institute of Medicine. (2002). *Report: Unequal treatment: Confronting racial and ethnic disparities in healthcare.* Retrieved from http://www.iom.edu

Johnson, C. D. (2009, November/December). Values: A personal and professional path to improving our workplace culture. *Audiology Today,* pp. 63–64.

Johnson, R. L., Saha, S., Arbelaez, J. J., Beach, M. C., & Cooper, L. A. (2004). Racial and ethnic differences in patient perceptions of bias and cultural competence in health care. *Journal of General Internal Medicine, 19*(2), 101–110.

Kasar, J., & Clark, E. N. (2000). *Developing professional behaviors.* Thorofare, NJ: Slack.

Kearney, N., Miller, M., Paul, J., & Smith, K. (2000). Oncology healthcare professionals' attitudes toward elderly people. *Annals of Oncology, 11*, 599–601.

Kohlberg, L. (1984). *The psychology of moral development: Essays on moral development.* San Francisco, CA: Harper & Row.

Latner, J. D., & Stunkard, A. J. (2003). Getting worse: The stigmatization of obese children. *Obesity Research, 11*, 452–456.

Luber, S. D., Fischer, D. R., & Venkat, A. (2008). Care of the bariatric surgery patient in the emergency department. *Journal of Emergency Medicine, 34*(1), 13–20.

Madan, A. K., Aliabadi-Wahle, S., & Beech, D. J. (2001). Ageism in medical students' treatment recommendations: The example of breast-conserving procedures. *Academic Medicine, 76*(3), 282–284.

Marrocco, A., & Stewart, D. E. (2001). We've come a long way, maybe: Recruitment of women and analysis of results by sex in clinical research. *Journal of Women's Health and Gender-Based Medicine, 10*(2), 175–179.

Martin, V. (2000). Developing team effectiveness. *Nursing Management, 7*(2), 26–29.

Mawn, B., & Reece, S. M. (2000). Reconfiguring a curriculum for the new millennium: The process of change. *Journal of Nursing Education, 39*(3), 101–108.

McGuire, T. G., Ayanian, J. Z., Ford, D. F., Henke, R. E. M., Rose, K. M., & Zaslavsky, A. M. (2008). Testing for statistical discrimination by race/ethnicity in panel data for depression treatment in primary care. *Health Services Research, 43*(2), 531–551.

McLaughlin, D., & Long, A. (1996). An extended literature review of health professionals' perceptions of illicit drugs and their clients who use them. *Journal of Psychiatric Mental Health Nursing, 3,* 283–288.

Moyers, P. A. (2005). The ethics of competence. In R. B. Purtilo, G. M. Jensen & C. B. Royeen (Eds.), *Educating for Moral Action* (pp. 21–30). Philadelphia, PA: F. A. Davis.

Musolino, G. M., & Mostrom, E. (2005). Reflection and the scholarship of teaching, learning and assessment. *Journal of Physical Therapy Education, 19*(3), 52–66.

Must, A., Spadano, J., Coakley, E. H., Field, A. E., Colditz, G., & Dietz, W. H. (1999). The disease burden associated with overweight and obesity. *Journal of the American Medical Association, 282,* 1523–1529.

Nicolette, J., & Jacobs, M. B. (2000). Integration of women's health into an internal medicine core curriculum for medical students. *Academic Medicine, 75*(11), 1061–1065.

Penner, L. A., Dovidio, J. F., Edmondson, D., Dailey, R. K., Makkova, T., Albrecht, T. L., & Gaertner, S. L. (2009). The experience of discrimination and black–white health disparities in medical care. *Journal of Black Psychology, 35,* 180–202.

Puhl, R. M., Moss-Racusin, C. A., Schwartz, M. B., & Brownell, K. D. (2008). Weight stigmatization and bias reduction: Perspectives of overweight and obese adults. *Health Education Research, 23*(2), 347–358.

Purtilo, R., & Haddad, A. (2007). *Health professional and patient interaction* (7th ed.). Philadelphia, PA: W. B. Saunders.

Rest, J. R. (1994). Background: Theory and research. In J. R. Rest & D. Navaez (Eds.), *Moral development in the professions: Psychology and applied ethics* (pp. 1–26). Hillsdale, NJ: Lawrence Erlbaum Associates.

Reyna, C., Goodwin, E. J., & Ferrari, J. R. (2007). Examining the relationship between contact, education, and ageism. *Journal of Gerontological Nursing, February, 33*(2), 50–55.

Rodts, M. F., & Lamb, K. V. (2008). Transforming your professional self: Encouraging lifelong personal and professional growth. *Orthopaedic Nursing, 27*(2), 125–135.

Ross, K. M., Shivy, V. A., & Mazzeo, S. E. (2009). Ambiguity and judgments of obese individuals: No news could be bad news. *Eating Behaviors, 10,* 152–156.

Rybarczyk, B., Haut, A., Lacey, R. F., Fogg, L. F., & Nicholas, J. J. (2001). A multifactorial study of age bias among rehabilitation professionals. *Archives of Physical Medicine and Rehabilitation, 82,* 625–632.

Schon, D. A. (1983). *The reflective practitioner: How professionals think in action.* New York, NY: Basic Books.

Schuster, M. A., Collins, R., Cunningham, W. E., Morton, S.C., Zierler, S., Wong, M., . . . Kanouse, D. E. (2005). Perceived discrimination in clinical care in a nationally representative sample of HIV-infected adults receiving health care. *Journal of General Internal Medicine, 20,* 807–813.

Schwartz, M. B., Vartanian, L. R., Nosek, B. A., & Brownell, K. D. (2006). The influence of one's own body weight on implicit and explicit anti-fat bias. *Obesity Research, 14,* 440–448.

Seo, W. S., & Chen, R. K. (2009). Attitudes of college students toward people with disabilities. *Journal of Applied Rehabilitation Counseling, 40*(4), 3–8.

Shortt, S. (2001). Venerable or vulnerable? Ageism in health care. *Journal of Health Services Research Policy, 6*(1), 1–2.

Sisola, S. W. (2000). Moral reasoning as a predictor of clinical practice: The development of physical therapy students across the professional curriculum. *Journal of Physical Therapy Education, 14*(3), 26–34.

Smart, J. (2008). *Disability, society and the individual* (2nd ed.). Austin, TX: ProEd.

Solheim, K., McElmurry, B. J., & Kim, M. J. (2007). Multidisciplinary teamwork in US primary health care. *Social Science and Medicine, 65,* 622–634.

Stepanikova, I., & Cook, K. S. (2008). Effects of poverty and lack of insurance on perceptions of racial and ethnic bias in health care. *Health Services Research, 43*(3), 915–930.

Suarez-Balcazar, Y., Rodawoski, J., Balcazar, F., Taylor-Ritzler, T., Portillo, N., Barwacz, D., & Willis, C. (2009). Perceived levels of cultural competence among occupational therapists. *American Journal of Occupational Therapy, 63*(4), 498–505.

Sumner, W. G. (1906). *Folkways,* Boston, MA: Ginn and Company.

Sumsion, T., & Smith, G. (2000). Barriers to client-centeredness and their resolution. *Canadian Journal of Occupational Therapy, 67*(1), 15–22.

Swisher, L. L. (2002). A retrospective analysis of ethics knowledge in physical therapy (1970–2000). *Physical Therapy, 82*(7), 692–706.

Thornicroft, G. (2008). Stigma and discrimination limit access to mental health care. *Epidemiologia Psichatria Sociale, 17*(1), 14–19.

Triezenberg, H. L., & Davis, C. M. (2000). Beyond the code of ethics: Educating physical therapists for their role as moral agents. *Journal of Physical Therapy Education, 14*(3), 48–48.

Trivedi, A. N., Zaslavsky, A. M., Schneider, E. C., & Ayanian, J. Z. (2005). Trends in the quality of care and racial disparities in Medicare managed care. *New England Journal of Medicine, 353,* 692–700.

U.S. Department of Health and Human Services. (2001). *Mental health: Culture, race, and ethnicity a supplement to mental health: A report of the surgeon general.* McLean, VA: International Medical Publishing.

U.S. Department of Health and Human Services. (2002). *Healthy people 2010* (2nd ed.). McLean, VA: International Medical Publishing.

U.S. Department of Health and Human Services. (2009). *Healthy people 2020.* Retrieved from http://www.healthypeople.gov/hp2020

Van Houtven, C. H., Voils, C. I., Oddone, E. Z., Weinfurt, K. P., Friedman, J. Y., Friedman, K. A., . . . Bosworth, H. B. (2005). Perceived discrimination and reported delay of pharmacy prescriptions and medical tests. *Journal of General Internal Medicine, 20,* 578–583.

Wang, P. S., Lane, M., Olfson, M., Pincus, H. A., Wells, K. B., & Kessler, R. C. (2005). Twelve-month use of mental health services in the United States: Results from the National Co-morbidity Survey Replication. *Archives of General Psychiatry, 62*(6), 629–640.

Webster, D. (2009). Addressing nursing students' stigmatizing beliefs. *Journal of Psychosocial Nursing, 47*(10), 34–42.

Whalley Hammell, K. (2009). Sacred texts: A skeptical exploration of the assumptions underpinning theories of occupation. *Canadian Journal of Occupational Therapy, 76*(1), 6–13.

Wharton, M. A. (2005). Enhancing professional accountability: Inquiry into the work of a professional ethics committee. In R. B. Purtilo, G. M. Jensen, & C. B. Royeen (Eds.), *Educating for moral action* (pp. 131–143). Philadelphia: F. A. Davis.

Williams, D. R., & Neighbors, H. (2001). Racism, discrimination and hypertension: Evidence and needed research. *Ethnicity and Disease, 11*(4), 800–816.

Williams, D. R., Neighbors, H. W., & Jackson, J. S. (2003). Racial and ethnic discrimination and health: Findings from community studies. *American Journal of Public Health, 93,* 200–208.

World Health Organization. (2010). *Social determinants of health.* Retrieved from http://www.who.int/social_determinants/en

# Multicultural Perspectives

Working in an inner-city clinic is challenging in more ways than I expected. I knew that many of the clients would be poor and have social difficulties, but I never realized how many different ethnic groups and cultures I would see. I used to think that all Asians or Latinos were the same and shared common values, beliefs, and traditions. Since starting my clinical rotation here, it is obvious that many different races and cultures are represented within each ethnic group. I learned that although people from China, Cambodia, or Vietnam may all be classified as Asian, they are different from one another and very different from me. My roommate says that I should treat everybody "the same," but I know that if I do, I'll offend people. If that happens, they won't trust me to care for them. I'm really confused about what to say and do.

*—From the journal of Susan Hancock, social work student*

The United States has been largely settled and developed by people who have emigrated from other countries. The first wave of settlers consisted of White Europeans, seeking religious or political freedom and economic opportunities. The culture and traditions they brought developed into what is currently the majority, or "American," culture. Some refer to this as Anglo-European culture. Newer immigrants continue to come to America for many of the same reasons as the early settlers, but it is also likely that some are escaping the impact of war, oppression, persecution, or other forms of violence. Recent immigrants are more likely to be from Asia, the Caribbean, or South and Central America than from Western Europe (Leavitt, 2010a).

Traditional wisdom held that the United States was a "melting pot" for immigrants, who would all assimilate, blending into a homogeneous "stew," with all individuals sharing the same culture and lifestyle. Today, the United States is more like a tossed salad, where each "ingredient" retains unique characteristics and maintains a highly visible identity (Brice & Campbell, 1999).

For this reason, health care providers must learn to understand, value, and respect racial, ethnic, or cultural differences.

In this chapter, we define culture and describe the many factors that contribute to an individual's cultural identity. While we must be aware and knowledgeable about our own and our clients' cultures, we must also be aware of the culture of medicine, as well as the culture of disability, and how it adds another variable to our interactions with others. Strategies for overcoming barriers and developing culturally competent practice are provided.

## RACE, ETHNICITY, AND CULTURE

The concepts of race, ethnicity, and culture are often confusing and defy simplistic definitions. Although race and ethnicity make a significant contribution to culture, they are not the only determinants. Race is generally perceived to be determined by genetically inherited traits that are identifiable by physical characteristics, such as skin color, facial features, and hair color or texture. Census surveys, college registration forms, and medical history questionnaires typically ask people to identify themselves as being members of a very short list of possible races. It is customary for people to be identified as the race they most resemble (i.e., anyone with a dark skin tone is called Black; someone who has fair skin is White). Race is difficult to determine and can be even harder to identify. With a global economy and people frequently immigrating from one part of the world to another, there are significant opportunities for individuals to intermarry and have children. Therefore, it appears that race is not a useful designation when trying to understand similarities or differences among people. Ethnicity is a more reliable concept than race in understanding people's values, beliefs, and behaviors.

Ethnicity, however, is also a complex and ambiguous designation. This concept is used to describe people of similar backgrounds, who identify with one another and choose to live or socialize together. This often occurs in response to the members' need to function in what might be perceived as a less than welcoming social environment (Spector, 2004). Characteristics that may be considered when defining ethnicity include geographic origin or residence; migration history; race; language or dialect spoken; religion or spiritual beliefs; shared traditions, values, or symbols; occupation; sexual orientation; socioeconomic status; and politics (Leavitt, 2010b; Loveland, 1999). Consider how an elderly woman who practices Buddhism and came to the United States on a crowded, leaky boat from Vietnam is ethnically different from a college student who is Japanese, Christian, and came to the United States with her father's economic support. Although both may be considered Asian, and both are immigrants, they are ethnically quite different.

Individuals who are not of Anglo-European descent may be called "people of color" or "minorities" because they are not White and are not from the majority culture in the United States. "People of color" is an inaccurate term, however, because people with fair skin can come from many racial or ethnic groups. People who look similar may, in fact, be racially or ethnically quite different. Further, the use of the term *minority* is quickly becoming outdated, as minority populations continue to swell. It is predicted that minority populations and new immigrants will become the majority of the population between the years 2030 and 2050 (U.S. Census Bureau, 2008). The term *minority* can be pejorative and imply that people who are not Anglo-European are "less than" the majority culture.

"Culture is a pattern of learned beliefs, shared values, and behavior; it includes language, styles of communication, practices, customs, and views on roles and relationships" (Davidson et al., 2007, p. 608). It cannot be defined by considering only one's race, ethnicity, or country of residence. A critical distinction between the concept of culture and race or ethnicity is that it is learned, not inherited. This learning occurs during the socialization process, beginning at birth. Culture produces material, or observable artifacts, with which we are all familiar, such as art, music, style of dress, and food preference. When we go to a historical museum, attend a Native American crafts show, or listen to an Italian opera, we are examining the material artifacts of a culture. Our food preferences, architecture, and holiday displays or decorations are also examples of material culture. It is easy to identify a person from a "foreign" or "minority" culture if he or she comes to the clinic wearing a sari or turban.

Culture also has nonmaterial aspects that describe intangibles, such as values, beliefs, attitudes, and feelings. Religious beliefs or spiritual practices, morals, ethics, and views about the roles of family members are examples of nonmaterial culture. These are not so easily observed. Nonmaterial culture provides individuals with paradigms that explain how the universe is ordered, including explanations for natural phenomena, such as health and illness. These ideas may be so deeply embedded that an individual is almost unaware that they exist and just assumes that this is how "everyone" thinks. Nonmaterial culture may be difficult to identify unless one asks respectful, nonjudgmental questions and is genuinely interested in learning about these beliefs and values.

Finally, culture provides a largely unconscious framework that we use for organizing our daily behavior. It determines *how* we interact with the world, and what physical, social, or cognitive behaviors are acceptable (Loveland, 1999). It defines the parameters of social relationships, such as gender and family roles, vocational and community relationships, and relationships with professionals. We can sometimes identify people from one social group or class from another by observing their behavior and listening to their choice of words. Individuals who share the same race can, however, have different cultural identities. Consider a middle-aged Black physician who lives in the suburbs and teaches at a prestigious medical school. His culture is much more likely to be similar to that of White professionals, living in similar circumstances, than it is to be like the culture of a Black adolescent attending an urban high school.

In America, we typically categorize individuals into groups by racial and ethnic features and historical and geographic origins. Although some variation is seen in how groups are identified and named, Americans with dark skin and origins in Africa are typically called African American or Black. Geographic origins in Africa and the experience of slavery serve as unifying themes. This grouping may also include people from the Caribbean islands, although some people from these regions might consider themselves Latino or Caribbean. Native American cultures encompass several hundred different tribes of people indigenous to North America. Older individuals prefer the term *American Indians*, whereas younger individuals prefer the term *Native American* (Broome & Broome, 2007). White or Caucasian individuals typically come from a European heritage and make up what is described as the mainstream or majority culture in America. They may also be referred to as Anglo or Anglo-European. Asian culture describes people who may come from China, Japan, Korea, Vietnam, or Eastern Asian countries, such as India, Pakistan, and Iran. Finally, individuals who are Latino or Hispanic share a common cultural origin (Spain) and language (Spanish) but more recently have likely emigrated from South America, Central America, or the Caribbean islands (Arredondo et al., 1996). The terms *Latino* and *Hispanic* may be preferred by different groups, depending on cultural identification.

Debate and controversy surround the naming or labeling of racial/ethnic groups. Issues of politics, stigma, and discrimination over the choice of these group names are significant in defining a culture. In addition, over time, group preferences change, and what was once considered an appropriate label may become unacceptable. We have chosen to use the terminology identified above because it is most consistently used in the current literature. The reader should understand that this does not imply universal acceptance of these terms.

Placing all Americans into only a few racial/ethnic groups seems contrary to a multifactorial approach to defining culture. Using only these broad categories to define human differences can lead to simplistic thinking about culture and stereotyping. Each large racial group listed above contains many subgroups or subcultures. For example, in the United States, there are more than 20 Latino or Hispanic subgroups and at least 18 Asian subgroups (Leavitt, 2010b). In addition, Irish people may be Irish Catholics or Irish Protestants. Some consider the United States to have a culture of disability, which is a subculture of the majority American culture.

Subcultures have much in common with a larger, more dominant culture but also have distinct characteristics that render them recognizably different (Loveland, 1999). They have their own sets of customs and beliefs that may differ from those of the larger culture. Unfortunately, some subcultures are viewed by mainstream culture as being odd, holding deviant beliefs, or engaging in unacceptable practices (Leininger, 1995). Individuals from a subculture may be unable to understand or relate to someone from a different subculture, even though both come from the same country (Erlen, 1998). For example, historically and culturally, India was a country with a rigidly stratified caste system. Someone from the Brahmin caste, at one end of the spectrum, would have virtually nothing in common with an individual who was considered an Untouchable, at the other end. The use of that restrictive social system is becoming more obsolete in much of India today.

Arredondo and colleagues (1996) have proposed a model for describing the dimensions of personal identity within a culture, which is still in use today. The largest, most prominent dimension is termed the *A Dimension,* which describes characteristics that are largely predetermined and difficult or impossible to change. *A Dimension* characteristics include age, ethnicity, gender, primary language, physical disability, race, and class. The *B Dimension* includes traits that are much more likely to be under the individual's control, including education, geographic location, income, religion, work experience, and hobbies or recreational interests. The *C Dimension* encompasses historical, political, and economic contexts that frame an individual's life experiences and opportunities. Although this model was designed to help professionals conceptualize the values and beliefs that are relevant to individual clients, these factors are also important for defining or describing various subcultures. In all interactions with clients and families, we must remember to identify the values and beliefs of the individual and not make assumptions based on stereotypes. We may use generalizations to alert us to *possible* similarities or differences between groups that provide a framework for closer examination. However, it is essential to explore these assumptions by observing the client's behaviors or asking respectfully about beliefs and preferences. We must not stereotype by assuming that any member of a group shares *all* the characteristics of that group.

## ACCULTURATION, ASSIMILATION, AND BICULTURALISM

One factor that affects an individual's cultural beliefs is the degree of acculturation. Following immigration to a new place of residence or country, a person ideally needs to adapt to the culture and lifestyle of the new home in order to survive and thrive. "Acculturation is the process through which people in subcultures adopt traits of the larger, or normative, culture" (Loveland, 1999, p. 19). This is necessary in order for immigrants to integrate and be a part of the new culture. During this process, the individual slowly leaves behind the language and the culture of origin to fully assume the beliefs and behaviors of the majority culture. It takes a significant length of time, typically more than one generation, for this to occur. Not everyone chooses to learn the language or learn it completely. In addition, many do not fully assume the beliefs and behaviors of the majority culture. Cultural practices and beliefs are strongly affected by the level of acculturation, which is not immediately evident to others.

This process is not easy and may cause significant stress and difficulty for those who are engaged in the change. Acculturation occurs across a spectrum of levels as norms and beliefs transition from the culture of origin to the new majority culture. As people acculturate, they slowly relinquish the "old ways" and begin to speak and behave in ways that are common for the majority culture. This can be hard to readily identify when a client wears Western-style clothing, speaks unaccented English, and eats a "typical" American diet in public. Health care providers may see these typical "American" behaviors and may expect that everyone will share *all* of their cultural beliefs and norms. Although there is some debate about the validity of expecting full acculturation to occur, the fact remains that at this time, not everyone accepts all the beliefs and behaviors of the majority culture (Spector, 2004). For example, regarding health beliefs, some clients may believe that an illness is a punishment for past behaviors, or that there is an imbalance between the body and the spirit. These clients may prefer traditional medicine over Western medicine or may wish to combine elements of the two systems.

The rate of acculturation can fluctuate and is affected by many factors. Perhaps the most significant variable is age, with younger individuals acculturating more quickly than older people. Some older people who immigrate never fully accept the culture of their new home and continue to speak their native language, practice traditional rituals, and socialize with others from their native culture. Other factors that affect the rate of acculturation include length of time in the new culture, place of residence (living with people from the native culture or the majority culture), language spoken at home, and amount of contact with the country of origin.

To determine the degree of acculturation, you can ask clients about the language spoken at home, the language of their media preference, their family roles, worldview, and frequency and type of social interactions with people from other cultural groups (Leavitt, 2001). Individuals may have strong connections to both the original culture and the majority culture. For example, they may dress, speak, and behave like others from the majority culture while at school or work. At home, however, they may speak their native language, eat traditional foods, and practice familiar rituals; that is, they are bicultural. Consider Mai Ling, who was born in China and came to the United States to attend college. She is now a college professor and fits in easily with her American peers at the university. However, she continues to feel that her cultural orientation is primarily Chinese. After many years away from China, she returned home for a visit. One day, her distraught mother confronted her and stated, "You are no longer Chinese! You do not behave like a proper Chinese daughter!" Mai Ling realized that she had become bicultural, neither fully American nor Chinese, but with strong values and beliefs from both cultures.

"Assimilation is different than acculturation in that the arriving group is totally absorbed into the dominant society. Their original culture is overridden by the dominant group" (Flaskerud, 2007, p. 543). In other words, the culture of origin has disappeared. Assimilation is most likely to occur when individuals are not physically different from the majority culture, when there is little contact with the native culture, and when there is little educational or physical segregation (Loveland, 1999). This would explain the lack of assimilation of the Hmong people from Southeast Asia, people from Puerto Rico, and Native Americans, who look physically different from the majority culture, tend to live in ethnically homogeneous settings, and maintain strong bonds with others from their culture of origin.

## ETHNOCENTRISM

Ethnocentrism is a belief in the superiority of one's culture or ethnic group. It creates a barrier to establishing relationships with those from other cultures whose beliefs or actions are perceived as odd, unacceptable, or even repugnant. The belief that your worldview and cultural practices are "correct" makes others inferior and less worthy of respect (Sue & Sue, 1999). When health providers interact with clients, ethnocentrism can present significant obstacles for effective practice. "It is exceptionally difficult to describe or comprehend the extent to which ethnocentrism and racism have been woven into the fabric of our health care system" (Tripp-Reimer, Choi, Kelley, & Enslein, 2001, p.14). The client's and family's ethnocentrism may also create barriers to effective health care delivery (Banja, 1996). People from Asian, Latino/Hispanic, African American, and Native American cultures may have health care beliefs that differ widely from those held by most Western medical practitioners. They, too, believe that their culturally defined understandings of health, illness, and appropriate healing behavior are the most appropriate. This may lead to refusal to seek health care from Western healers or to client nonadherence with the recommended treatment (Canlas, 1999; Stell, 1999; Sung, 1999).

## WORLDVIEW

The aspects of culture that involve values, beliefs, and the way members of a group understand the world around them can be summarized under the concept of *worldview*. This concept refers to the internalized and largely invisible values people use to form a cohesive picture of the world around them (Leininger, 1995). People from cultures with different worldviews may find each other's behavior bewildering or even offensive. Before beginning to interact with clients, it is necessary to determine how their belief systems affect the way they structure their social interactions and how they make important life decisions. In other words, it is important to assess their worldview and adjust your interventions accordingly. Failure to do this may result in dissatisfaction and lack of adherence with suggested treatments. Worldview consists of several dimensions: (1) social organization and relationships, (2) time orientation, (3) activity orientation and levels of environmental control, (4) use of space, and (5) communication between people. Worldviews can be divided into two broad categories: collectivist and individualist. Individuals in each of these categories have differing orientations on the dimensions listed above. See Table 3–1 for a comparison of these two different belief systems.

### Social Organization and Relationships

The majority culture in the United States and other Western cultures is individualistic and places importance on the values of autonomy, that is, self-determination. Each person has the primary responsibility for his or her actions. Personal autonomy is highly valued and rewarded (Sue & Sue, 1999). Within this philosophy, the nuclear family is viewed as the most important social unit. We expect our young people to sleep in their own beds, live apart from parents and other family members as adults, and be financially independent. They are also encouraged to make decisions regarding careers, marriage, and living arrangements that best suit their own needs, without

**Table 3–1**    Comparison of Cultural Value Systems or Worldview

|  | Collectivist Cultures | Individualistic Cultures |
| --- | --- | --- |
| **Racial/Ethnic Groups** | • Most typically seen in Latino, African American, Asian, and Native American cultures | • Traditionally seen in mainstream American and Anglo-European cultures |
| **Time** | • Past or present oriented<br>• Respect for elders<br>• "Lose" control of time | • Future oriented<br>• Precise time is important<br>• Plans are made, appointments are kept |
| **Activity Orientation/ Environmental Control** | • Fate<br>• Just "being"<br>• Human interactions dominate<br>• Cooperation<br>• Harmony with others and nature | • Personal control over the environment and outcomes<br>• Doing, working, achieving<br>• Taking charge<br>• Self-help<br>• Competition |
| **Social Organization** | • Group welfare<br>• Harmony<br>• Hierarchy | • Privacy, self-achievement<br>• Autonomy<br>• Independence<br>• Equality |
| **Communication** | • Low context<br>• Indirect<br>• Low eye contact<br>• Formal | • High context<br>• Direct<br>• High eye contact<br>• Informal |

*Source:* The work of Purnell & Lattanzi (2006) and Leavitt (2010b).

consideration of the impact on the extended family, kinship group, or tribe (Sue & Sue, 1999). Medical determinations are also personal decisions, and while family involvement is valued, these decisions are made independently of the family. People expect to be provided with all relevant information and to provide fully informed consent. Direct communication is valued, and communication with strangers is easily established (Brice & Campbell, 1999).

For people who are of racial/ethnic cultures other than Anglo-European, the orientation is collectivist in nature. Although there is great variability among the many cultural traditions that ascribe to this belief system, the primary value is that the needs of the group supersede the needs of the individual. Uniformity and conformity are the ideals rather than individualism and freedom of choice (Crabtree, 2006). Information about health is more often widely shared with many people involved in making decisions about treatments. Within this orientation, the extended family is the psychosocial unit, with dependence and connectedness to the group strongly valued (Brice & Campbell, 1999). People do not make decisions based on what is good for the individual but rather on what is best for the larger family or social group. In this tradition, health decisions are not made alone but within the extended family. Some cultures may have a designated person, such as the husband, who decides for the wife and children, or the oldest son, who decides for the family. The principles of confidentiality and informed consent may not apply in the same way in collectivist cultures, where the family unit may be much broader than the nuclear family and include aunts, uncles, cousins, or tribal elders (Davidson et al., 2007).

Although the individualistic majority of Americans values solving problems directly, collectivist cultures take a different approach. Problems are solved indirectly by suggestion or guidance. Confrontation is not only avoided, it is considered unacceptable. In Japanese culture, "the nail that sticks out gets hammered down." In contrast, in American culture, we believe that "the squeaky wheel gets the grease."

## Time Orientation

People from various cultures may have vastly different orientations to time. Some are present oriented, whereas others focus primarily on the past or future (Spector, 2004). In the United States, people from the Caucasian majority culture are strongly focused on the future. They value precise "clock time," and being on time for appointments is expected (Leininger, 1995). This future orientation also affects our expectations for health care behavior. We expect our clients and colleagues to plan ahead, make and keep appointments, and take steps to maintain health or prevent future problems (Spector, 2004). Cultures with a focus on the future also tend to delay immediate pleasure to work for future gratification (Brice & Campbell, 1999; Sue & Sue, 1999).

Other cultures do not necessarily share this future orientation. People who are part of some African American or Native American cultures, for example, tend to be present oriented (Sue & Sue, 1999). Because they may perceive time as "circular" or "flowing," dividing time into artificial segments becomes meaningless. Making and keeping schedules may also be construed as unimportant or disruptive. In addition, people who are present oriented may value youth and beauty and choose to live in the moment, rather than planning or sacrificing for the future (Brice & Campbell, 1999; Davidhizar, Dowd, & Newman-Giger, 1997).

In contrast, people of cultures that focus on the past tend to value elders and honor traditions. Changes in traditional practices, beliefs, and behaviors are strongly discouraged. In Asian cultures, for example, people often have a past-orientation and rely on traditional healing practices, such as herbal treatments, acupuncture, and the use of traditional healers (Spector, 2004). The advice of elders is precious; they are considered to have gained great wisdom.

## Activity Orientation/Environmental Control

Culture influences the level of control people believe they have over their environment and how much they can affect their destinies. The majority culture in the United States is extremely action oriented, with an emphasis on environmental control. Individuals are expected to master nature, overcome all obstacles, and control their own future. The Protestant work ethic dictates an achievement-oriented outlook, based on a belief that all problems have solutions (Sue & Sue, 1999). This may help explain why Americans tend to view themselves as a "can-do" society, where people who face challenges or adversity are expected to "pull themselves up by their bootstraps." Every problem is perceived as being solvable, if you work hard or long enough. We do not often consider that some people have no "boots," let alone "bootstraps."

People from other cultures, particularly Asian, Latino, and Native American, sometimes reflect a feeling of powerlessness over nature (Sue & Sue, 1999). Harmony with the universe, rather than mastery or control of it, is valued. Behaviors that Caucasian Americans view as passivity, noncompetitiveness, stoicism, or being "unmotivated" may actually be associated with serenity or inner peace with one's place in the universe. For example, people in the Latino culture may believe that one's status in life is predetermined and that one cannot be held accountable for it because this is the state into which a person is born. For Native Americans, harmony with nature is a core value.

Incompatibility of beliefs between health care providers and clients can lead to significant conflict if they hold opposing ideas about the optimal level of activism and environmental control (Gannotti, Handwerker, Groce, & Cruz, 2001). Consider Emilio, a young child with cerebral palsy, living in a traditional Puerto Rican family home. The medical staff believes that it is important for the family to perform daily exercises with Emilio, practice new skills, and encourage him to work hard to maximize function. They are frustrated by the family's apparent lack of motivation and follow-through with their recommendations. The family decides to discontinue medical care with their facility because they feel uncomfortable with the health care providers' emphasis on their taking control of the situation.

## Use of Space

Cultural space refers to the ways different cultures use the body and regard visual, territorial, and interpersonal distance to others (Leininger, 1995). Health care professionals must often cross clients' physical boundaries in order to examine or treat them. We may innocently assume that everyone maintains the same boundaries that we do or that all clients will accept the suspension of boundaries in order to receive care. This is not so. For example, a young female health care provider was assigned to treat a gentleman who practiced Islam. When she extended her hand to greet him, he politely declined and did not make eye contact with her. The therapist asked him if he would prefer a male therapist to treat him, and he gratefully accepted the offer.

*Territorial space* describes the larger area that is occupied or defended by a group or about which that group holds strong emotional ties (Leininger, 1995; Spector, 2004). Some people, who have immigrated from Iran refer to themselves as Persians, using an earlier name for their homeland. *Personal space* refers to the space immediately surrounding the body. What is comfortable for one person may be unacceptable for another. In the majority American culture, the intimate zone extends to about 18 inches from the body and allows individuals to have very close personal contact. In other cultures, the zone of personal comfort can be more or less. Only close personal associates are allowed to enter this space. Violating personal space preferences can lead to stress, anger, and conflict. Entering without permission may be viewed as an act of aggression (Leininger, 1995; Spector, 2004; Sue & Sue, 1999).

## Communication

Communication, as described in Chapter 5, forms the basis for human interaction. There is a strong reciprocal relationship between culture and communication, with each exerting a powerful influence on the other. The language we use is influenced by our culture, and the words that are available in our language help to shape perceptions of reality and convey ideas. The language that we acquire as children influences our worldview and our beliefs (Brice & Campbell, 1999). As our culture develops, words and phrases arise or are "coined" to describe new phenomena. For example, the rapid growth in the use of computers and other technical devices has spawned a new language of technology-related words and acronyms.

Unfortunately, many health care providers in the United States speak only English, while clients from other cultures may have limited English skills. Differences in the structure and formation of language can make it difficult or impossible for direct translation of ideas or social reality. Clients who are bilingual may be assumed to have good English proficiency, but they may have difficulty with complex medical terms or be unable to describe their symptoms accurately. In the United States, where everyone "shares" the English language, it is assumed that we all understand each other, but this may not be so.

$M$r. Chang, who is Chinese, is my newest client, and I just can't seem to figure out how to communicate with him. He has chronic obstructive pulmonary disease and is coming to our center for rehabilitation. His family seems very supportive, and his wife and daughter often come to his appointments with him. They seem very interested in his health, sitting quietly in the room, while he goes through his program. However, I don't have a clue whether anyone understands a word I'm saying! They always seem to listen attentively, nod, and smile.

When I ask if they understand, they politely say "yes" and never ask any questions. Mr. Chang doesn't seem to be improving, and I suspect that he is not following his exercise program at home. However, when I ask if there are any problems or if they would like me to make some changes, they state that everything is fine. I wish I could figure out what to do differently.

*—From the journal of Sean Murphy, exercise physiology student*

In the above journal entry, there are many possible explanations for the client's and family's behavior. They may not be sufficiently proficient in English to understand what is being explained. In Chinese culture, protecting one's honor is highly valued. The client and his family may have been too embarrassed to admit their lack of comprehension. Respecting others, especially those in positions of authority, is important, and asking questions is considered a sign of disrespect. In Asian cultures, health care providers are considered to hold positions of high esteem and authority. They may have been respecting the honor of the health care professional by not wanting to embarrass him for not clearly explaining what was expected of them. The student could have provided pictures, diagrams, or instructions in the client's native language. Asking the client to demonstrate the exercises would be another way to assess understanding. Chinese families traditionally maintain a high level of involvement in health care situations, and the student may be able to find a way to tactfully engage them in supporting Mr. Chang's treatment.

Language and communication differences present significant barriers to providing effective health care to clients and families from minority cultures (Choi & Wynne, 2000). In a study of Latino parents, 26 percent stated that language problems were the greatest barrier to obtaining health care for their children. Many families indicated the wrong diagnosis was made, or incorrect treatment was received because the health care provider and the client did not understand each other (Flores, Abreu, Olivar, & Kastner, 1998). See Chapter 5 for additional information regarding this topic.

Although language is a significant component of communication, it is not the only factor. The style and content of interactions are also significant. An important concept used to describe the culturally mediated style of communication is the designation of a culture as having a high or low context. *Context* refers to the level of environmental or social cues that are available to help frame the exchange of information. "Low-context communication relies little on the surrounding context for interpretation" (Brice & Campbell, 1999, p. 86). It tends to be explicit and highly descriptive. Low-context communication also assumes that words must be used to explain everything because little is implicitly understood. Because little can be taken for granted, much must be explained. This communication is most commonly seen in individualistic cultures that prefer a very direct style of communication. For example, in a university community, the students, faculty, and staff come from diverse backgrounds. In this setting, people must explicitly explain what they mean. One cannot merely say "look this over." Some would interpret that to mean literally glance at it; others would give it a light reading; and yet others would study it carefully.

High-context communication is found in cultures that are rich in tradition and often highly structured. It is dependent on nonverbal interactions, strong group identification, and understanding of the rules of interaction. It relies on shared group experiences, history, and customs to express ideas, rather than verbal communication. Nonverbal cues and messages are used extensively to convey meaning. This type of interaction is most often seen in collectivist cultures (Sue & Sue, 1999). For example, African American cultures tend to be high context. Members of these cultural groups often use body movements, facial expressions, and culturally relevant phrases to express ideas, using few words. Asian cultures also tend to be high context. Communication is very indirect, with individuals rarely stating exactly what they mean or what they want. Instead, meaning is conveyed from subtle clues within the context of the situation. Consider a sports team in which the members participate daily for several hours over many months. Using a word or phrase, or perhaps stating someone's name or a team name, can send the group into gales of laughter, as the group members recall a situation they all experienced together. "Outsiders" may often miss important information.

Low-context language tends to be logical and linear, whereas high-context communication is indirect and less explicit. It is easy to see how cultural misinterpretations can occur. Members of low-context cultures may view individuals who use high-context forms of expression as being less intelligent, less educated, or less interested because they use fewer words. Individuals who prefer high-context communication can be offended by overly direct statements made by those who use a low-context communication style. They prefer suggestion and guidance rather than forceful declarations.

## Disability

Race, ethnicity, gender, sexual orientation, religion, language, age, and social class are typically cited as salient contributors to an individual's culture and personal identity. However, the effect of having an impairment or disability also contributes to one's cultural identity and should be added to the list of contributors to cultural identity. Indeed, some would go so far as to say there is a disability culture or, at least, a disability subculture (Eddey & Robey, 2005; Leavitt & Roush, 2010). This idea is controversial, and many do not support it. Those who are opposed to the concept of a disability culture believe that, for many reasons, people with disabilities (PWD) are not alike. For example, Eddey and Robey have explained that while each PWD has an impairment significant enough to be disabling, there is a broad range of impairments and disabilities. Some are visible, whereas others are not, and some cause more distress than others. Further, disabilities are spread across all racial and ethnic groups, so PWD may have very different cultures of origin. On the surface, it would appear that they share few common features aside from their disability status. They do not acquire this culture from previous generations of family and friends and, in fact, may be the only person in the family to have a disability. Finally, PWD have been and continue to be isolated and marginalized, so there are fewer opportunities for meeting, socializing, and developing a culture.

As noted in Chapter 10, people with disabilities represent the largest minority group in the United States, standing at 54.4 million people (U.S. Census Bureau, 2008). Further, it is a cultural group that is eliciting increased awareness from health care providers. Disability culture and disability studies (the study of disability culture) are quickly becoming important bodies of knowledge for rehabilitation providers (Leavitt & Roush, 2010). Grassroots advocates who joined the disability rights movement when it first began in the 1980s see themselves as a part of a culture.

They have shared goals, frustrations, and experiences related to the lack of civil rights faced by people with disabilities in comparison to the general population. In addition, PWD have developed shared beliefs, values, attitudes, and coping strategies. These cultural attributes can extend to include family, friends, caretakers, and other advocates (Eddey & Robey, 2005; Fleisher & Zames, 2001). From their shared worldview, PWD have joined together to form a community based on cultural norms, centered around collective goals, but use various means and ways of expression to meet these goals (Peters, 2000).

Brown (2002) further argues that PWD generate cultural artifacts, such as art, music, literature, humor, and other expressions of their experience of disability. "Distinctive disability press and publications are numerous" (Peters, 2000, p. 590). Most importantly, they feel proud of themselves as people with disabilities. Table 3–2 contrasts the differences in worldviews between the culture of people with disabilities and the majority U.S. culture.

For many, the experience of living with a disability is an essential determinant of status and identity based on many factors, including the perception of prejudice, discrimination, and oppression (Leavitt & Roush, 2010). As a culturally distinct group, people with disabilities have reported shared, negative experiences when interacting with health care professionals, and the evidence seems to support their perceptions. One study examined health professional students'

**Table 3–2** Comparison of Worldviews of Disability versus Nondisability Cultures

| Disability Culture | Nondisability Culture |
|---|---|
| • Positive orientation toward helping and being helped<br>• Skill in managing multiple problems | • Achievement oriented |
| • Will share the same norms as nondisabled groups<br>• High-context communication with other people who have disabilities<br>• Finely tuned capacity for interpersonal communication<br>• Additional factors may be present, such as hearing and visual impairments, having altered verbal communication, different levels of cognition, and differing physical ability, that affect communication | • High- and low-context communication<br>• Direct communication is preferred in standard "American" culture |
| • Flexible, adaptive, resourceful approach to tasks and problems<br>• Understanding that needs are different, depending on abilities | • Activity oriented<br>• Mastery over the environment |
| • Tolerance for dealing with the unpredictable<br>• Present oriented | • Future oriented |
| • Interdependence (collectivist) | • Independence (individualistic) |
| • Acceptance of human differences | • Autonomous/individualistic |
| • Produces artifacts | • Produces artifacts |

*Source:* Gill (1995).

attitudes about people with disabilities and found that all students' attitudes were less positive than the established norms produced for the assessment tool. Among all health professions' students, nursing students held the least positive opinions. There were no attitudinal differences by gender. Students with a background in disability held more positive attitudes, and years of experience and hours worked with this population predicted comfort with challenging rehabilitation situations (Tervo & Palmer, 2004).

## HEALTH BELIEFS AND PRACTICES

Although culture strongly influences the health beliefs and practices of clients, there are multiple variations within each culture. Clients integrate cultural, personal, family, and "popular" beliefs, personal experiences, and biomedical information to explain health and illness. "Personal experiences, family attitudes, and group beliefs interact to provide an underlying structure for decision-making during illness" (Pachter, 1994, p. 690).

Culture profoundly influences health and responses to illness. It determines how people define health and illness, explains the causes of illness, and describes how to maintain health and how to restore health when illness occurs (Spector, 2004; Vanderhoff, 2005). The ways people behave when they are ill are also culturally determined, as are the expected behaviors of health care providers. Clients may appear in the medical setting complaining of "high blood," "nerves," "wind," "evil eye," or "soul loss." The provider may inaccurately assume the clients are ignorant or lack education and, therefore, need to be taught about the facts and true nature of their health problems. Instead, these are culture-bound syndromes, which can alert the provider that the individual may be someone who maintains traditional health care beliefs and prefers traditional practices.

To illustrate some salient health beliefs and practices, we discuss those held by the four largest minority cultures in the United States: Native American, Asian, Latino/Hispanic, and African American. Although each of these cultures is unique, and each subculture within the larger culture even more unique, several important beliefs tend to be consistent among groupings. These beliefs must be recognized and understood because, in many cases, they are strikingly different from those held by practitioners of Western medicine. We will be making the assumption that the reader is already familiar with the majority culture's views on health and illness, with a reliance on Western medical practices.

Health beliefs held by racial or ethnic minorities *may* include:

- Health is believed to result from a harmony of mind, body, and spirit *or* health results from harmony from within the family *or* harmony with natural or spiritual forces.
- Disharmony will result in illness.
- Healing practices are based on restoring balance or harmony.
- The role of the health care provider is to restore this balance.
- Illness may be a punishment for past or current behaviors.
- Illness may result from the malignant intent of others, such as the "evil eye," curses, or voodoo.
- The personality or social style of the health care professional is extremely important.
- Great value is placed on traditional medical practices, such as herbs, teas, chants or prayers delivered by traditional healers, special tokens and amulets, and acupuncture.

Healers who practice Western medicine may find it difficult to understand these beliefs or practices, but it is essential to maintain an open mind and a curious attitude, while approaching each health belief with respect.

## Native American Cultures

Native Americans are the original indigenous people of North, South, and Central America. Currently, they make up 1.5 percent of the American population (Broome & Broome, 2007). Many estimates hold that between 1500 and 1900, their numbers decreased by 90 to 95 percent, through forced relocation, disease, alcohol, slavery, and warfare. Thus, "historical trauma and unresolved grief are a legacy that many Indian people struggle with today" (Weaver, 1998, p. 204). Distrust and suspicion are a common result of this experience. Currently, the United States recognizes more than 500 tribes (Broome & Broome, 2007), each with its own unique cultural traditions and ways of living. We cannot make assumptions or generalizations about the beliefs of the numerous tribes. These individual differences are best discovered from the tribe members themselves (Weaver, 1998). It is distressing that 25 percent live in poverty and experience significant health disparities that lead to poorer health outcomes than those encountered by Caucasian Americans.

Many beliefs *are* shared across tribes. Members of Native American cultures share a belief in spiritual forces and the traditions of their ancestors. Medicine and healing are closely tied to religion and bound by sacred religious narratives and rituals. Because each person has three dimensions—mind, body, and spirit—all must be treated in order for healing to occur. The spirit is considered to be the most important element in Native American cultures, and spiritual distress is manifested by physical symptoms. The mind links the body and spirit, and wellness is achieved when all three are in harmony (Pichette, Garrett, Kosciulek, & Rosenthal, 1999). While acquired disabilities may be perceived to be balanced by a strong mind, congenital conditions are believed to occur because of immoral behavior of the individual, negative spirits, or sorcery (Broome & Broome, 2007).

Native Americans do not traditionally speak about illness, disability, or death, because it is believed that this may cause the spirit to manifest the problem in the body. This belief has significant implications for Western health care practitioners, who are trained to educate clients by explaining diseases and treatments in great detail. They perceive that the healer's power is closely tied to his or her spirituality, and there must be a connectedness before healing can occur (Broome & Broome, 2007). Health care interactions are further complicated by the fact that people of these cultures typically use few words, avoid smiling, and believe that making eye contact is a sign of disrespect. These factors may lead health care providers to believe that the client is disinterested or nonadherent.

## Asian Cultures

People from Asian cultures have been immigrating to the United States since the 1800s. They come from places as diverse as the Far East, Southeast Asia, and the Indian subcontinent and represent many countries, such as China, Japan, Vietnam, India, Pakistan, and the Philippines. They are the third largest emerging culture, with the largest percentage being people from China (Spector, 2004).

Similar to people of Native American cultures, those from traditional Asian cultures also believe that health results from a harmony between the body and the spirit. They view the universe as an indivisible whole, with each person interconnected to all others in a state of harmonious balance. In the Confucian value system, practiced by many Asians, it is believed that loyalty and harmony within the family lead to harmony with the environment and within the self. This harmony is the foundation for good health and well-being, and a disruption will lead to illness. Hierarchy and respect for elders are essential. Children are expected to be well behaved and achieve in school because it will bring honor to the family and maintain harmony. "Saving face," protecting one's honor, and "giving face," showing respect for others, are also highly valued behaviors. Being disrespectful is not tolerated (Brice & Campbell, 1999).

Many Asians believe that a disruption of this state of balance or harmony leads to illness. For example, people who are Chinese believe there must be a balance between the forces of yin and yang that are found within each person. Yin signifies forces that are static, internal, downward, dull, or low activity. In contrast, dynamic, external, upward, and brilliant forces manifest yang. Imbalance or predominance of either force, yin or yang, causes specific, identifiable diseases, treated by restoring balance (Spector, 2004).

As discussed earlier, Asian cultures value authority figures and expect the medical practitioner to provide the "best" treatment. They are the experts and should tell the clients what the best course of treatment is, rather than discussing options and offering choices. People of Asian cultures tend to be reserved, and it is unusual to openly discuss feelings or display emotions. Unfortunately, this may lead to the mistaken notion that they have a high tolerance for pain, when in fact, they may be too embarrassed to admit having pain or too polite to ask for pain medication when it is not offered. In addition, Chinese clients often prefer to use traditional healing techniques, such as acupuncture or herbs, rather than, or in addition to, Western health interventions (Tang & Cheng, 2001).

## Latino/Hispanic Cultures

People from Latino or Hispanic cultures are originally from Mexico, South and Central America, and the Caribbean islands. Some are directly descended from Spanish explorers (hence, the term Hispanic), whereas others are from various groups from Latin America (Latino). In different geographic areas, one term might be preferred to another. At this time, people of Latino descent are one of the largest minority groups in America (12.5 percent of the population), with the largest ethnic group being from Mexico (Hatcher & Whittemore, 2007).

Latinos as a group tend to have strong religious beliefs. Good health is regarded as good luck or a gift from God. Poor health is the result of fate and is not under the active control of the client or family. Disease or disability may also be perceived as punishment for sins or transgressions or as a result of negative spiritual forces, such as the "evil eye." Similar to the other cultures discussed, people from Latino cultures do not separate the natural and spiritual worlds and, therefore, body and soul are not separate entities (Salimbene, 2000). For example, *susto* (soul loss) is an illness that can develop after a serious fright or trauma and occurs when the soul leaves the body and wanders freely. The symptoms of this disorder are similar to depression or anxiety and include disruptions in sleep patterns, as well as loss of energy, interest, and weight (Spector, 2004).

An essential element in providing care is *respeto* (respect). All people, regardless of age, education, or social class, expect to be treated equally, with regard to dignity, formality, and respect. The personality and social skills of the health care provider are extremely important to the Latino client. A warm, caring personality, *personalismo,* is also expected. Health professionals are expected to shake clients' hands, warmly greet them, make eye contact, and show a genuine interest in the individuals and their families. The value of using empathetic, yet informal, interactions with personal stories cannot be overemphasized (Evans, Coon, & Crogan, 2007). Latino culture is highly collectivist, with extended family expected to be present and included in all encounters. They tend to be involved in the clients' medical care and expect to be included in decision making. It may be alarming for health professionals to see so many family members participate in medical appointments or visits during recovery, providing noisy and enthusiastic support for the clients (Leavitt, 2001; Nava, 2000; Salimbene, 2000). Many Latinos use traditional healing techniques, such as eating special food, using herbs, or calling in a spiritual healer. Western medicine is also used and may be combined with traditional healing methods.

## African American Cultures

The first Black people who were brought to America from Africa were sold as slaves. Families were disrupted, native cultures destroyed, and human rights ignored. Other Black Americans are people who are descended from slaves but have lived in the Caribbean and came here voluntarily. Although more than 150 years have passed since the United States' Civil War and the emancipation of the slaves, the experiences of 400 years of slavery, and the discrimination that followed, continue to exert powerful influences on the African American community. Racial discrimination has decreased substantially since the Civil Rights movement began in the 1960s, but many African American people continue to be disadvantaged and feel powerless. This has caused many to distrust individuals from other cultures, especially Caucasian Americans, and to have an expectation that discrimination is still present (Coleman, 2009). These concerns promote wariness and a reluctance to seek health care for anything but the most serious conditions. Health care professionals need to acknowledge and appreciate these concerns (Spector, 2004). Traditional healers and healing techniques, such as folk remedies, are often used as alternatives to the formal medical system. For many individuals from African American cultures, entering the formal medical care system is avoided at all costs, and care is only sought when the situation is severe.

People from African American cultures have deep spiritual beliefs and strong religious practices. These "spiritual beliefs and practices are a source of comfort, coping, and support and are generally the most effective way to influence healing" (Johnson, Elbert-Avila, & Tulsky, 2005, p. 711). It is believed that God is responsible for all spiritual and physical health. Further, only God has the power to make decisions about who shall live or when someone shall die. Prayer is used as a healing technique because divine intervention can occur, and miracles can and do happen.

This belief in the power of prayer to effect a positive change may lead a person to refuse to accept a diagnosis of a terminal illness or an incurable disease. Because only God can decide that it is time for the client to die, aggressive treatment of illness is likely to be requested, and hospice and advance directives are rarely used. Doctors are seen as the instruments of God, who are expected to help prolong life as long as possible. This can cause conflict between care providers and the client or family (Johnson et al., 2005).

## THE CULTURE OF MEDICINE

I have been doing a lot of thinking lately about the people from different ethnic groups and cultures that I have been seeing on my clinical rotation. Some people have been here for generations but still have cultural values that I don't understand. Others are recent immigrants, and their beliefs are even more different than my own. In school, I have been taking science courses and learning about all the great new medicines and treatments that we have available to treat so many illnesses. There is so much that we have to offer people, and everyone works so hard and seems to care so much. I don't understand how some people don't value this.

> Even so, it is frustrating for me so see how many of the clients behave. They're often late to appointments, and sometimes, they bring in the whole family. Frequently, they don't seem to respect us and barely speak or look us in the eye. But the worst part is when they either refuse our treatments or say they will do them, and then don't. Why don't the clients understand that we have the best health care system in the world? Why don't they respect us enough to show up on time and follow the rules?
>
> —*From the journal of Johannes Fryeberg, physician assistant student*

In the Western medical system, health care providers are trained in a biomedical approach to health care. Sickness is viewed as a biological process gone awry, with scientific explanations for the various disorders and their treatments. As children, we are socialized by our families to acquire the norms, beliefs, values, rituals, language, and practices that are consistent with our culture of origin. During the educational process to become health care providers, we are trained to acquire the beliefs and attributes of the Western health care system. We set aside the health-related beliefs of our native culture and families, as we learn to identify ourselves as health care providers and become socialized into the culture of medicine. In the context of the work setting, health care providers share many common beliefs and practices. We have rigid expectations for our own professional behaviors and also have a set of expectations for "appropriate" behavior for clients (Spector, 2004). Typical values that health professionals share include:

- A core of scientific knowledge that defines health, describes disease, identifies causes of illness, and prescribes acceptable treatment methods, such as medicines, surgery, or exercises
- A common language (medical terminology and jargon) that is not understood by outsiders; a reliance on English as the language of choice in client interactions
- Rituals, such as hand washing, sterile procedure, bed making, charting, and performing the physical exam
- A formalized style of interaction that is governed by rules of communication and professional behavior
- Values and norms, such as promptness, cleanliness, compliance, orderliness, and a hierarchy of responsibility
- Ethical beliefs based on such things as autonomy, confidentiality and justice (Pachter, 1994; Royeen & Crabtree, 2006; Spector, 2004).

Health care providers in the United States are socialized in Western medicine, as taught and practiced in medical schools, universities, and hospitals, to provide the answers to meet everyone's health care needs (Spector, 2004). This belief, however, is not shared by all clients, even if the client and clinician are otherwise culturally similar. Therefore, every medical encounter has three potential cross-cultural components: (1) the native culture of the health care provider, (2) the native culture of the client, and (3) the culture of the majority health care system. Health care providers must be continuously aware of the potential for conflicts among one or more of these cultural intersections. The complexity and sensitivity of our interactions with clients present opportunities for misunderstanding and miscommunication. Health practitioners may believe that poor adherence or "disrespect" for health professionals is solely the clients' problem. However, failure to present the medical problem and its treatment in a manner that is congruent with the clients' beliefs is the providers' problem (Tripp-Reimer et al., 2001). We must learn to be flexible and open to learning about the type of health care the client desires and do our best to match our treatments to what is acceptable to them. Ethically, it is our responsibility to develop sensitive and effective practices that respect these cultural differences (American Physical Therapy Association, 2010). To do so, it is important to remember that biomedical ethics are based on Western philosophy and beliefs. Our clients may come from other cultures with different values regarding autonomy of decision making and other ethical beliefs that are held sacred. For example, we need to determine who is the decision maker in the family. Individuals from many cultures, including Asian, African American, Mexican, and Middle Eastern, do not consider the client autonomous, and decisions are made jointly by the family (Davidson et al., 2007).

## Cultural Considerations and Health Disparities

Poverty and minority status play a significant role in determining who will get sick and how they will respond when they become ill (Freeman, 2004). These two conditions often coexist because people from minority cultures are more likely to live below the poverty line than people who are Caucasian. According to 2010 data, the rate of poverty was 12.3 percent for Caucasian Americans, 33 percent for African Americans, 30 percent for Latinos, and 20 percent for people in other categories (Kaiser Family Foundation, 2010). It is important to remember that a family of four earning $22,050 is considered to be at the poverty line (U.S. Department of Health and Human Services, 2009). Poverty and the consequences of living in poor neighborhoods compound the cultural differences between ethnic/minorities and medical care providers who are predominantly middle–class Caucasians.

A study of barriers to health care for children from families of Latino origin provides evidence of cultural factors that limit access to quality medical care (Flores et al., 1998). In this study, most families were not fluent English speakers. Spanish was the primary language spoken at home in 86 percent of the families. Significant barriers to health care included lack of a common language, followed by long waits at the doctor's office, and no insurance or difficulty paying for care. Although 11 percent of the families stated that language and cultural barriers kept them from bringing their children in for care, transportation was listed as the *most* significant reason why they did not keep medical appointments.

Poor inner-city neighborhoods have higher levels of crime, drug use, and single-parent households. People who are poor are less likely to have insurance. The combined effects of poverty and race can marginalize residents and create barriers to assimilation and movement into the mainstream culture and better paying jobs (Williams, 1999). Lack of education and poor job skills present significant barriers to good jobs, upward mobility, high-quality housing, and good neighborhoods. For example, education and social infrastructures, such as affordable day care, job training, and access to jobs with insurance, are usually unavailable to women attempting to make a transition from public assistance to stable employment (Anderson, Halter, & Gryzlak, 2004). It is important for health providers to understand that poverty and race are powerful predictors of health behaviors and adherence to health regimens, resulting in health disparities due to access barriers to high-quality medical care. In addition, PWD have poorer health than those who are not disabled. Research now demonstrates that, just as there are racial and ethnic disparities in health for individuals without disabilities, there are also racial disparities in the health of people who do have disabilities. In fact, disability compounds race as a factor for poor health. Therefore, PWD who are ethnic minorities have worse outcomes and higher disparities than any other population (Jones & Sinclair, 2008).

Davidson and coauthors (2007) have identified several ways in which the lack of cultural competence on the part of health providers and agencies can lead to disparities in health outcomes:

- Clients lack trust in the health care system.
- Health providers lack knowledge and skills, including cultural awareness, knowledge of clients' beliefs and values, and how to perform a cultural assessment.
- Providers are unable to acknowledge and respect clients' spiritual, cultural, and health beliefs.
- Providers who lack cultural competence have an inability to establish effective relationships with clients.
- Providers fail to provide appropriate and acceptable care for clients with diverse health beliefs.
- Communication between clients and providers is ineffective.
- The number of interpreters is insufficient.

The lack of skill demonstrated by these behaviors poses significant barriers to providing appropriate health care to people from different cultures who have conflicting beliefs. Clients intuitively believe that when health care providers reject their views of health and illness, they are also rejecting all of the clients' cultural beliefs (Sung, 1999). Further, lack of awareness and respect for the health practices and beliefs of clients can lead to emotional pain and embarrassment with a provider who is perceived to be insulting or discriminatory (Coleman, 2009). The result is withdrawal from the health provider or nonadherence with treatment. Most health providers are committed to providing high-quality care to all clients and treating them with dignity and respect. However, unless the provider has been trained in culturally sensitive care practices, he or she may feel unintentional bias or disrespect for certain cultural health beliefs or practices. The client may be aware of the provider's feelings, regardless of how well he or she attempts to appear nonjudgmental. Effective clinical encounters are based on trust, and when this trust does not exist, the likelihood of an effective relationship is negatively affected (Thomas, 1999). Therefore, health care providers need to learn how to assess the cultural beliefs and practices of clients, so that services can be delivered in a manner that is both sensitive and respectful of cultural norms.

## CREATING SOLUTIONS FOR CULTURALLY COMPETENT PRACTICES

Solutions to improving effective cross-cultural health care are both simple and complex. The key to eliminating fear and distrust by people of other cultures is to develop knowledge about, and respect for, their traditions (Canlas, 1999). This includes using many frames of reference when interacting with others and understanding that there is no one "right" way to provide health care. This ability to embrace and effectively use multiple cultural paradigms has been termed *cultural competence*. "Cultural competence is defined as a set of congruent behaviors, attitudes, policies, and structures that come together in a system or agency or among professionals and enable the system, agency, or professionals to work effectively in cross-cultural situations. . . . For the individual, it entails being capable of functioning effectively in the context of cultural difference" (Flaskerud, 2007, p. 121). These skills are not static but are fluid and evolving (White, Hill, Mackel, Rowley, Rickards, & Jenkins, 2007). Attaining this competence is a journey that cannot be accomplished quickly or without some missteps. Culturally competent care needs to happen not only on an individual level but at an agency or organizational level, in order for truly unbiased care to occur. In this section, we briefly discuss cultural competence at the level of the provider.

At a foundational level, we need to move beyond ethnocentrism and recognize the importance of respecting culturally different health beliefs as valid beliefs for the client. One way to

---

**BOX 3–1  Questions to Ask to Elicit Health Beliefs**

1. How is our medical care different from what you or your family typically use?
2. Do you try to prevent or treat illness using herbs, spices, special foods or diets, or other sources, such as vitamins?
3. Do you or your family consult someone other than a doctor for your medical care? Perhaps a religious or community leader?
4. To provide the best care for you, what would you like us to know about your culture or your health preferences?
5. Are we doing anything that you or your family are not comfortable with?
6. Who makes the health care decisions in your family? Who would you like me to talk to? How much information would you like me to provide to the client?

*Source:* Mahan (2006).

---

elicit the health beliefs of a client or family is to ask the questions presented in Box 3–1. Every individual has perceptions of illness, disease, and causality that are culturally defined and potentially different from our own. These need to be accepted as the legitimate health care preferences of the client (Ahmann, 2002). Belief systems influence health practices and the use of both traditional and Western approaches to health care. It is essential that health care providers strive to develop cultural competency in order to be able to establish trusting relationships with clients. This will diminish discomfort with the traditional medical system, increase client satisfaction and adherence, and, ultimately, help to eliminate health disparities. All care must be acceptable to the client (Ahmann, 2002; White et al., 2007).

Cultural competency is more than just attaining knowledge about cultural groups. It also involves being able to communicate with individual clients to understand their specific beliefs. These may vary according to the ethnic groups with which the clients identify, as well as their age, gender, sexual orientation, social background, level of education, and disability. Without this detailed and specific information, knowledge of various cultures can lead to stereotypical assumptions (Jirwe, Gerrish, Keeney, & Emami, 2009). A study reported in the *Journal of Bone and Joint Surgery* states that 80 percent of orthopedic surgeons believe that treating all patients the same, using a courteous, friendly, approachable manner and simple words, would be effective for all clients. In fact, using the same approach with all clients is exactly the wrong thing to do (White et al., 2007).

Culturally competent health care providers recognize that it is necessary to alter natural communication styles to be accepted by clients from minority cultures. Demonstrating respect in our interactions may include learning to use an indirect rather than a direct style. We can learn to use conversational styles that are comfortable to the clients, such as extended greetings, expressing concern about the family, altering the speed or pacing of the conversation, and valuing silence (Tripp-Reimer et al., 2001). Body language, such as the use of personal space and eye contact, are other issues that may need to be altered.

It is unwise to assume that all people from a particular neighborhood, ethnic group, or culture have the same values or feel comfortable with the same health care practices. Therefore, it is important to carefully assess the cultural beliefs and behaviors of each client and family. Chapter 5 includes questions to determine how clients perceive their illnesses, which must be determined prior to developing a plan of care. We need to understand how the client and family would like us to interact with them and what practices are comfortable. For example, we can ask the family of the client, "Who makes the health care decisions in the family? Who would you like us to address? How much information should the client be given?" (Simpson, Mohr, & Redman, 2000). It may not feel "right" to us to ask the family's permission to give information to the client, but it may be right for them. It is important to attentively listen to the messages family members are giving. Carefully assess the client and family understanding of the illness and the plan of care you are recommending. Ask them to explain it to you in their own words or demonstrate the technique (Wilson & Robledo, 1999).

It may also be useful to ask the client and family about the health care practices they use at home. You may mention that you have met other clients who call their condition _____ and treat it by using _____. You can follow by asking if this is what they call the illness or if this is a treatment they would use. The effect of a traditional measure can be a powerful adjunct to care. If folk remedies are benign, they can be included in the client's treatment plan, but the health care provider first needs to be knowledgeable about potential outcomes. If possible contraindications for use of a folk remedy are explained respectfully and the negotiations are handled sensitively, clients will often accept the care provider's recommendations,. It may also be appropriate to incorporate or accept folk healers into the overall plan of care. The health care provider can support the clients' practices, while educating them about the benefits of adding Western medical interventions (DiCaprio, Garwick, Kohman, & Blum, 1999; Wilson & Robledo, 1999).

When conflict arises about the most effective form of treatment, the health care provider is obligated to determine what components of the intervention are absolutely essential and be prepared to compromise everything else. For example, taking antibiotics to treat an infection may save the client's life, but the wisdom of drinking large volumes of water and resting may be of lesser importance. Encouraging clients to engage in practices they traditionally use, such as massage, acupuncture, or herbal treatments, in addition to Western medical treatments, demonstrates respect for their beliefs and facilitates collaboration. At times, hope can be nurtured and supported by incorporating traditional practices into Western care (Brice & Campbell, 1999; Fadiman, 1997). This strategy may take more time than seems available, but an inability to listen and compromise sends the message that information is not important and diminishes the provider's credibility. In reality, this becomes time well spent as client adherence and satisfaction improve.

## Summary

In this chapter, we summarized important concepts in providing sensitive, effective care to clients from other cultures. The concepts of worldview and characteristic beliefs or behaviors were described. Examples were provided to facilitate understanding of how people from various cultures can respond differently to similar events. We also presented information about the culture of medicine and the values and beliefs that we accept as we acculturate as health care professionals.

Barriers to providing effective health care to people from minority cultures were presented. Many of these barriers arise from ethnocentrism and our lack of awareness of our own cultural beliefs and biases. Strategies were offered to help readers begin to develop cultural competence. The key concept is our responsibility to be open to and respectful of all cultural practices during interactions with clients.

## Reflective Questions

1. In what racial or ethnic group do you consider yourself to be?
   a. Do you think others would recognize you as a member of this group?
   b. Do you consider yourself part of a culture or subculture?
   c. What traits or characteristics do you think identify you as part of this group?
   d. Describe the derivation of your name.
2. What beliefs, attitudes, and practices have you acquired from your family's cultural heritage regarding:
   a. religious or spiritual beliefs?
   b. holiday traditions?
   c. environmental/activity control?
   d. social organization and relationships?
   e. Are you past, present, or future oriented? How does this affect you?
3. Think about your cultural communication style.
   a. Is it high context or low context? Provide examples.
   b. Is it direct or indirect? Provide examples.
4. Describe your personal health beliefs.
   a. What is health? What is illness? What is death?
   b. Do you have any interest in using traditional or complementary interventions? If so, which ones?
   c. What do you do to stay healthy? What do you do when you become ill?
   d. How could you show respect for a client who had very different health beliefs than you do?
5. Consider working with clients from a culture different from your own.
   a. What specific actions can you take to increase your knowledge of this culture?
   b. How can you improve your effectiveness in working with people from diverse cultures?
   c. What questions can you ask or what behaviors can you use to develop a good relationship with clients from cultures that are different than your own?

## Case Study

Mark Stillman is a therapist who works in an urban home care setting, treating many clients who are recent immigrants to the United States, including Mrs. Mendoza, who is from Mexico. She is living with her son, daughter-in-law, and grandchildren, who treat her with great respect and patience, even though her stroke has made her care challenging. Mark speaks limited Spanish, and the family speaks limited English.

On occasion, the family is not ready for Mark when he arrives, or at other times, no one answers the doorbell or telephone, and he is unsure whether or not they are home. When they do connect, Mark wants to get to work right away because of his busy schedule, but the family always offers him coffee and food and talks with him, in limited English, about things that have nothing to do with Mrs. Mendoza. They ask what Mark considers to be personal questions and talk about many things, except for matters for which he is there. Sometimes it is hard for him to actually perform his treatments because it is a small home, and many family members are always present. After initially assessing Mrs. Mendoza, Mark had developed a plan of care for her, and he is surprised that although the family shows her love and tenderness, no one seems particularly interested in or adherent to his program, including his client.

1. What role do you think spoken language and other communication factors play in Mark's care for Mrs. Mendoza?
2. Consider some general guidelines about cultural norms of people from Latino cultures.
   a. What might be some of the differences between Mark's beliefs about personal behavior and theirs?
   b. What barriers might these differences create?
3. What value do you think the Mendoza family might place on medical intervention to improve the health or independence of Mrs. Mendoza?
4. How might Mark modify his interventions, attitude, and behavior to create a more positive collaboration with this family?

# References

Ahmann, E. (2002). Developing cultural competence in health care settings. *Pediatric Nursing, 26*(3) 133–137.

American Physical Therapy Association. (2010). *Code of ethics.* Retrieved from htto://www.apta.org

Anderson, S. G., Halter, A. P., & Gryzlak, B. M. (2004). Difficulties after leaving TANF: Inner-city women talk about reasons for returning to welfare. *Social Work, 49*(2), 185–194.

Arredondo, P., Toporek, R., Brown, S. P., Jones, J., Locke, D. C., Sanchez, J., & Stadler, H. (1996). Operationalization of the multicultural counseling competencies. *Journal of Multicultural Counseling and Development, 24,* 42–78.

Banja, J. D. (1996). Ethics, values, and world culture: The impact on rehabilitation. *Disability and Rehabilitation, 113*(6), 2279–2284.

Brice, A., & Campbell, L. (1999). Cross-cultural communication. In R. L. Leavitt (Ed.), *Cross-cultural rehabilitation* (pp. 83–94). London, United Kingdom: W. B. Saunders.

Broome, B., & Broome, R. (2007). Native Americans: Traditional healing. *Urologic Nursing, 27*(2), 161–174.

Brown, S. E. (2002). What is disability culture? *Disability Studies Quarterly, 22,* 34–50.

Canlas, L. G. (1999). Issues of health care mistrust in east Harlem. *Mount Sinai Journal of Medicine, 66*(49), 257–258.

Choi, K. H., & Wynne, M. E. (2000). Providing services to Asian Americans with developmental disabilities and their families: Mainstream service providers' perspective. *Community Mental Health Journal, 36*(6), 589–595.

Coleman, J. J. (2009). Culture care meanings of African American parents related to infant mortality and health care. *Journal of Cultural Diversity, 16*(3), 109–119.

Crabtree, J. L. (2006). Ethics of culture in rehabilitation. In M. Royeen & J. L. Crabtree (Eds.), *Culture in rehabilitation: From competency to proficiency* (pp. 59–63). Upper Saddle River, NJ: Pearson.

Davidhizar, R., Dowd, S. B., & Newman-Giger, J. (1997). Model for cultural diversity in the radiology department. *Radiologic Technology, 68*(3), 233–239.

Davidson, J. E., Powers, K., Hedayar, M., Tieszen, M., Kon, A., Shepard, E., .Armstrong, D. (2007). Clinical practice guidelines for support of the family in the patient-centered intensive care unit. American College of Critical Care Medicine Task Force 2004. *Critical Care Medicine, 35*(2), 605–622.

DiCaprio, J. J., Garwick, A. W., Kohman, C., & Blum, R. W. (1999). Culture and the care of children with chronic conditions. *Archives of Pediatrics and Adolescent Medicine, 153*(10), 1030–1037.

Eddey, G., & Robey, K. (2005). Considering the culture of disability in cultural competence education. *Academic Medicine, 90,* 706–712.

Erlen, J. A. (1998). Culture, ethics and respect: The bottom line is understanding. *Orthopedic Nursing, 17*(6), 79–83.

Evans, B. C., Coon, D. W., & Crogan, N. L. (2007). *Personalismo* and breaking barriers: Accessing Hispanic populations for clinical services and research. *Geriatric Nursing, 28*(5), 289–296.

Fadiman, A. (1997). *The spirit catches you and you fall down.* New York, NY: Farrar, Straus, and Giroux.

Flaskerud, J. H. (2007). Cultural competence column: Acculturation. *Issues in Mental Health Nursing, 28,* 543–436.

Fleisher, D, & Zames, F. (2001). *The disability rights movement: From charity to confrontation.* Philadelphia, PA: Temple University Press.

Flores, G., Abreu, M., Olivar, M. A., & Kastner, B. (1998). Access barriers to health care for Latino children. *Archives of Pediatrics and Adolescent Medicine, 152,* 1119–1125.

Freeman, H. P. (2004). Poverty, culture, and social injustice. *CA Cancer Journal Clinics, 54,* 72–77.

Gannotti, M. E., Handwerker, W. P., Groce, N. E., & Cruz, C. (2001). Sociocultural influences on disability status in Puerto Rican children. *Physical Therapy, 81*(9), 1512–1523.

Gill, C. J. (1995) A psychological review of disability culture. *Disabilities Studies Quarterly, 15,* 16–19.

Hatcher, E., & Whittemore, R. (2007). Hispanic adults' beliefs about type 2 diabetes: Clinical implications. *Journal of the American Academy of Nurse Practitioners, 19,* 536–545.

Jirwe, M., Gerrish, K., Keeney, S., & Emami, A. (2009). Identifying the core components of cultural competence: Findings from a Delphi study. *Journal of Clinical Nursing, 18*(18), 2622–2634.

Johnson, K. S., Elbert-Avila, K. I., & Tulsky, J. A. (2005). The influences of spiritual beliefs and practices on the treatment preferences of African Americans: A review of the literature. *Journal of American Geriatric Society, 53,* 711–719.

Jones, G. C., & Sinclair, L. B. (2008). Multiple health disparities among minority adults with mobility limitations: An application of the ICF framework and codes. *Disability and Rehabilitation, 30*(12–13), 901–915.

Kaiser Family Foundation. (2010). *State health facts.* Retrieved from http://www.statehealthfacts.org

Leavitt, R. L. (2001). Special considerations when working with individuals of Hispanic origin. *GeriNotes, 7*(6), 20–23.

Leavitt, R. L. (2010a). Introduction. In R. L. Leavitt (Ed.), *Cultural competence: A lifelong journey to cultural proficiency* (pp. 1–19). Thorofare: NJ: Slack.

Leavitt, R. L. (2010b). Exploring cultural diversity. In R. L. Leavitt (Ed.), *Cultural competence: A lifelong journey to cultural proficiency* (pp. 51–77). Thorofare, NJ: Slack.

Leavitt, R., & Roush, S. E. (2010) Disability across cultures. In R. L. Leavitt (Ed.), *Cultural competence: A lifelong journey to cultural proficiency* (pp. 77–98). Thorofare, NJ: Slack.

Leininger, M. (1995). *Transcultural nursing: Concepts, theories, research and practices.* New York, NY: McGraw-Hill.

Loveland, C. (1999). The concept of culture. In R. L. Leavitt (Ed.), *Cross-cultural rehabilitation: An international perspective* (pp. 15–26). London, United Kingdom: W. B. Saunders.

Mahan, V. (2006). Challenges in the treatment of depression. *Journal of the American Psychiatric Nurses Association, 11*(6), 366–370.

Nava, Y. (2000). *It's all in the frijoles.* New York, NY: Fireside Books.

Pachter, L. P. (1994). Culture and clinical care: Folk illness beliefs and behaviors and their implications for healthcare delivery. *Journal of the American Medical Association, 271*(9), 690–694.

Peters, S. (2000). Is there a disability culture? A syncretisation of three possible world views. *Disability & Society, 15*(4), 583–601.

Pichette, E. F., Garrett, M. T., Kosciulek, J., & Rosenthal, D. A. (1999). Cultural identification of American Indians and its impact on rehabilitation services. *Journal of Rehabilitation, 65*(3), 3–8.

Purnell, L. D., & Lattanzi, J. B. (2006). Introducing steps to cultural study and cultural competence. In J. B. Lattanzi & L. D. Purnell (Eds.), *Developing cultural competence in physical therapy practice* (pp. 21–37). Philadelphia, PA: F. A. Davis.

Royeen, M., & Crabtree, J. (Eds.). (2006). *Culture in rehabilitation: From competency to proficiency.* Upper Saddle River, NJ: Pearson Prentice Hall.

Salimbene, S. (2000). *What language does your patient hurt in?* Rockford, IL: EMC Paradigm.

Simpson, G., Mohr, R., & Redman, A. (2000). Cultural variations in the understanding of traumatic brain injury and brain injury rehabilitation. *Brain Injury, 14*(2), 125–140.

Spector, R. (2004). *Cultural diversity in health and illness.* Upper Saddle River, NJ: Pearson Prentice Hall.

Stell, L. K. (1999). Diagnosing death: What's trust got to do with it? *Mount Sinai Journal of Medicine, 66*(4), 229–235.

Sue, D., & Sue, D. W. (1999). *Counseling the culturally different.* New York, NY: Wiley.

Sung, C. L. (1999). Asian patients' distrust of Western medical care. *Mount Sinai Journal of Medicine, 66*(4), 259–262.

Tang, S. H., & Cheng, S. Y. (2001). Chinese culture and health practices. *GeriNotes, 7*(6), 15–16.

Tervo, R. C., & Palmer, G. (2004). Health professional student attitudes toward people with disabilities. *Clinical Rehabilitation, 18*(8), 908–915.

Thomas, L. M. (1999). Trusting under pressure. *Mount Sinai Journal of Medicine, 66*(4), 223–228.

Tripp-Reimer, T., Choi, E., Kelley, L S., & Enslein, J. C. (2001). Cultural barriers to care: Inverting the problem. *Diabetes Spectrum, 14*(1), 13–26.

U.S. Census Bureau. (2008). Retrieved from http://www.census.gov

U.S. Department of Health and Human Services. (2009). *Federal Register, 74*(14), 4199–4201.

Vanderhoff, M. (2005). Patient education and health literacy. *PT—Magazine of Physical Therapy, 13*(9), 42–46.

Weaver, H. N. (1998) Indigenous people in a multicultural society: Unique issues for human services. *Social Work, 43*(3), 203–211.

White, A. A., Hill, J. A., Mackel, A. M., Rowley, D. L., Rickards, E. P., & Jenkens. B. (2007). The relevance of culturally competent care in orthopaedics to outcomes and health care disparities. *Journal of Bone and Joint Surgery, 89*(6), 1379–1384.

Williams, D. (1999). Race, socioeconomic status, and health: The added effects of racism and discrimination. *Annals of New York Academy of Science, 896,* 173–188.

Wilson, A. H., & Robledo, L. (1999). Listening to Hispanic mothers: Guidelines for teaching. *Journal of the Society of Pediatric Nurses, 4*(3), 125–127.

# 4

# Spirituality

I went into the intensive care unit today for the first time to see my new client, Jennifer. She was in a very serious motor vehicle accident. She broke several bones, including her neck, and it looks like she will have a very high level of quadriplegia and be ventilator dependent for the rest of her life. I have to admit I was a little uncomfortable with the complexity of Jennifer's diagnosis and all of the tubes, sounds, and smells in the ICU, but it was what happened after my supervisor excused herself to find a nurse that truly overwhelmed me. Jennifer asked me if I would pray with her! I reflexively said "yes," but then realized I wasn't really sure what to do. I awkwardly asked her if she knew the Lord's Prayer, and she nodded, so I quickly recited it and finished up her treatment as fast as I could. As I was saying goodbye, she got my attention, smiled, and thanked me for taking the time to pray with her. She said it meant a lot. I thought I was on pretty shaky ground, but that made me feel like I did the right thing. Later, I realized it was probably the cross that I wear around my neck that made her comfortable enough to ask me to pray with her.

*—From the journal of Lucinda Pean, occupational therapy student*

The onset of serious illness or disability is frequently associated with a heightened sense of spirituality (Branch, Torke, Brown-Haithco, 2006; McClain, Rosenfeld, & Breitbart, 2003; Puchalski, 2004). Many clients rely on their personal belief systems to make sense of their circumstances or to provide them with mechanisms for coping with the uncertainties and changes associated with altered health (Giaquinto, Spiridigliozzi, & Caracciolo, 2007). Health care professionals need to acknowledge this aspect of their clients' experiences, which can enable them to access helpful inner resources or become aware of potentially harmful beliefs or practices that could be detrimental to their health and healing (VandeCreek & Burton, 2001). This approach honors clients as whole, integrated persons and acknowledges their right to make medical decisions that are based on the fundamental beliefs they use to order their lives (Bush & Bruni, 2008; Cohen, Wheeler, & Scott, 2001).

In spite of potential benefits, addressing spirituality in health care settings today is a challenging proposition. Until the latter part of the 20th century, shared social values were derived from a Judeo-Christian foundation, and the terms *spirituality* and *religion* could be used interchangeably. Society is now characterized by ever-increasing cultural and religious diversity, creating a need to redefine the concept of spirituality for secular applications (Lee, 2002). The contemporary meaning of spirituality, and the one used in this chapter, refers to each person's interpretation of the entity that provides them with direction, meaning, and purpose in life (Cohen et al., 2001). This concept of spirituality is a broad one that is inclusive of, but not limited to, religious affiliation and belief in God.

Until the early 1900s, spirituality was an intrinsic component of medical care in the United States. Although influential leaders in the fields of medicine and theology defended the importance of this linkage (Cabot & Dicks, 1936), growing emphases on scientific objectivity led to a clear delineation between these two entities. The spiritual aspects of care became progressively more marginalized from the practice of medicine as the importance of scientific rigor increased (Cohen et al., 2001; Daaleman, 2004).

The biomedical model that emerged is appropriately applauded for impressive scientific and technological advances, but it is also associated with the high levels of dissatisfaction among clients and health care providers that characterize health care today (Broom & Tovey, 2007; Graber & Johnson, 2001). The objective nature of science, which is at the heart of evidence-based medicine, has left little room for the "softer side" of health care. Current evidence suggests that a return to more spiritually sensitive care could enhance the experience for everyone involved, including clients, their loved ones, and health care providers. For example, parents of children who received end-of-life care in pediatric intensive care units indicated that they knew they were in good hands when they received clear, honest communication; felt that the staff really cared; saw sincere signs of compassion for both parents and children; and had their spiritual needs met (Meyer, Ritholz, Burns, & Truog, 2006). Interestingly, the health professionals who provide care also seem to benefit when clients are treated in a compassionate, spiritually sensitive manner because of the personal fulfillment associated with altruism and belonging to a caring community (Chiu, Emblen, Van Hofwegen, Sawatzky, & Meyerhoff, 2004; Graber & Johnson, 2001).

Just how important are these concepts to the American public? The results of a 2008 Gallup Poll found that 78 percent of the U.S. population believes in God, another 15 percent believes in a "universal spirit/higher power," and only 6 percent deny belief in either. Another study, designed to investigate the use of complementary and alternative health practices, revealed that prayer was the most common complement to biomedical treatment among respondents. Forty-three percent reported praying for their own health, 24.4 percent had someone else praying for their health, and 9.6 percent participated in prayer groups for their own health (Barnes, Powell-Griner, McFann, & Nahin, 2004). Given the apparent importance of spirituality in the lives of the population we serve, this chapter discusses the controversy that exists about the integration of spirituality in health care, presents evidence to support such integration, and provides strategies to help health professionals decide when and how to open a dialogue about spirituality with their clients.

## THE CONTROVERSY

During the past decade, increasing numbers of physicians, nurses, social workers, psychologists, and other health professionals have begun to address spirituality during health care encounters, a practice about which there is some debate. Opinions range from those who strongly support it to those who strongly oppose it. Proponents see this as a natural extension of compassionate care that responds to a growing body of evidence about important linkages between spirituality, health, and clients' ability to cope with difficult circumstances (Craigie & Hobbs, 1999; Koenig & Cohen, 2002; Puchalski, 2009). Others are uncertain. Although they might appreciate the potential value of discussing spirituality with their clients, they are reluctant because of the fear of being intrusive and the risk of saying or doing the wrong thing. In addition, there are perceived limits of time, reimbursement, and training (Ellis, Campbell, Detwiler-Breidenbach, & Hubbard, 2002; Vance, 2001). In today's health care reimbursement system, there is reason to believe these concerns are valid.

Another faction of clinicians adamantly opposes the involvement of anyone other than chaplains and clergy in the spiritual care of clients. They believe that it is unethical to be involved in this aspect of patient care, because doctors, nurses, and other clinicians run the risk of exceeding professional practice boundaries, proselytizing, or appearing coercive (Sloan, 2009; Sloan & Bagiella, 2001; Sloan, Bagiella, & Powell, 1999).

No one denies the important role of health care chaplains, who are trained to help clients access their own inner resources to assist them in coping with illness or disability. Like other health professionals, chaplains are required to earn a graduate degree and complete a full year of clinical education to demonstrate clinical competency. They adhere to a code of professional ethics, profess a commitment to attend to the spiritual needs of all clients, and are not permitted to proselytize (VandeCreek & Burton, 2001).

Unfortunately, pastoral care departments rarely receive the administrative resources or recognition they need to maintain services at a level that is essential to meet the needs of all clients (Feudtner, Haney, & Dimmers, 2003; Massachusetts General Hospital, 2003; McCarthy, 2000). In fact, many smaller hospitals rely solely on the services of local clergy, volunteer laypersons, and clinicians to offer their clients spiritual support (Associated Press, 2004; Driscoll, 2003; Perkins, 2003). Although this approach is well intended, the use of nonprofessional spiritual-care providers can be problematic, because this practice can leave clients vulnerable to proselytizing or coercion (White, 2003).

In response to ethical concerns about clinicians helping to meet the spiritual needs of clients, experts in the field have developed preprofessional and continuing education curricula to guide clinical practices via relationship-centered models of care. Whereas traditional practice guidelines call for professional relationships that avoid interactions that could be misconstrued as friendly or social, relationship-centered care encourages providers to care and to show that they care (Ventura, 2005). Strict professional boundaries need to be relaxed *to a point*. Puchalski (2009) describes the ethical dimension of relationship-centered care as "intimacy with formality" (p. 805). This acknowledges the power differential between professionals and their clients, while allowing clients to share concerns of a more intimate nature with their professional caregivers. She recommends following the lead of clients in discussions related to spirituality and cautions that it is unethical to either ignore spiritual concerns or to try to address those that extend beyond one's level of professional expertise or comfort. "Intimacy with formality" permits open and honest dialogue with clients to demonstrate honor and respect for their beliefs and values, while simultaneously honoring professional codes of ethics. These codes require health professionals to balance their obligations to clients, themselves, and the health care system. The latter requires attention to time, practicing within one's own area of expertise, and appropriate referral to other health professionals, as indicated.

Each health care discipline has its own set of ethical guidelines. It is our duty to carefully consider these and any other applicable codes of conduct to ensure that client–professional relationships are not breached. Our clients are dependent on us in many ways. They must never feel that the care to which they are entitled is dependent on meeting some unstated, but perhaps implied, expectation of the health care provider.

## THE EVIDENCE

The body of knowledge that supports the integration of spirituality in health care has an early foundation dating back to medieval times. Even then, health care providers understood that the mind, body, and spirit were inseparable (Chopra, 1993; Newman, 1998). Hildegard of Bingen, a 12th-century nun and health care practitioner, was a proponent of a low-fat diet, rich in fresh fruits and vegetables, whole grains, and seafood, no sugar, and minimal salt and alcohol. Prescribed treatment regimens consisted of fasting, herbal remedies, and other detoxifying techniques. Meditation, introspection, and prayer were essential components of treatment (Newman, 1998).

The techniques of St. Hildegard were not unlike those that formed the basis of Ayurveda, the ancient Indian medical science (Chopra & Doiphode, 2002). Ayurveda stems from the Vedas, India's ancient books of knowledge. The literal translation of the term *Ayurveda* is life (Ayu) science (Veda) (Chauhan, 1998). Control of one's own physiology is gained through the use of herbs, diet, massage, exercise, music, and meditation. These ancient traditions form the basis of the practice of Deepak Chopra, an endocrinologist who is the founding director of The Chopra Center for Well-Being in Carlsbad, California. The Chopra Center boasts an exceptionally high rate of spontaneous cancer remission. Critics of the practice are quick to point out that this high rate may simply be due to the fact that the center is looking for and measuring this phenomenon, while other practice sites do not necessarily collect this information (Chopra, 1993). Clients often visit Chopra's center as a last resort. When they learn that a cure may be possible, it comes into the realm of believable. The belief and expectations generated by the relationship between client and care provider are intended to influence the outcome and, apparently, they do. Chopra believes that success in the program depends on the client's ability to activate the internal "pharmacy" and natural defenses of the body. By achieving a balance in and awareness of connection of the mind, body, and spirit, clients learn how to control bodily functions. Among the many reported benefits of his program are control of heart rate, blood pressure, gastric acid secretion, and bowel motility.

Herbert Benson has been teaching the relaxation response to his clients for many years (Benson, 2000). He incorporates several of the same concepts that Chopra uses in his practice. Benson describes his model of care as a three-legged stool. One leg is based on the use of medications. The second relies on the use of medical procedures, including surgery, to correct physical problems. The third leg of the stool represents self-care practices. Clients are taught the importance of managing their stress, eating well, and exercising (Benson & Stuart, 1992). An important aspect of Benson's self-care program is the client's inner belief system and its ability to promote healing.

Benson and Chopra agree that the *placebo effect* may play an important role in clients' responses. The placebo effect is based on the expectations of both the client and the health care provider that the treatment will actually help. A significant amount of scientific evidence supports the relevance of client and practitioner belief systems in the overall care of clients. The placebo effect is one of the most powerful techniques available to us. It is an indication that the client has been able to activate his or her own internal "pharmacy," a source that is much more accurate and effective than externally administered drugs (Benson & Stuart, 1992; Chopra, 1993; Stefano, Fricchione, Slingsby, & Benson, 2001).

One important component of practicing self-care is daily stress management. Benson teaches clients to meditate once or twice daily for 20 minutes. Jon Kabat-Zinn (1990), founding director of the Center for Mindfulness in Medicine, Health Care, and Society in Worcester, Massachusetts, also incorporates daily meditation in his practice. Although meditation practices vary, three essential features are common to all forms of meditation (Benson, 2000). First, the person must sit or lie in a quiet and comfortable place. Second, the person must clear his or her mind of all thoughts, ideas, worries, and distractions. Finally, the individual uses a focal point, such as a word, sound, or phrase. Another technique is to focus on the breath (Kabat-Zinn, 1990). Yoga, t'ai chi, karate, and qi qong have all been described as moving meditation and are believed to have the same beneficial effects (Chen & Snyder, 1999; Ross, Bohannon, Davis, & Gurchiek, 1999).

The common denominator in all of these practices is clearing the mind of all stresses. Hans Selye, often referred to as the "father of stress," was a pioneer in psychosomatic medicine. He described stress as an integral element in any living being (Selye, 1974). Responding to stress may be part of our biological makeup, but it is also healthy to keep it balanced. Clearing the mind of stressful thoughts elicits the relaxation response (Benson, 1996), which turns off the arousing effects of the sympathetic nervous system. The body returns to a calmer state, improving immune system function and cardiovascular health, and diminishing anxiety and depression (Benson, 1996; Kabat-Zinn, 1990; Koenig, 1999; Ornish, 1990).

Researchers have demonstrated that the active practice of prayer, along with a positive attitude, healthy lifestyle, and substantial physical and emotional support of the community, significantly improves medical outcomes (Benson, 1996; Koenig, 1999; Matthews, 1998; McCullough & Larson, 1999; Meyers, 1999; WHOQOL SRPB Group, 2006). Although the studies are too numerous for our discussion, the following list highlights the wide range of documented health benefits that have been found among adults who practice spiritual beliefs on a regular basis:

- Significantly reduced blood pressure
- Stronger immune systems
- Fewer health problems
- Fewer hospitalizations
- Shorter lengths of stay when hospitalized
- Stronger social support systems
- Stronger family ties
- Stronger and healthier marriages
- Stronger sense of well-being and acceptance
- Lower rates of depression.

Although many clients believe positive outcomes are the result of divine intervention, scientists offer alternative explanations. Koenig and Cohen (2002) indicated that deep spiritual belief and regular attendance at religious services are generally accompanied by positive health habits, including healthy eating, regular wellness care, compliance with medical advice, and abstinence from drinking, smoking, and unsafe sexual practices. In addition, the social support offered by a religious community prevents isolation and may even provide physical or financial support for those in need (Cohen, 2002). The health benefits of regular spiritual practices are not limited to adults. Adolescents who practice their spirituality are significantly less likely to consider suicide, use drugs or alcohol, or engage in delinquent behaviors or in early sexual activity (Ritt-Olson et al., 2004; Wong, Rew, & Slaikeu, 2006).

Some researchers argue that it is the healthy lifestyle that is responsible for all of the measured health benefits. Certainly, a healthy lifestyle can strengthen the immune system, lower stress levels, decrease the sympathetic nervous system response, and promote early detection of illness. Whether the positive benefits can be explained in scientific or spiritual terms, it is clear that the inner peace of a deep, personal faith is beneficial to many of our clients (Koenig, 1999; Matthews, 1998; Waite & Lehrer, 2003; Yanek, Becker, Moy, Gittelsohn, & Koffman, 2001).

## CONNECTIONS OF THE MIND, BODY, AND SPIRIT

I had a really amazing experience today. If I hadn't seen it for myself, I would have thought somebody was making this stuff up—or at least really exaggerating. As part of my clinical rotation, I am assigned to the Wellness Clinic, affiliated with the hospital. I have been attending the Stress Management class, which met once a week for seven weeks. The clients learned many different techniques: meditation, mindfulness, exercises, diet, etc. There was even some discussion about the role of prayer.

Last night was the last session of the class, and the clients were talking about what changes they had made since they started attending. It was incredible. One woman had lowered her blood pressure 10 points. Another had decreased her neck pain from 8 down to 2, on a scale of 1 to 10. Someone else is now able to fall asleep without using medication. I guess this stuff really works! I'd really like to know how. It seems like the activities are so simple, but the effects are so powerful.

*—From the journal of Fred Morris, nursing student*

The essential connection between the mind, body, and spirit exists in the limbic system, which lies deep in the brain at the level of the midbrain and brainstem (Koenig & Cohen, 2002). Attempts to understand the intricate interfaces that are mediated by the limbic system have given rise to a relatively new interdisciplinary field of study known as *psychoneuroimmunology*, which is concerned with complex interactions that occur between the central nervous system (CNS) and the immune system (Adler, 2000). These interactions are bidirectional. That is, the CNS mediates both physical and psychological control mechanisms. This affects the immune system, and the immune system affects the CNS (Kiecolt-Glaser, McGuire, Robles, & Glaser, 2002). Box 4–1 provides a summary of functions associated with the limbic system.

The mechanisms that control psychoneuroimmunological responses are quite complex and intricately connected to emotional health. The limbic system is the region of the brain where emotional memories are stored and emotional responses are mediated (Whybrow, 1997). Two very important emotional functions occur here. One function allows us to make emotional attachments and bond with other people. This includes our ability to respond to others in a nurturing way. The limbic system also monitors all sensory information received and interprets it for emotional content. It is through this process that we decide what to think and feel about new information based on our prior experiences, which influence our perception of new information. Does the current situation appear to be pleasant and something we want to approach? Is there a potential threat or harm we need to avoid? Based on our appraisal of the situation, we decide how

BOX 4–1     The Limbic System Is Responsible for Physical and Emotional Survival

**Memory and Cognition**

- Stores memories with a social or emotional connection
- Monitors incoming information and "decides" what to remember
- Compares incoming information to previous information and "decides" how to respond
- Provides motivation for action

**Emotions, Mood, Social Skills**

- Regulates emotional state and mood
- Organizes social behaviors
- Facilitates self-concept and self-esteem
- Develops attitudes and opinions about the external world

**Autonomic System**

- Heart rate, blood pressure, breathing
- Hunger, thirst, digestion, elimination, fluid regulation
- Temperature regulation, sweating
- Attention, arousal, alertness, focus, concentration
- Muscle tone, posture, readiness to act
- Controls level of sensory stimulation allowed

to respond. The final perception of any situation causes a corresponding output from the autonomic nervous system (ANS). Whether or not our perceptions are valid, outcomes are based on these perceptions.

The ANS has two complementary subsystems, the sympathetic nervous system (SNS) and the parasympathetic nervous system (PNS). In a healthy person, these two systems act collaboratively to maintain a steady state, as well as to ensure the efficiency of our automatic survival skills (Umphred, 1995). The SNS responds to rapid or unexpected change. Fear, anger, or arousal of any kind will stimulate the SNS to become active. All systems of our body are affected. This generalized response has been described as a "fight-or-flight response." Identified by Walter Cannon of Harvard Medical School in the early 1900s, this response involves involuntary physiological changes. When an individual perceives a situation as challenging, the sympathetic response occurs automatically (Cannon, 1929).

Once activated, the SNS causes constriction of blood vessels in the brain and the gut and an increase in blood pressure, heart rate, and respiratory rate. The pupils dilate, and the threshold of sensory receptors is lowered. Blood is shunted away from the brain and digestive system and directed to the muscles. Muscle tension is increased. We become hypervigilant, prepared for any change in the environment. In this heightened state of arousal, we may be unable to concentrate or focus on other ideas. Sleep is difficult or impossible.

This response is so powerful that people have been known to lift cars off victims in order to save lives. Without the assistance of the SNS, such feats of valor and strength would not be possible. Many of the stresses faced in daily life, however, are ongoing and continuous. It is generally not healthy to maintain the response over time. It activates the release of three hormones by the adrenal glands: epinephrine, norepinephrine, and cortisol. Epinephrine and norepinephrine produce the "adrenaline rush" that we feel when we are angry, afraid, or aroused. Cortisol initially produces anti-inflammatory effects, but when released over time, it acts to suppress the immune system. This can leave the body susceptible to infectious, autoimmune, and neoplastic diseases (Rabin, 2002).

Whereas the SNS is responsible for mediating fight-or-flight reactions, the PNS supports the opposite responses. A calm, unchanging, nonthreatening environment allows the PNS to decrease the blood pressure, heart rate, and respiratory rate. Blood is shunted away from the muscles and directed to the brain and digestive system. Tension and muscle tone are reduced (Umphred, 1995). We no longer feel the need to escape from danger, so we can concentrate on learning and social activities. We are able to sleep. The contrasting functions of the SNS and PNS are outlined in Table 4–1.

It is important to realize that *perceived* stress, threat, or danger can trigger a SNS state. For example, for most adults, the sight of a young child rushing into the street in front of a car will trigger a SNS response and all of its uncomfortable sensations. The sight of a friendly dog could trigger the same SNS response if the person has a fearful memory of dogs. Conversely, when there is a perception of safety, the PNS maintains the bodily functions at a level that supports a calm, yet alert, state.

Both the SNS and PNS are needed to maintain homeostasis and to support our ability to respond appropriately to changes in the environment. The optimal healthy state is achieved when there is a balance between the two systems. The person is able to focus attention on the matters of everyday life but has a healthy readiness to react to stress. In our stressful, stimuli-filled culture,

| Table 4–1  The Autonomic Nervous System | |
|---|---|
| **Sympathetic—Stimulating** | **Parasympathetic—Relaxing** |
| Arousal, fight-or-flight response<br>Stimulus: fear, excitement, anger, pain | Relaxation, focused attention<br>Stimulus: safe, familiar, trust, lack of change |
| Sensory overload or bombardment overload | Lack of stimulation or sensory overload |
| *Possible Responses:*<br>• Increased respiratory rate<br>• Increased heart rate and blood pressure<br>• Blood gets shunted to muscles<br><br>• Increased glucose levels and energy<br>• Alert, aroused, focused on environment<br>• Cannot sleep<br>• Quick responses, impulsiveness<br>• Enhanced sensory input<br>• Survival responses to change<br>• Happy, angry, aroused, excited, afraid<br>• Agitated, irritable, aggressive<br>• Hyperactive<br>• Disorganized responses | *Possible Responses:*<br>• Decreased respiratory rate<br>• Decreased heart rate and blood pressure<br>• Blood gets shunted to brain and digestive system<br>• Decreased glucose levels and energy<br>• Calm, relaxed, content<br>• Fatigue, enhanced sleep<br>• Maintained attention, concentration<br>• Filtered-out sensory input<br>• Slow, thoughtful responses<br>• Focused, emotionally bonded<br>• Bored, withdrawn, apathetic<br>• Lethargic, shut down, confused<br>• Coma, catatonic |
| *Sensory Input:*<br>• Quick, fast, light, bright colors<br>• Loud, fast-changing, movement<br>• Hot, cold, forceful, unexpected, rough | *Sensory Input:*<br>• Slow, maintained, dull, pleasant<br>• Quiet, soft, smooth, warm, firm, rhythmic<br>• Moderate, unchanging, predictable |

the SNS seems to be chronically overactive. Over time, this can create a constant state of hyper-vigilance and chronic stress, leading to an increased susceptibility to illness (Kabat-Zinn, 1990).

Modern medicine is able to offer a variety of interventions that are capable of reducing stress and the associated immunosuppressive substances that accompany a stress response. Interventions that have been assessed to document their ability to reduce immunosuppressive activity include, but are not limited to, psychotherapy for post-traumatic stress disorder (Olff, deVries, Güzelcan, Assies, & Gersons, 2007); mindfulness meditation to increase the rate of healing skin lesions associated with psoriasis (Kabat-Zinn et al., 1998); regular participation in a spiritual community and routine practice of meditation or prayer (Koenig, 1999); and the administration of client-controlled pain medication to decrease healing time following surgery (Beilin et al., 2003).

Recognizing the benefits that accompany stress reduction and the important role that spirituality can play, the next section of this chapter offers some clinical guidelines and recommendations.

## CLINICAL APPLICATIONS

Today, I had the weirdest experience. I was doing an intake evaluation on this client, Dick. He recently experienced a right cerebrovascular accident and now has a significant left hemiplegia. He told me that twelve years ago, he had been diagnosed with terminal pancreatic cancer. His only symptom was that he had become jaundiced. When he went to the doctor, he was given a full workup, which resulted in his being rushed into surgery for a Whipple procedure. The surgeon had to close him right back up because the cancer had completely consumed his pancreas and had spread to the surrounding organs. He was given six to eight weeks to live.

Now, here's the strange part. He mentioned that he just prayed and prayed—he knew that he could beat the cancer. He opted to have chemotherapy and radiation to "extend his life." There was no promise for a cure. After nearly dying from the treatment, he has done reasonably well. His last MRI, done three years ago, showed that he is cancer-free! I don't know too much about cure rates in cancer, but it was my understanding that pancreatic cancer is usually terminal.

Now, he's had a fairly massive stroke. What makes it difficult for me is that he thinks his prayers will cure him once more. I've seen a few other clients who have had strokes. Although they did get some return of function, none were actually "cured," especially when they also had arteriosclerosis as bad as this client's. While I don't want to discourage him from his beliefs, I don't want to mislead him either. I wonder if it would be wrong for me to pray with him. I have a fair amount of faith myself, but I'm unsure how much I should incorporate this into our time together.

—*From the journal of Tom Chisholm, social work student*

Clients' spiritual strength can help them overcome the limitations and disappointments inherent in situations of illness and injury. In spite of significant advances in medicine, there are still many diseases and conditions that cannot be cured, and many treatment options are accompanied by serious side effects. Diabetes, arthritis, mental illness, spinal cord injury, and AIDS, for example, cannot yet be cured, but the process of healing can be facilitated. Healing restores the person to a sense of wholeness, even if the disease or condition remains present. Clients who are able to draw effectively on their spirituality can greatly benefit from this in their healing process. Anything that buffers stress or provides emotional support is important (Benson, 1996; Koenig, 1999; McColl et al., 2000).

It is appropriate for us to use all available therapeutic agents to help our clients recover. We commonly encourage good nutrition, exercise, stress-reduction techniques, and adequate sleep. Knowing that spirituality can positively influence healing, we must also address this. We can begin by determining how each client nourishes his or her spirit. Some may rely on the serenity of an afternoon walk on the beach; others may find peace in prayer or meditation, and still others may need to reconnect with a certain community for support or encouragement. The evidence shows that clients, especially those who become seriously ill, disabled, or experience chronic pain, expect their health care providers to address spiritual themes, and it is our duty to do so (Barnes et al., 2004; Ben-Arye, Bar-Sela, Frenkel, Kuten, & Hermoni, 2006; Ehman, Ott, Short, Ciampa, & Hansen-Flaschen, 1999).

Approaches to addressing clients' spirituality vary and depend on the level of comfort that health care providers have with their own spirituality, as well as their knowledge and understanding of other forms of spiritual expression (Anandarajab, 2008; Anandarajab & Hight, 2001; Puchalski & Romer, 2003). Clinicians and clients may find it easiest to engage in discussions about spirituality with those who share their own spiritual beliefs. However, it is always important for clinicians to ensure that the focus remains on the understandings and needs of the client. The purpose of any discussion between the clients and care providers is to gather information about the clients' health and well-being from their own frame of reference. Therefore, the best approach to obtaining information about spirituality is to encourage clients to tell you about issues that define who they are, their purpose in life, and their dreams for the future (Craigie & Hobbs, 1999; Ventura, 2005).

The role of the clinician is to be a facilitator who helps clients discover their own answers, resources, and understanding by asking questions about the meaning clients attach to the experiences of life, illness, or disability. Alternatively, one can simply ask clients what motivates, excites, or helps them get through trying times. It may be helpful to explore who or what in their lives can provide support or contribute to their healing, whether that is family, friends, spiritual communities, or the higher power of their belief system. This approach signals a genuine concern and lets clients know that their beliefs and values are being respected. Heartfelt questions may prompt clients to reflect on the importance of spirituality in their lives, reminding them about helpful resources that they can access to assist in healing. When it is done well, a dialogue about the client's spiritual well-being offers an opportunity to create a meaningful connection with the client.

As discussed in Chapter 8, clients' coping strategies will vary depending on their experiences with grief and loss, their personalities, and other factors. When the onset of serious illness or disability makes it difficult for clients to cope with their changing circumstances, clinicians can help by recognizing coping strategies that are meaningful to the client and providing assistance where possible. Consider the client who has sustained a cervical level spinal cord injury, whose spiritual practice involves weekly attendance at a local church. Physical accommodations, such as ramps or physical assistance to overcome stairs, would be relatively easy to arrange. However, if the client is experiencing anger as part of the grieving process or fear of facing the community with a new, fragile, and altered sense of self, the issues are more complex. As in every aspect of clinical practice, the purpose of examining clients' spiritual needs is to establish possible solutions for identified problems. At times, we can help the client accomplish the problem-solving necessary. Other times, it is appropriate to make referral to a chaplain, the client's own clergy member(s), or other sources of spiritual support who are better trained to deal with spiritual concerns. Knowing the difference and having the necessary resources are key to positive outcomes.

## Summary

This chapter discussed the importance of viewing our clients as whole beings. The interrelatedness of the mind, body, and spirit is well documented and has been summarized here. The benefits of addressing each of these health dimensions can lead to significantly improved outcomes.

## Reflective Questions

1. What practices do you use to help yourself feel calm in a crisis or to overcome feelings of sadness or loss?
2. Do you use any of the spiritual practices discussed in this chapter?
   a. If yes, how often do you use these practices?
   b. If yes, describe them and their effect on you.
   c. If not, why not?
   d. If not, would you consider using them in the future?
3. a. Would you consider addressing your clients' spiritual beliefs and practices with them?
   b. If yes, under what circumstances?
   c. If not, why?
4. a. How do you think you might respond to someone whose beliefs or spiritual practices are different from your own?
   b. What if you found the beliefs or practices to be offensive?
5. What would you do if a client asked you to pray with him or her?

## Case Study

Ruth Parker is a 54-year-old woman who faces many stressors in her life, both at work and at home. She presents with a host of physical problems, including headaches, hypertension, generalized anxiety, and insomnia. Her physician has recommended medications, but she is reluctant to use any of them. Instead, she asks if other alternatives are available.

1. a. What is there about Mrs. Parker's life circumstances that might be contributing to her health problems?
   b. Provide a physiological rationale for your response.
2. What interventions could you recommend for Mrs. Parker that do not include medications?
3. Provide a rationale for each intervention you identified in question 2.
4. Mrs. Parker tells you that her neighbor uses copper bracelets and magnets to treat her arthritis and asks whether this might be helpful for her. How might you respond?

## References

Adler, R. (2000). On the development of psychoneuroimmunology. *European Journal of Pharmacology, 405*(1–3), 167–176.

Anandarajab, G. (2008). The 3 H and BMESEST models for spirituality in multicultural whole-person medicine. *Annals of Family Medicine, 6*(5), 448–458.

Anandarajab, G., & Hight, E. (2001). Spirituality and medical practice: Using the HOPE questions as a practical tool for spiritual assessment. *American Family Physician, 63*(1), 81–88.

Associated Press. (2004). Hospitals rule an obstacle to clergy. *The Boston Globe.* Retrieved from http://www.boston.com/news/local/rhode_island/articles/2004/04/12/hospital_rule_an_obstacle_to_clergy?mode=PF

Barnes, P. M., Powell-Griner, E., McFann, K., & Nahin, R. L. (2004). Complementary and alternative medicine among adults: United States, 2002. *Seminars in Integrative Medicine, 2*(2), 54–71.

Beilin, B., Shavit, Y., Trabekin, E., Mordashev, B., Mayburd, E., Zeidel, A., & Bessler, H. (2003). Pain management on immune response to surgery. *Anesthesia & Analgesia, 97*(3), 822–827.

Ben-Arye, E., Bar-Sela, G., Frankel, M., Kuten, A., & Hermoni, D. (2006). Is a biopsychosocial-spiritual approach relevant to cancer treatment? A study of patients and oncology staff members on issues of complementary medicine and spirituality. *Supportive Care in Cancer, 14*(2), 147–152.

Benson, H. (1996). *Timeless healing: The power and biology of belief.* New York, NY: Scribner.

Benson, H. (2000). *The relaxation response.* New York, NY: Harper Collins.

Benson, H., & Stuart, E. (1992). *The wellness book: The comprehensive guide to maintaining health and treating stress-related illness.* New York, NY: Fireside.

Branch, W. T., Torke, A., & Brown-Haithco, R. C. (2006). The importance of spirituality in African-Americans' end-of-life experience. *Journal of General Internal Medicine, 21*(11), 1203–1205.

Broom, A., & Tovey, P. (2007). The dialectical tension between individuation and depersonalization in cancer clients' mediation of complementary, alternative, and biomedical cancer treatments. *Sociology, 41*, 1021–1039.

Bush, T., & Bruni, N. (2008). Spiritual care as a dimension of holistic care: A relational interpretation. *International Journal of Palliative Nursing, 14*(11), 539–545.

Cabot, R. C., & Dicks, R. L. (1936). *The art of ministering to the sick.* New York, NY: Macmillan.

Cannon, W. B. (1929). *Bodily changes in pain, hunger, fear and rage.* New York, NY: Appleton.

Chauhan, P. S. (1998). *Ayurveda: The traditional Indian medical science. Ayurvedic.* Retrieved from http://www.ayurvedic.org

Chen, K. M., & Snyder, M. (1999). A research-based use of tai chi/movement therapy as a nursing intervention. *Journal of Holistic Nursing, 17*(3), 267–279.

Chiu, L., Emblen, J. D., Van Hofwegen, L., Sawatzky, R., & Meyerhoff, H. (2004). An integrative review of the concept of spirituality in the health sciences. *Western Journal of Nursing Research, 26*(4), 405–428.

Chopra, A., & Doiphode, V. V. (2002). Ayurvedic medicine: Core concept, therapeutic principles, and current relevance. *Medical Clinics of North America, 86*(1), 75–89.

Chopra, D. (1993). *The healing mind: Ancient wisdom, modern insights* [Videotape]. Lancaster, MA: The Maharishi Ayurveda Health Center.

Cohen, C. B., Wheeler, S. E., & Scott, D. A. (2001). Walking a fine line: Physicians' inquiries into patients' religious and spiritual beliefs. *The Hastings Center Report, 31*(5), 29–39.

Cohen, S. (2002). Psychosocial stress, social networks, and susceptibility to infection. In H. G. Koenig & H. J. Cohen (Eds.), *The link between religion and health: Psychoneuroimmunology and the faith factor* (pp. 101–123). New York, NY: Oxford University Press.

Craigie, F. C., Jr., & Hobbs, R. F., III. (1999). Spiritual perspectives and practices of family physicians with expressed interest in spirituality. *Family Medicine, 31*(8), 578–585.

Daaleman, T. P. (2004). Religion, spirituality, and the practice of medicine. *Journal of the American Board of Family Practice, 17*, 370–376.

Driscoll, J. J. (2003). HIPAA calling the question: Is the chaplain a health care professional? *Vision, 13*(5), 4–5.

Ehman, J. W., Ott, B. B., Short, T. H., Ciampa, P. C., & Hansen-Flaschen, J. (1999). Do patients want physicians to inquire about their spiritual or religious beliefs if they become gravely ill? *Archives of Internal Medicine, 159*, 1803–1806.

Ellis, M. R., Campbell, J. D., Detwiler-Breidenbach, A., & Hubbard, D. K. (2002). What do family physicians think about spirituality in clinical practice? *Journal of Family Practice, 51*(3), 249–254.

Feudtner, C., Haney, J., & Dimmers, M. A. (2003). Spiritual care needs of hospitalized children and their families: A national survey of pastoral care providers' perceptions. *Pediatrics, 111*(1), e67–e72. Retrieved from http://pediatrics.aappublications.org/cgi/reprint/111/1/e67

Gallup Poll. (2008). *Majority of Americans believe in God.* Retrieved from http://www.gallup.com/video/109111/Majority-Americans-Believe-God.aspx

Giaquinto, S., Spiridigliozzi, C., & Caracciolo, B. (2007). Can faith protect from emotional distress after stroke? *Stroke, 38*, 993–997.

Graber, D. R., & Johnson, J. A. (2001). Spirituality and health care organizations. *Journal of Health Care Management, 46*(1), 39–50.

Kabat-Zinn, J. (1990). *Full catastrophe living: Using the wisdom of your body and mind to face stress, pain, and illness.* New York, NY: Delta.

Kabat-Zinn, J., Wheeler, E., Light, T., Skillings, A., Scharf, M. J., Cropley, T. G., . . . Bernhard, J. D. (1998). Influence of a mindfulness meditation-based stress reduction intervention on rates of skin clearing in clients with moderate to severe psoriasis undergoing phototherapy (UVB) and photochemotherapy (PUVA). *Psychosomatic Medicine, 60*, 625–632.

Kiecolt-Glaser, J. K., McGuire, L., Robles, T. F., & Glaser, R. (2002). Psychoneuroimmunology: Psychological influences on immune function and health. *Journal of Consulting and Clinical Psychology, 70*(3), 537–547.

Koenig, H. G. (1999). *The healing power of faith: Science explores medicine's last great frontier.* New York, NY: Simon & Schuster.

Koenig, H. G., & Cohen, H. J. (Eds.). (2002). *The link between religion and health: Psychoneuroimmunology and the faith factor.* New York, NY: Oxford University Press.

Lee, S. J. (2002). In a secular spirit: Strategies of clinical pastoral education. *Health Care Analysis, 10*(4), 339–356.

Massachusetts General Hospital. (2003). Learning the language of pastoral care. *Caring Headline: MGH Patient Care Services.* Retrieved from http://pcs.mgh.harvard.edu/Caring_Headlines/Archive/PDF/2003/July%2017,%202003.pdf

Matthews, D. A. (1998). *The faith factor: Proof of the healing power of prayer.* New York, NY: Penguin Books.

McCarthy, M. P. (2000). Health care reform: Analysis of narrative responses from directors of pastoral care departments. *Journal of Health Care Chaplaincy, 10*(1), 19–36.

McClain, C. S., Rosenfeld, B., & Breitbart, W. (2003). Effect of spiritual well-being on end-of-life despair in terminally-ill cancer clients. *Lancet, 361*(9369), 1603–1607.

McColl, M. A., Bickenback, J., Johnston, J., Nishihama, S., Schumaker, M., Smith, K., . . . Yealland, B. (2000). Changes in spiritual beliefs after traumatic disability. *Archives of Physical Medicine and Rehabilitation, 81*(6), 817–823.

McCullough, M., & Larson, D. (1999). Religion and depression: A review of the literature. *Twin Research, 2,* 126–139.

Meyer, E. C., Ritholz, M. D., Burns, J. P., & Truog, R. D. (2006). Improving the quality of end-of-life care in the pediatric intensive care unit: Parents' priorities and recommendations. *Pediatrics, 117,* 649–657.

Meyers, D. G. (1999, December). The pursuit of personal and social healing: What role for spirituality? In H. Benson (Chair), *Spirituality and healing in medicine.* Symposium conducted at the meeting of Harvard Medical School, Department of Continuing Education and Mind/Body Medical Institute, and CareGroup, Beth Israel Deaconess Medical Center, Boston.

Newman, B. (1998). *Voice of the living light: Hildegard of Bingen and her world.* Berkeley: University of California Press.

Olff, M., deVries, G. J., Güzelcan, Y., Assies, J., & Gersons, B. P. R. (2007). Changes in cortisol and DHEA plasma levels after psychotherapy for PTSD. *Psychoneuroendocrinology, 32*(6), 619–626.

Ornish, D. (1990). *Dr. Dean Ornish's program for reversing heart disease.* New York, NY: Random House.

Perkins, A. (2003). Healing patients' spirits. *Eagle Tribune.* Retrieved from http://www.eagletribune.com/news/stories/20030209/LN_002.htm

Puchalski, C. (2004). Spirituality in health: The role of spirituality in critical care. *Critical Care Clinics, 20*(3), 487–504.

Puchalski, C. (2009). Ethical concerns and boundaries in spirituality and health. *American Medical Association Journal of Ethics, 11*(10), 804–806.

Puchalski , C., & Romer, A. L. (2003). Taking a spiritual history allows clinicians to understand clients more fully. *Journal of Palliative Medicine, 3*(1), 129–137.

Rabin, B. S. (2002). Understanding how stress affects the physical body. In H. G. Koenig & H. J. Cohen (Eds.), *The link between religion and health: Psychoneuroimmunology and the faith factor* (pp. 43–68). New York, NY: Oxford University Press.

Ritt-Olson, A., Milam, J., Unger, J. B., Trinidad, L., Teran, L., Dent, C., & Sussman, S. (2004). The protective influence of spirituality and "health-as-a-value" against monthly substance use among adolescents varying in risk. *Journal of Adolescent Health, 34*(3), 192–199.

Ross, M. C., Bohannon, A. S., Davis, D. C., & Gurchiek, L. (1999). The effects of a short-term exercise program on movement, pain, and mood in the elderly. *Journal of Holistic Nursing, 17*(2), 139–147.

Selye, H. (1974). *Stress without distress.* New York, NY: J. P. Lippincott.

Sloan, R. P. (2009). Why patient's religion is not their doctors business. *American Medical Association Journal of Ethics, 11*(10), 811–814.

Sloan, R. P., & Bagiella, E. (2001). Spirituality and medical practice: A look at the evidence. *American Family Physician, 63*(1), 33–34.

Sloan, R. P., Bagiella, E., & Powell, T. (1999). Religion, spirituality and medicine, *Lancet, 353,* 664.

Stefano, G. B., Fricchione, G. L., Slingsby, B. T., & Benson, H. (2001). The placebo effect and relaxation response: Neural processes and their coupling to constitutive nitric oxide. *Brain Research Reviews, 35,* 1–19.

Umphred, D. (1995). *Neurological rehabilitation* (3rd ed.). St. Louis, MO: Mosby.

Vance, D. L. (2001). Nurses' attitudes towards spirituality and patient care. *Medical Surgical Nursing, 10,* 264–274.

VandeCreek, L., & Burton, L. (Eds.). (2001). A white paper. Professional chaplaincy: Its role and importance in health care. *Journal of Pastoral Care, 55*(1), 81–97.

Ventura, S. H. (2005). *A middle-range theory to guide the promotion, support, or improvement of spiritually sensitive care in hospital settings* (Doctoral dissertation). Available from ProQuest Dissertations & Theses database. (UMI No. 3171582)

Waite, L. J., & Lehrer, E. L. (2003). The benefits from marriage and religion in the United States: A comparative analysis. *Population and Development Review, 29*(2), 255–276.

White, L. J. (2003). *Federal funding partially preserved for CPE programs.* Retrieved from the Association for Clinical Pastoral Education, Inc., website: http://www.acpe.edu/medicare_update.htm

WHOQOL SRPB Group. (2006). A cross-cultural study of spirituality, religion and personal beliefs as components of quality of life. *Social Science & Medicine, 62*(6), 1486–1497.

Whybrow, P. C. (1997). *A mood apart: The thinker's guide to emotion and its disorders.* New York, NY: HarperPerennial.

Wong, Y. J., Rew, K. D., & Slaikeu, B. A. (2006). A systematic review of recent research on adolescent religiosity and mental health. *Issues in Mental Health Nursing, 27*(2), 161–183.

Yanek, L. R., Becker, D. M., Moy, T. F., Gittelsohn, J., & Koffman, D. M. (2001). Protect joy: Faith based cardiovascular health promotion for African American women. *Public Health Report, 116*(Suppl. 1): 68–81.

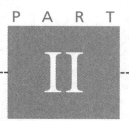

P A R T

II

# Making Connections

# Communication

Patrick was late again! In frustration, I asked the nurse why he was never down in physical therapy (PT) for his scheduled appointments. She said, "He's the most impossible amputee I've ever worked with. Come with me, and you'll understand." As we approached his room, she shouted, "Patrick, get out of bed!" and threw up the shade. Depressed and angry, he shouted obscenities at the nurse and pulled the covers over his head.

I was absolutely appalled at her lack of sensitivity and compassion. No wonder he refused to have PT that day. I determined another strategy was in order. The following morning, I entered his room, smiled, and said, "Patrick, it's time to get up for PT. Your appointment is in 30 minutes. Will that work for you?" He nodded, and I left. One-half hour later, on the dot, he wheeled his chair into the clinic.

—*From the journal of Lindsay Cushing, physical therapist student*

"Communication is the interpretation of meaning from interpersonal interactions and extends far beyond verbal information to include elements of body movement, expressions, and subconscious mechanisms" (Davis, 2009, p. 78). Health care providers are required to communicate on a daily basis with clients, clients' families and friends, third-party payers, equipment vendors, and other health care professionals. Effective and timely communication is key to providing successful client- and family-centered health care and achieving optimal health outcomes. It enables providers to understand individual needs, helps clarify complicated issues, and promotes client adherence to complex treatment regimens. It is especially important when working with clients who have limited or no English proficiency skills, those with limited health literacy, and clients whose cultural backgrounds are not well understood by providers (Saha, Beach, & Cooper, 2008).

First and foremost, communication is the means by which we establish a therapeutic relationship with each client. There is strong support for including core communication studies and other professional behaviors, such as caring and empathy, in health care curricula and continuing education programs to better prepare client- and family-centered practitioners (Ang, 2002; Bonvicini et al., 2008; Greenfield, Anderson, Cox, & Tanner, 2008; Henkin, Dee, & Beatus, 2000; Raica, 2009; Taylor, Wook Lee, Kielhofner, & Ketkar, 2009). Learning experiences that promote the use of open-ended inquiries, active listening, reflective practice, empathy, and other caring behaviors can better prepare novice clinicians for the transition from the classroom to the clinic (Greenfield et al., 2008).

Although clients consider a provider's demonstration of caring and empathy to be extremely important to them, such demonstrations are often lacking in many medical encounters (Bonvicini et al., 2008). Unless providers are able to display these qualities to clients, interventions may be ineffective, regardless of the providers' clinical skills (Charon, 2001). Empathy is the ability to identify with and understand someone's situation, feelings, and emotions and recognize that the client is someone's mother, daughter, wife, or sibling. This includes imagining what it feels like to "be in the clients' shoes," to actually see things through their eyes, to not only hear what they are saying but to absorb their verbal and nonverbal cues (Davis, 2009; Fox et al., 2009).

In a study of general practitioners who had been patients, participants stated, "You never really appreciate what it's like being a patient until you are a patient . . . suddenly you realize that you feel very small and that you don't have much of a voice and you don't feel very powerful . . . you feel very vulnerable and you can get very emotional, and you cannot be very rational about things" (Fox et al., 2009, p. 1582). Other participants indicated feelings of anxiety, shock, and loss of control. Waiting for a medical procedure, one participant indicated that being an "insider" in the health care system gave her the ability to be seen more quickly than other patients who lacked such power. While she still felt anxious and some sense of disempowerment, she recognized that her feelings were tempered because of her professional medical status. Respondents indicated that, as a result of their experiences, they developed a better understanding of and enhanced emotional connection with future patients. Recognizing their own disempowering feelings, they worked harder to empathize with patients, to recognize their emotions, and to empower them in clinical decision making.

Studies show that an empathetic approach to client care leads to improvements in the quality of client–provider relationships, enhanced treatment outcomes, and enrichment of practitioners' own lives (Davis, 2009; Greenfield et al., 2008). The first step in developing empathy is to practice effective communication skills. Good communication skills allow health care providers to focus on the person, not the disease; to build a therapeutic alliance that improves both the client's and provider's perspectives; and to achieve more appropriate therapeutic goals (Saha et al., 2008; Teal & Street, 2009).

Health care professionals agree that they must possess effective communication skills to motivate clients, promote adherence with treatment protocols, and ensure appropriate, cost-efficient outcomes (Pettrey, 2003; Vanderhoff, 2005). Studies show that poor communication often results in negative consequences. If information is not relayed adequately, inaccurate diagnoses can result (Sutcliffe, Lewton, & Rosenthal, 2004). Clients may grow dissatisfied and frustrated with health care providers, become nonadherent with treatment plans, or seek alternative care, resulting in higher medical costs. In addition, practitioners can also become frustrated and develop symptoms of burnout. To prevent the latter, it is helpful for providers to recognize their own limitations, know that they cannot *cure* everyone, and practice stress management strategies to help balance work and family life (Greenfield et al., 2008).

Although individuals may believe they are clearly conveying messages to others, receivers may not always hear the message senders thought they were conveying. The opening journal entry in this chapter provides a good example. The nurse thought she was helping Patrick prepare for therapy, but he responded to her approach as an unwelcome interruption to his sleep. In addition, her behavior suggested disapproval and judgment. In contrast, Lindsay reframed the situation, giving Patrick the opportunity to take control and "save face." As a result, she was successful in motivating him. A health professional's role is to provide clients with factual information that helps them formulate their own decisions, not offer value judgments. In this chapter, we discuss the components of effective communication and their importance in conducting a client-centered patient interview.

## ELEMENTS OF EFFECTIVE COMMUNICATION

Communication begins when the sender expresses an idea, either verbally or nonverbally. Verbal messages are influenced by paralanguage cues, such as tone of voice, pitch, volume, and speed. Nonverbal messages may be sent intentionally or unintentionally. They include facial expression, touch, proxemics, and behavior. The receiver interprets the message within a context that is mediated by these influencing factors. The receiver's understanding of the meaning of the message is further affected by what he or she perceives and feels. People's perceptions may vary depending on social role, literacy level, cultural background, personal needs, age, and prior life experiences. The physical context in which a discussion takes place, the time of day, the individual's mental status, and other factors occurring in one or more of the participants' lives may also influence the communication process (Barringer & Glod, 1998).

Communication between health care providers and clients differs from day-to-day social interactions with friends or family members. Individuals choose their friends but not necessarily their clients. Social relationships are based on enjoyment and mutual satisfaction, whereas professional affiliations exist for the benefit of the client. A health professional may elect to end a friendship based on another individual's unacceptable social responses but may be obligated to continue treating a client who behaves similarly. During social interactions, individuals share problems and experiences, whereas in therapeutic situations, the focus is solely on the client's concerns. In social surroundings, people often speak without thinking beforehand about what they are going to say or how it will influence others. In health care settings, communication should be planned in advance, whenever possible, to help facilitate accurate communication. To ensure that messages are being correctly interpreted by both sender and receiver, health care professionals need to continuously observe and analyze their interactions with others (Vanderhoff, 2005). Providing feedback and paraphrasing messages may help ensure clarification.

### Levels of Communication

Communication occurs at four levels. It starts at the *intrapersonal level,* as we absorb information from our environment and begin to develop and formulate our thoughts and ideas. Once we decide to send a message to another person, we start to communicate at the *interpersonal level.* Here, the opportunity for misinterpretation begins. A higher level of communication takes place when we participate in a *small group discussion* with more than one other individual. This frequently occurs at team and family meetings. People enter with differing goals, objectives, and backgrounds, and the chances of misinterpretation or conflict increase. Finally, *organizational communication* takes place when *several groups* within a facility meet to discuss problems or establish policies. Egos, personal agendas, and professional differences may all interfere with the exchange. Everyone needs to strive to keep the channels of communication open and effective (Davis, 2006).

## DEVELOPING CLIENT–PRACTITIONER RAPPORT

As health care professionals, we might neglect to think about the culture shock that clients experience when they encounter the health care setting. Clients enter with their own concerns, anxieties, and value systems. They have their personal routine and may be accustomed to privacy. In an inpatient setting, they may have an unknown and unwanted roommate. We socialize them into *our* world. We often require them to wear particular attire and eat at preset times. They select what they are eating from limited menus. In addition to coping with their illness, disease, or disability, we expect them to value our expertise and follow our instructions. Is it any wonder why clients may feel dependent, vulnerable, or afraid?

Studies confirm that practitioners who adopt a friendly and reassuring manner are more effective than those who do not. In fact, in one study of empathy and its relationship to the common cold, researchers found that clinician empathy, as perceived by patients, significantly decreased illness duration and severity associated with immune system changes (Rakel et al., 2009). The adage that a picture is worth a thousand words may seem almost too basic to mention, but a perceived inhospitable health care environment can damage an impression before the provider even begins to speak. Facial expressions and postures may be the first "picture" or impression the client receives, depending on his or her learning style, cultural context, and other factors. Explaining who you are and why you are there can establish a therapeutic foundation, and a smile can be very comforting. Pulling up a chair to sit at eye level with a client who is seated or reclining can make the health professional seem open to communication and collaboration rather than authoritative and distant. Taken together, these simple measures demonstrate a willingness to spend the time needed for clients and providers to get to know each other. Evidence shows that when providers use these techniques, clients' psychological well-being and their ability to recall information at a later date both improve (Stiefel et al., 2010).

Prior to entering a client's room or greeting a client in the clinic or home setting, providers should clear their thoughts in order to be mindful and focused on the person they are about to meet. By taking time to practice this simple strategy, practitioners make themselves ready to be truly present in each and every experience. The process involves practitioners becoming aware of their thoughts and reflecting on their biases and expectations, which enables them to remain nonjudgmental and ready to listen intently to what the client has to say (Epstein, 1999; Hutchinson, 2005). Therapists who are aware of their own thoughts and feelings and who are oriented toward the interpersonal aspects of client interactions achieve more effective therapeutic relationships and better outcomes. In occupational therapy, this concept is referred to as "use of self." It involves the therapist's use of his or her own personality, perceptions, and judgments as part of the therapeutic process (Taylor et al., 2009).

Health care professionals often work with very distressed people, whose emotional strain can affect their ability to communicate. Our attempts to deal with difficult situations can affect our own ability to communicate and be compassionate (Halstead, 2001). In a busy health care setting, providers are frequently under stress. It may be easy to fall into the habit of concentrating on the illness, disease, or injury rather than on the client as a person. Although this may be an appropriate response in the emergency department, it is not appropriate in most other cases. Before we can effectively treat a client, we must develop a good relationship or rapport (Schneider, Kaplan, Greenfield, Li, & Wilson, 2004).

In our efforts to be empathetic and compassionate, though, we need to be genuine and not offer false reassurances. "I know how you feel" is not authentic—we do not know how they feel. Instead, we might say, "This must be difficult for you," "Tell me how this is affecting you," or

"How are you feeling?" Similarly, we may not be able to tell them that "everything will be all right." Clients have a right, and often a need, to express their emotions regarding their illness or disability. The provider's role is to listen and be empathetic (Halstead, 2001).

It is important for providers to ask clients about their health practices. Do they eat a balanced diet? Do they exercise regularly? Do they use seat belts? Do they consume drugs or alcohol? As clients talk, providers can practice active listening skills by leaning toward the client, nodding, and asking clarifying questions. Keep in mind that some clients find touch comforting; others do not. It may be appropriate for providers to touch a client's arm or shoulder to demonstrate caring. If the client withdraws or appears uncomfortable, responsive providers will withdraw their touch and avoid unnecessary touch in the future.

Before beginning to examine or treat clients, providers can let clients know what to expect to help build a sense of trust and respect and allay anxiety. The extra minutes it takes to develop this sense of rapport is well worth the effort as the treatment program progresses. Consider the case of Donnie, a physical therapist student completing an internship in a skilled nursing facility. On his way to meet a new client who was admitted following a stroke, he stopped by the nurses' station to review her medical record. A staff member said, "Good luck with Mrs. Benson. She is in a bad mood today and refuses to do anything." Donnie approached the room with trepidation. As he entered, he took time to note the pictures and personal items on the bedside table. He introduced himself to the client and said, "From your pictures, I see that you like to dance." She responded, "I was quite a dancer in my day." As Donnie developed a therapeutic relationship with her, she allowed him to proceed. Following an evaluation, he asked her if she would like to dance with him. A few minutes later, the staff was amazed as they saw Donnie and Mrs. Benson smiling and *waltzing* down the corridor.

As health care professionals, we need to develop an awareness and ability to reflect on our own attitudes, styles, and approaches to clients. Rather than assuming that a client is "difficult," it is important to question our own attitudes and develop more effective strategies. Taking the time to view clients as the "experts" in *their individual situations* and allowing time for them to express their desires, values, and emotions may improve therapeutic relationships and lead to better client outcomes (Beach & Inui, 2006; Greenfield et al., 2008). This is especially important in a health care environment in which clients are quickly discharged. In addition to treating the client, the health care provider must play the roles of educator and facilitator, helping clients become independent in their own care as quickly as possible (Vanderhoff, 2005).

## Client-Sensitive Language

As Martin (1999) noted, "language shapes thought" (p. 44). Thinking about clients as their illness or disability reinforces emotional detachment. For some, the person *becomes* the diagnosis, which frames the context in how we connect. Focusing on the individual enables us to see his or her abilities, needs, desires, and goals rather than the impairments. For example, the common expression of "confined to a wheelchair" promotes a negative connotation of being limited, even imprisoned. The wheelchair, in fact, is just the opposite. It is liberating, providing a means of mobility, of accessing the world. Refer to Table 5–1 for other examples of diminishing and empowering language.

In addition to empowering clients, we show respect by using "people-first" language. The terminology we use reflects how we think about clients (Martin, 1999). Consider how the nurse in Lindsay's journal referred to Patrick as "the most impossible amputee." Patrick is not the amputation. He is a person who has undergone a surgical amputation of his lower limb.

| Table 5–1 | Examples of Diminishing and Empowering Terminology |

| Diminishing Terminology | Empowering Terminology |
| --- | --- |
| • Stroke victim | • Person who has had a stroke |
| • Stricken with polio | • Person who has polio |
| • Afflicted with cerebral palsy | • Person with cerebral palsy; diagnosed with cerebral palsy |
| • Suffers from Parkinson's disease | • Person who has Parkinson's disease |
| • Mute; dumb | • Person who is unable to speak |
| • Confined to a wheelchair | • Uses a wheelchair |
| • The handicapped; impaired; disabled; crippled; deformed | • Person with a disability or impairment |
| • Normal (as though a person with a disability is not normal) | • Person without a disability |
| • The blind | • Person who is visually impaired; person who is blind |
| • Epileptic | • Person with epilepsy; person with a seizure disorder |
| • Schizophrenic | • Person with schizophrenia |
| • Alcoholic | • Person with alcoholism |
| • Fits | • Seizures |
| • Victim of … | • Survivor of … |
| • Suffering from | • Diagnosed with |

We often hear health care workers using terminology such as "that CVA," "the shoulder," or "the arthritic client." People are not their impairments, functional limitations, or disabilities, but rather the person with a stroke, the woman with a shoulder problem, the client with arthritis. Acknowledging their individuality and totality is part of a therapeutic outcome. Providers need to be aware of this and encourage others to avoid referring to clients by their diagnoses or body parts.

Similarly, choice of words, tone, and volume can communicate certain messages, even when they are unintended. For example, by referring to older clients as "honey" or "dear," health providers may inadvertently transmit messages of dependence or incompetence to older adults by infantilizing them, using what has become known as *elderspeak* (Williams, Kemper, & Hummert, 2004, p. 17).

## MINDFULNESS: BEING PRESENT IN THE MOMENT

Today, I had an experience that made me very sad. I've been on my rotation at the hospital for three months, and my supervisor seems very pleased with my skills. I have a lot of independence and am responsible for my own caseload. A therapist was out sick with the flu today, and I was asked to pick up two of her clients on top of my own. Boy was I overwhelmed! I only had time to skim the charts and then rush in and do the best treatment I could with very little time.

Later, I was scheduled to examine Ms. Jones, a newly admitted client. She's a 23-year-old woman who was in a car accident that caused a fracture-dislocation at the lumbar 4-5 level of the spinal cord. At this time, she has paraplegia, with no sensation in her lower extremities. I was feeling so rushed that I just barged into her room and quickly introduced myself before I started bombarding her with questions about her past medical history and current status. Then I began running through the items on the evaluation form as quickly as I could. She started crying and then shouted, "You're just like all the others! I'm a person." I felt so terrible. I realized I was not treating her as a client, but as an object. I quickly apologized and fled the room. I immediately recognized my mistake. I had let my frustration take over, and as a result, I failed to be there for her when she needed me.

—*From the journal of Mark Smart, occupational therapy student*

Today, the need to be highly productive places significant demands on health care practitioners. The ability to simultaneously perform multiple tasks is expected. While running from client to client, it is easy to forget that each person is a unique human being. What messages does this behavior convey? When providers work with one client but are preoccupied with others, they risk giving the client the impression that he or she is "in the way" and "unimportant." To avoid this, providers should practice mindfulness. This requires that we fully attend to each task (Epstein, 1999; Epstein & Street, 2007; Hutchinson, 2005; Kabat-Zinn, 1994; Kearney, Weininger, Vachon, Harrison, & Mount, 2009; Mead & Bower, 2002; Mentgen, 2001; Teal & Street, 2009).

How do providers become mindful in the midst of a chaotic health care environment? Studies show that mindful practitioners develop self-awareness, clearing their minds of mental clutter, so that they are able to focus on the present moment. Mindfulness involves self-assessment, the ability to be aware of one's own opinions, prejudices, and expectations. Practitioners must understand and respect what the client is feeling and distinguish the client's feelings from their own. The mindful practitioner welcomes uncertainty, and difficult patients become interesting (Epstein & Street, 2007; Hutchinson, 2005; Kabat-Zinn, 1994; Kearney et al., 2009; Mead & Bower, 2002; Mentgen, 2001). Whereas all practitioners rely on academic knowledge, the mindful practitioner also relies on knowledge of the self and client. Barriers to mindfulness include emphasis on explicit rather than tacit knowledge, time constraints, and the desire to maintain emotional distance from clients. To develop mindfulness, practitioners learn to actively listen to their clients and observe and learn from mentors in clinical settings. In addition, practitioners may want to practice meditation (Epstein, 1999) or maintain a personal journal of their client encounters to reflect on and learn from their actions in practice (Epstein, 1999; Schon, 1983; Wainwright, Shepard, Harman, & Stephens, 2010).

It only takes a minute to focus and give complete attention to the client. This small intervention can greatly enhance the effectiveness of the treatment. Clients are aware of the state of mind we bring to the interaction. Had Mark, the occupational therapy student, been able to eliminate the distractions and fully attend to Ms. Jones, he might have developed a rapport with her and been more successful in eliciting information. She might have become a partner in her care and been spared feeling like a "victim" of *his* distress.

## VERBAL COMMUNICATION

### Vocabulary

It is important to match your chosen communication technique as closely as possible to the preferred style of the client, which may mean adjusting your typical approach. For example, you may need to speak more slowly or more loudly, consider how you make eye contact, and, perhaps, not ask too many questions of a client who comes from a culture that uses indirect language skills. This is information that may not be readily apparent and can only be identified by carefully observing a client's response to you.

As stated earlier, communication involves sending a message to a receiver (an audience). When sending a message, it is important for the sender to keep in mind the needs of the audience. First, consider the importance of vocabulary. When talking to another health care professional who shares our common language, providers should use medical terminology. However, when speaking with a client, providers need to use words that the client understands; for example, you would use a different language with an adult who has undergone a heart transplant than with a child who has a developmental delay. Sometimes, clients nod and smile, apparently signaling that they understand, even when they do not. Checking with clients to determine what they have heard helps avoid misunderstandings. Providers can ask them to repeat the information or ask questions to determine clarity of understanding.

Using medical terminology may unknowingly frighten clients. For example, suggesting that a client go to a short-term care facility for rehabilitation following surgery may be routine to the provider, but the client may hear, "I am being sent to a nursing home and will never go home again." To avoid such miscommunication, observe clients' nonverbal responses. If they appear upset by something said, ask questions to clarify misconceptions or concerns prior to moving on to new topics or activities. Whatever vocabulary providers choose, it is essential to speak with clients at their level of understanding (Vanderhoff, 2005). Words are building blocks, but they are only a part of verbal communication.

### Paralanguage

Paralanguage, an important component of verbal communication, includes pitch, tone, speed, volume, emotional quality, stress, and accent (Purtilo & Haddad, 2007). The phrase "It's not what you say but how you say it that counts" illustrates the idea that what one says can be interpreted many different ways. Sometimes, especially when we are stressed, busy, or impatient, what we planned to say comes out sounding all wrong.

When we are in a hurry, we tend to talk faster. When we are excited or angry, we talk louder. If we are nervous, the listener may detect a higher pitch or tone. Accents may be difficult for some to understand. When communicating with clients, it is important to appear calm and concerned. Maintain an appropriate tone and volume to convey a sense of trust and interest. Take time to emphasize key words so the listener "hears" them and recognizes their importance. Volume should vary depending on the size of the room and the hearing capabilities of the audience.

### Active Listening

Active listening is an essential evaluation tool (Jensen, Gwyer, Shepard, & Hack, 2000). The onus falls on the health care provider to intently listen to clients' stories, understand their needs within the context of their lives, create a plan of care in collaboration with clients and significant others, and teach clients and significant others the skills they need to carry out the plan of care

(Vanderhoff, 2005). Although hearing implies the ability to perceive sound, *active listening* involves being alert and receptive to both verbal and nonverbal communication cues. Whenever possible, eliminate the physical and mental distractions that may hinder communication. Strive to appear relaxed and interested in what clients have to say. Listen to their stories. This is not the time to spend reviewing the medical record and previous documentation. Although making some notes may be appropriate, ignoring the client while taking copious notes is not effective (Davis, 2009).

Florence Nightingale is reported to have said, "We must not talk to them [clients], not at them, but with them" (Attewell, 1998). Active listening shows clients that you are fully present in the moment, grasping the meaning of what they are saying. One difference noted between "expert" and "novice" physical therapists (Jensen et al., 2000) relates to the importance of listening. Skilled clinicians claim that they "got much more information from listening than from structuring questions" and that "if you go in and listen to the clients, they will tell you" (p. 33). It is very powerful for the client to feel your complete presence.

Active listening skills are also relevant in other situations and can clarify miscommunication and de-escalate conflict. Consider this scenario: A busy phlebotomist enters a client's room to draw blood and discovers the speech-language pathologist in the midst of treatment. Knowing how many clients he still needs to see, he demands emotionally, "You'll have to stop for a minute. I need to draw blood immediately. I'm in a hurry." Although the therapist may have the urge to respond in kind, anger will not resolve the situation and may even inflame it. The potential conflict may be diffused by a process of active listening, which includes a three-step framework: restatement, reflection, and clarification (Davis, 2006). Through this process, listeners let speakers know they were heard and understood: "I understand that you're in a hurry and want to see this client immediately." Listeners then describe how they think the speaker feels and gives him or her the opportunity to clarify feelings: "It sounds like you're having a hectic day and are upset." Finally, the listener summarizes the situation and asks for a potential solution: "We can stop for a moment or two and let you draw some blood" or "We'll be done in about fifteen minutes, if you want to come back." Either response would reduce conflict and allow both health care providers to proceed with client care, always a primary concern. Ask yourself: What are the medical priorities? What would most benefit the client at this time? Active listening is a challenging skill to develop and requires practice. When used effectively, it can improve therapeutic interactions as well as diffuse angry situations, leading to effective solutions.

It is not always easy for providers to be "therapeutic" in their approach, especially when they are the target of disappointment, frustration, and blame. Expert clinicians do not judge or categorize clients as difficult or nonadherent. Instead, they evaluate the challenge and accept the responsibility of developing alternate communication solutions (Jensen et al., 2000). Consider Joyce, a woman with multiple sclerosis, who bellowed at the occupational therapist, "When I came here, they told me that I would be able to dress myself within a week. Well, I can't. It's all your fault! If I had a better therapist, I would be home by now." Although the therapist might reflexively respond defensively, it is therapeutically beneficial to take a different approach. In this case, the occupational therapist could say, "I understand that when you first came to this hospital, you thought you'd be able to take care of yourself. You now see that this will take more time and be more involved than you anticipated. You sound frustrated. Unfortunately, there are no quick solutions. We have to work on your balance and strength so that you're able to be more independent."

How will you react the next time you are confronted by an angry client or colleague? Keep in mind that clients sometimes just need to talk to express their fear, anger, or frustration with their illness, injury, or disability. Providers may be called on to listen therapeutically, without responding, to affirm that what clients are experiencing is normal and understandable, even if the clients need to repeat the story multiple times to everyone with whom they come in contact (Halstead, 2001).

Clinicians should be aware that when they are under stress they may be tempted to respond inappropriately. When emotionally upset, providers should recognize their feelings, take responsibility for their actions, and not blame others. Not all situations will work out the way we would like, even for expert clinicians. People are emotional; they may become angry and frustrated and verbally "strike out" when they feel they cannot control a situation. Providers must do their best to maintain a level head and respond appropriately to clients, family members, and other health care professionals. If, however, a health care professional says something inappropriate, a well-timed apology is in order. These strategies not only improve communication capabilities but also allow health care professionals to provide more effective client care.

On occasion, professional caregivers may feel anger or resentment toward their clients. Recognize that this is a normal reaction. To be compassionate with our clients, we need to recognize and respond to our own feelings and needs (Halstead, 2001). Studies have shown that health providers who practice meditation, mindfulness, and/or participate in reflective writing are less likely to lose perspective or experience burnout on the job. They are also more likely to be engaged with their clients and coworkers, be less judgmental of themselves and others, be more empathetic, have a greater sense of self-actualization, and be better appreciated by their clients (Kearney et al., 2009).

## NONVERBAL COMMUNICATION

Although verbal communication is important, people also convey messages without saying a word. It is imperative to "tune in" to the nonverbal cues we give and receive. If we are unaware of the nonverbal signals we send to clients, we may inadvertently jeopardize our therapeutic relationships. Open to ambiguous interpretation and not always easy to understand, nonverbal communication strongly influences the perceived meaning of messages. For example, a provider enters a client's room and finds him in tears. Should the clinician immediately assume the client is depressed about his condition? Should the health care provider leave and avoid interacting? Instead, he opens a dialogue and discovers that these are tears of joy over news of a new grandchild. This information may motivate him to achieve the goal of returning home. It is important to verify assumptions and not accept seemingly pat conclusions. By reading body language, tone of voice, pacing of speech, and other forms of paralanguage, we can better hear the message and "read between the lines" (Coulehan & Block, 2001).

### Facial Expressions

Facial expressions are important because they convey emotions. Following a biopsy, a frightened client is alert to the expression on the doctor's face as she walks into the room to announce the diagnosis. Is the news good or bad? Afraid and lacking information, we attempt to learn what we can by watching people. Research shows that fear, sadness, and anger are identified by looking at one's eyes, whereas happiness and disgust are best identified by looking at an individual's mouth (Ekman, 1999). What do the health care providers' facial expressions convey to clients? What do clients' expressions convey to the health care provider?

When treating a client, it is important to be aware of the expression on the person's face. Consider the adage, "The eyes are the mirror of the soul." Is the person in pain? Does he or she wince when moved from the bed to the chair? Some clients will report when they feel pain; others are stoic and silent. Observing facial expressions and nonverbal language and communicating with clients assists providers in better understanding what clients may be thinking and feeling.

## Touch

Touch is another form of nonverbal communication. In health care settings, providers touch clients to examine, evaluate, treat, and comfort them. In fact, as health care professionals, we often have intimate contact with clients that otherwise would be restricted to their significant others.

There are several forms of touch. *Procedural* or *instrumental* touch occurs when our hands come in contact with clients, as we carry out interventions, such as moving a client into bed, performing range-of-motion exercises, or drawing blood. *Expressive* or *caring* touch involves contact that is meant to convey emotional support. This may include resting a hand on a client's arm or shoulder (Barringer & Glod, 1998; Routasalo, 1999). Although expressive or caring touch may be "therapeutic," it should not be confused with the complementary/alternative approach known as *therapeutic touch.* This is a technique in which a health care practitioner combines mindfulness, intent, and hand movements to promote healing by balancing energy fields. Hands may be placed directly on the skin, over clothing, or several inches above the client's body (Hayes & Cox, 1999; Herdtner, 2000; Monroe, 2009; Umbreit, 2000).

Health professionals' touching style is influenced by their cultural backgrounds, previous experience, and education. Although many studies show that touch has a calming and comforting effect on clients, individual responses to touch vary, depending on age, gender, parts of the body being touched, physical environment, cultural heritage, prior experience, and personal interpretation of the meaning of the touch (Monroe, 2009; Routasalo, 1999).

Like verbal communication, the true meaning of a touch may be misinterpreted by either a client or health care provider. Touch that is intended to be comforting may be perceived as controlling or as a sexual advance (Schacher, Stalker, & Teram, 1999). Therefore, it is important to inform clients about what you are going to do and the reason for it. Touch should be firm enough to let the client feel safe and secure but should not be so firm as to cause unnecessary discomfort. We constantly need to assess how clients are responding to our touch. Do they withdraw? Do they appear physically or emotionally uncomfortable? If so, clarify the response with them. Keep the lines of communication open.

## Spatial Distances/Proxemics

Spatial distances also convey nonverbal information. Sitting down to speak with someone seated in a wheelchair puts you at the same level as the client and conveys equality and respect. Standing over clients and talking down to them may convey a message of superiority. Standing in a doorway to talk to clients may imply that you are too busy to interact with them or do not really care what they have to say. Moving closer to clients sends a positive message that, as a health care provider, you are interested.

The concept of *proxemics* represents another aspect of spatial distances. Proxemics identifies the distances we maintain while communicating with others. As discussed in Chapter 3, these distances may vary depending on culture. However, according to Davis (2009), proxemics generally involves four different zones of space: intimate, personal, social, and public. Interactions within different spaces may evoke different meanings for clients, varying from feelings of comfort to those of discomfort, depending on the individual's previous experiences and the relationships with health care providers. When providing health care interventions, we frequently enter intimate or personal zones, and this should be done with great sensitivity. For example, one could say, "May I please hold your arm so that I can obtain your blood pressure?"

### Distracting Behaviors

Constantly checking your watch, answering telephone calls, responding to pagers, or talking with others while you are with clients conveys a message that you are really too busy to be with them, have other things to do, or are disinterested. Clients may become uncomfortable and feel unimportant. They may fail to relay valuable information because they do not want to "hold you up" or think you do not care. Although there are times when clinicians need to respond to outside distractions, these need to be prioritized and limited.

It is important to remember that clients and families do not always share the perspective or priorities of health care providers (Woltersdorf, 1998). Whereas the latter are usually goal centered, clients and family members tend to be emotionally centered. Through listening, observing, and avoiding distracting behaviors before speaking, providers can learn about clients' emotional needs and discover how best to help them.

## WRITTEN COMMUNICATION

Written communication is extremely important in the health care setting. For example, letters are written to doctors to describe client progress, to third-party payers to justify treatments and request equipment, and to other health care professionals who are collaborating in client care. In addition, information is recorded in the medical record, and written instructions are given to clients to assist them in following recommended suggestions and home care programs.

One advantage of written over verbal communication is that printed material is more permanent (Vanderhoff, 2005). Providers can refer to notes to review client progress. Clients can refer to the written word to remind them, for example, about what medications to take and when. They can review the information at their own pace, as often as necessary. However, when preparing written information, the target readers must be kept in mind. Many studies have identified incongruities in the reading levels of written health care materials and the literacy skills of the intended audience (McCray, 2005). Write to your audience; use appropriate, culturally sensitive terminology; and ensure that the information is accurate, clear, concise, understandable, and legible.

### Electronic Communication

The media is a significant shaper of values and attitudes. It is becoming increasingly more common for health care professionals and clients to provide and/or access information via television and radio broadcasts and Internet websites rather than through print media such as newspapers, magazines, and bulletins. Electronic communication is transforming the way health care professionals and clients gather information and interact with one another. Clinical decision-making software and online sources of medical information that clients explore are two examples. Rapid Internet access and inexpensive web cameras have made videoconferencing possible, and that same technology allows professionals to assess situations, such as the status of a wound, without additional clinic visits (Jadad & Delamothe, 2004).

An important consideration for using electronic forms of communication is that transmissions can be intercepted by unintended audiences, thereby making confidentiality a paramount concern. In addition, clients may obtain information from websites that present inaccurate data.

You can provide an important professional service by instructing clients about the best ways to assess the quality and reliability of medically related websites.

Many clients and practitioners now prefer to communicate by electronic mail (e-mail), a trend that is becoming more prevalent because it allows individuals to ask or answer questions any time of the day or night (Kummervold, Trondsen, Andreassen, Gammon, & Hjortdahl, 2004). Because there is no opportunity to read nonverbal cues through e-mail, it is important to ensure that messages are as clear as possible. Utilize professional communication skills with formal salutations and closings, appropriate terminology, correct punctuation, and dictionary spelling for all words. Read your message prior to sending, and correct any errors or potential sources of misinterpretation. Remember that e-mail communications become an official part of clients' medical records as well as an important indication of your professionalism and clinical abilities.

Electronic communication can be a detriment or boon for people with disabilities and those who are aging. Not everyone is computer literate or has access. Helping clients to gain access to electronic aids such as print magnifiers, talking computers, and other forms of assistive technology can provide flexibility and improve access to information that can be used to improve health and wellness.

## USING HUMOR TO COMMUNICATE

Many strategies are used to assist in developing relationships with clients. When used appropriately, humor can be one of them. It may open the lines of communication, decrease stress, and establish a sense of camaraderie. Humor has been shown to be an effective coping strategy for clients and their family members, as well as health care providers. In addition, it has been shown to increase job productivity (Wanzer, Booth-Butterfield, & Booth-Butterfield, 2005) and decrease the number of malpractice claims filed (Levinson, Roter, Mullooly, Dull, & Frankel, 1997). Effective use of humor has also been shown to lead to more positive perceived or actual outcomes (Cann, Zapata, & Davis, 2009). Although humor does not *solve* problems, it can diminish their impact.

Laughter involves every major system in the body. When you laugh, you enjoy yourself, blissfully unaware of the release of catecholamine, which will boost your alertness and enhance your ability to solve problems. You probably are not focusing on how your dilated blood vessels, increased heart rate, and circulation are spreading a high-density lipoprotein throughout your body, which may lower your risk of heart disease. Your lungs expand, bringing in more oxygen and expelling more carbon dioxide than you did before you laughed. Your muscular tension is released, as you exercise your diaphragm, facial, upper extremity, thoracic, and abdominal muscles, and stress hormones are lowered (Hassed, 2001).

Schmitt's (1990) research indicated that most clients welcome laughter. The majority of clients in her survey strongly agreed with its benefits, stating, "Laughing helps me get through difficult times," "Sometimes, laughing works as well as a pain pill," "When I laugh, I feel better," "I appreciate an opportunity to laugh when I feel sad," and "Rehabilitation hospitals should encourage laughter to help clients feel better about their stay" (p. 145). Clients perceive that nurses who laugh with them are being therapeutic.

When used inappropriately, however, humor may interfere with communication or offend others (Cann et al., 2009). At its extreme, it may even cause psychological harm. Struggling to maintain his sitting balance, a 25-year-old man with a traumatic brain injury wildly threw a ball, which landed far from the desired target. The recreation therapist responded, "Well, we won't be picking *you* to pitch on the center's team." Although she was trying to lighten his mood, the client, a former semiprofessional baseball player, took this message to heart and became quite depressed. He refused to "try again," thus setting back his progress.

Inappropriate humor may antagonize and alienate people. Once this has occurred, it can be difficult or impossible to reestablish a therapeutic relationship. Make sure you know and understand your client prior to injecting humor into your conversation. If a client appears offended by something you said, apologize, assure the client that you meant no disrespect, and be sure to avoid such topics in the future. Attempt to reestablish a sense of rapport and mutual respect with the client. If, over time, you believe that is impossible, the client may benefit by having his or her care transferred to someone else.

Think about the potential impact of humor. Try to put yourself in the position of the client, friend, or family member. Does the humor have the same effect on you as it did before? Clients are in a vulnerable position when they come to you. Although humor can be an excellent communication tool when used in a therapeutic manner, it can also have undesirable effects. You may be unaware of where sensitive areas lie. Avoid jokes related to gender, politics, religion, culture, or sexual orientation. When integrating humor into health care interactions, it is wise to proceed with caution.

## BARRIERS TO EFFECTIVE COMMUNICATION

### Role Uncertainty

Communication can be negatively affected by a number of factors, including role uncertainty. Clients may not know what we expect of them and not know what to expect from us. For example, older clients may expect health professionals to be somewhat paternalistic and willingly hand over the responsibility for their health and well-being to their health care providers. More commonly, clients and health professionals expect to work collaboratively in treatment planning. This may be uncomfortable for older clients, who want to be told what to do and may be reluctant to ask questions. They may appear passive to a younger generation of clinicians. It is important to encourage them to assume a more active role in their health care.

In an inpatient setting, clients often have contact with many different professionals during the course of a day. Team members may have different expectations for them, providing them with conflicting information, further contributing to their role uncertainty. Another complicating factor is that everyone is in a hurry, which may confuse clients, who may hesitate to ask questions or discuss physical or psychosocial concerns because they do not want to bother their providers (Northouse & Northouse, 1998).

### Sensory Overload

Sensory overload may adversely affect both receptive and expressive communication (Purtilo & Haddad, 2007). Are directions understandable, amidst a frightening environment of intravenous poles and buzzing machines? Institutional smells, distracting visual stimuli, and unfamiliar touch can bombard clients' senses. As a result, they may become unable to organize their thoughts to effectively communicate and may leave a health care provider's office not really understanding what the provider said or knowing what they are expected to do next. People process information at varying rates. Instructions to a client may seem abundantly clear to us, but they may not be easy for others to fathom. Providers can help diminish sensory overload by meeting clients one on one in a quiet room and eliminating distractions.

## Voice and Word Choice

It is important to give clear, simple instructions using a tone and volume that are easy to hear and comprehend. Whenever possible, provide clients with written instructions, including pictures, if this enhances understanding. Providers may ask the client to repeat directions or demonstrate a task. If the instructions are for home use, ask, "Can you picture yourself doing this on your own at home?" If the client says no, ask why not. This creates an opportunity to promote understanding and allow clients to voice questions or concerns in a safe environment. Whenever possible, give clients a period of time to think about the instructions. Review them at the next session and ask for a demonstration to determine whether the client truly understands or has any questions.

## Physical Appearance

Consider the saying "First impressions are lasting." People often judge others based on their appearance, which may include height, weight, hairstyle, clothing, skin color, piercings, tattoos, accessories, and physical attractiveness. As discussed in Chapter 2, we tend to gravitate to individuals who are similar to ourselves and may have overt or covert biases against those who differ from us. Providers need to recognize that seeing the client as being "similar to" or "different from" themselves may affect their emotional and cognitive responses to a situation (Garden, 2008). Health care professionals need to be aware of their own biases and refrain from making judgments about clients based on physical appearances. Conversely, providers should realize that their first impression of clients may affect relationships. Uniforms, stethoscopes, and other tools of the trade convey messages. Although a professional appearance may help inspire trust and confidence in clients and allay a measure of anxiety, it may create a barrier for others.

　Sometimes health providers misinterpret the functional impact of apparent physical limitations. One study examined people who were blind or visually impaired to determine barriers to effective health care (O'Day, Killeen, & Iezzoni, 2004). The two barriers the researchers identified were (1) the assumption made by health providers that clients who are blind or visually impaired would not be able to fully participate in their own care, and (2) the failure of providers to have written materials available in alternative formats, including Braille, large print, or audiotape. Failure to accommodate different abilities in health care, such as providing wheelchair-accessible examination rooms and alternative forms of communication, demonstrates a bias toward "ableism," which can cause people with disabilities to feel unwelcome. Conversely, developing universally accessible services demonstrates respect for differences and facilitates access and participation for all clients.

## Gender Differences

Differences in communication styles between men and women can lead to misinterpretation of messages (James & Cinelli, 2003). In general, women like to talk to others when they have a problem or need to make a decision, whereas men like to keep their problems to themselves. Women tend to be relationship oriented and want to connect with others more so than men do. To men, status and dominance are often more important than relationship building. Women tend to ask questions to build rapport, whereas men like to tell others what to do and provide information rather than asking questions. When women are involved in disagreements, there is great potential for disruption of the relationship that exists between the opposing parties. When men disagree, they tend to express their disagreement, move on to other topics, and forget about it. Disagreements rarely impact other aspects of their relationships. As listeners, women tend to nod their heads to indicate they are listening, whereas men only nod their heads when they agree with the speaker (Lieberman, 2010).

Loscalzo (1999) studied the communication styles of men and women who were being treated for cancer. He found that women tend to be better communicators than men, who tend to compartmentalize their lives. During times of stress, women want to talk about what is happening, while men would rather not. What seems to help men is to have a plan for solving problems and getting on with life. Whereas most women enjoy communicating about problems and joining support groups, men want health care providers to help them identify problems and come up with solutions. Loscalzo also found that women generally cope with a cancer diagnosis better than men, both as clients and as caregivers. Men are frequently unwilling to join support groups, and when they do, they use the group for educational purposes only. Conversely, women use support groups to share experiences and encourage one another.

Although certain characteristics of communication are attributable to men and others to women, it is important to realize that most people are able to adapt communication styles to fit specific needs. Very few people use one style all of the time. This concept is demonstrated in health care through the practice of *safety culture*. Safety culture refers to a set of professional behaviors designed to deliberately avoid the influence of status, gender, and other social or cultural norms in favor of "best practices" for communication in health care (Carney, West, Neily, Mills, & Bagian, 2010).

Students and health care professionals will most likely find differences in communication styles between men and women, as well as between those of different professions. Recognizing your own communication style and adapting it to meet the existing circumstances are of utmost importance to ensure positive client outcomes. Whereas women may be more comfortable making decisions via consensus, and men may be more comfortable giving orders, each may need to move out of his or her comfort zone and communicate using a less familiar style to ensure effective communication. Table 5–2 provides an overview of male versus female communication styles.

## Cultural Barriers

As stated earlier, individuals are usually more comfortable with people from a similar culture. They may even inadvertently be biased and treat people from other cultures differently. In fact, a review of the literature on cultural differences in medical communication revealed that during

| Table 5–2    Gender Differences in Communication | |
| --- | --- |
| **Male Communication Style** | **Female Communication Style** |
| Give information/report | Collect information/gain rapport |
| Talk about things (sports, business) | Talk about people |
| Focus on facts, reason, and logic | Focus on feelings, senses, and meaning |
| Thrive on competition | Thrive on harmony and relating |
| "Know" by analyzing and figuring things out | "Know" by intuition |
| Assertive | Cooperative |
| Seek intellectual understanding | Empathize |
| Focused, specific, and logical | Holistic—"wise angled" |
| Comfortable with rules, order, structure | Comfortable with fluidity |
| Want to think | Want to feel |

*Source:* Simon & Pedersen (2005).

doctor/patient encounters, White doctors behaved less effectively when interacting with patients from minority groups than with those who were White, and patients from minority groups were less expressive or assertive during the medical encounter than their White counterparts (Schouten & Meeuwesen, 2006).

In today's multicultural environment, language barriers affect one's ability to communicate effectively. If a client speaks a different language, it is important to provide a professional interpreter to assist with the communication process. Family members are usually not the most appropriate resource. Clients do not always want to discuss their concerns in front of family. In certain cultures, for example, men prefer not to reveal their problems to their wives or children. In addition, well-intentioned family members may edit or misinterpret messages being translated (Misra-Hebert, 2003).

Beyond language, other cultural influences affect communication, including differences in values, beliefs, emotions, and nonverbal cues. People from some cultures are encouraged to cry when they feel pain; individuals from other cultures are discouraged from doing so and may, in fact, hide their pain. This could certainly affect treatment interventions. In cross-cultural encounters, providers need to understand the client's interpretation of authority figures, the use of physical contact, communication style, and the role of gender, sexuality, and the family in decision making. Failure to appropriately interpret this information can adversely affect health outcomes (Misra-Hebert, 2003).

Ideally, administrators should recruit and hire health professionals who share languages and cultures with the people who live in the communities being served. However, this may not be feasible due to lower representation of minority cultures in health care professions. Therefore, health providers are advised to learn as much as possible about the cultures and languages of the communities they serve. In all settings, the use of clear, culturally appropriate written instructions, complete with pictures or videotapes/DVDs and available in various languages, greatly enhances communication between clients and providers (Thompson et al., 2007).

Improving the cultural competence of health care providers is one way of responding to the demographic changes in the United States and decreasing health disparities (Teal & Street, 2009). Research has shown that culturally competent communication skills can be taught and, when implemented in the clinical setting, improve patient care (Misra-Hebert, 2003). It has also been suggested that courses on communication skills training, which include role-playing and facilitation by experienced trainers, should be required in all health professional education programs (Stiefel et al., 2010).

## CONFLICT

Health care providers interact daily with clients, families, colleagues, insurance providers, and others. Everyone brings his or her background, culture, beliefs, and goals into the workplace, and viewpoints vary. Even when people share similar goals, they may have different perspectives and priorities regarding those goals. Conflict becomes inevitable (Xu & Davidhizar, 2004). Although some people seem to thrive on conflict, many are uncomfortable with it and either try to avoid it or handle it poorly. To manage conflict effectively, we need to change our own behavior or alter the situation.

Despite the negative connotations of conflict, it has both positive and negative elements. Managed appropriately, conflict can lead to positive changes, such as decreased stress levels, improved staff cohesiveness, job satisfaction, and creative problem solving. Ignored, avoided, or poorly managed conflict negatively affects all people involved. It can permeate an organization, group, or relationship, decreasing everyone's ability to work effectively (Lipcamon & Mainwaring, 2004). Sometimes, coworkers are able to adequately resolve their issues independently. At other times, the assistance of managers, supervisors, or neutral third parties is required.

Conflict involves tension or disagreement between two or more opposing forces. It is a process in which one party perceives that its interests are being opposed or negatively affected by another. Once that occurs, people need to decide how to deal with the situation, even if their choice is to do nothing. If they respond emotionally, actions will lead to reactions and conflict is under way.

In the health care system, individuals work both independently and interdependently. Opinions about the most appropriate form of care may differ. In one study of clinical decision making in intensive care units, physicians and nurses identified conflict during patient management discussions (Coombs, 2003). In another study with more than 200 patients in intensive care, doctors and nurses documented 248 conflicts concerning vital matters of patient care, as well as disputes between teams and families, among team members, and among family members (Studdert et al., 2003). Time constraints and limited resources influence decision making. As health professionals work together to provide client-centered care, roles may overlap and lines of authority for ultimate decision making may blur. Conflict is often a by-product. Consider the conflict described in this case:

> My supervisor reprimanded me this morning in front of a client and his daughter. I was so embarrassed! I became so nervous that my hands were shaking as I tried to continue with the treatment. I knew Mr. Chen had lost all confidence in my abilities. He looked as if he feared I was going to hurt him. His daughter asked me if I was sure I knew what I was doing. Finally, my supervisor suggested I leave and finish up some paperwork while he completed the treatment. I left the room and ran to the ladies' room in tears to compose myself. Later in the day, my supervisor acted as if nothing had happened. We continued to treat other patients. I was anxious and afraid I would make another mistake, but I didn't say anything to him.
>
> Tonight, I talked with my roommate. She told me that I should meet with my supervisor first thing in the morning and discuss the situation. I know she's right. I can accept constructive criticism, but I think he handled it inappropriately. He could have directed me to correct my error and then talked to me later in the staff room, away from the client and his daughter. The client's safety wasn't at risk. As much as I hate confrontation and would like to pretend this never happened, I know my roommate is right. If I don't say something, I'll always be afraid that he'll do this to me again, and my ability to learn will be in jeopardy. He probably doesn't even know how he made me feel.
>
> —*From the journal of Shannon Sullivan, nursing student*

Although Shannon would have preferred to ignore this situation, she realized that strategy would not solve her problem and could negatively affect her educational experience and her ability to treat clients effectively. If she is able to discuss her feelings and situation with her supervisor, she may be able to develop a better working relationship with him. Together, they could develop learning objectives and discuss appropriate feedback mechanisms. Shannon might be more at ease treating clients in the presence of her supervisor, and she could learn how to improve her nursing skills from him.

## Levels of Conflict

Conflict can occur at personal, interpersonal, intragroup, or intergroup levels, as discussed in the following sections.

**PERSONAL CONFLICT**   At the personal level, conflict occurs within an individual (Dove, 1998). He or she may receive pressure from colleagues to do something that is not in accordance with his or her personal value system. For example, a supervisor may suggest that an occupational therapist delegate portions of a client's treatment to an occupational therapy assistant in order to increase productivity. The occupational therapist may believe that the client requires the attention and skills of a therapist and that it is inappropriate to delegate this part of the care. As a result, the occupational therapist may feel internal personal conflict and have to decide whether to adhere to the supervisor's suggestion or confront the supervisor to discuss the situation. The ultimate decision will be influenced by how strongly the occupational therapist feels about the level of care needed, the experience of both the occupational therapist and the assistant, and the conflict-management style the occupational therapist uses in this situation.

An individual may also experience interrole conflicts at a personal level. Consider Tim Gallagher, a nurse in the intensive care unit in a large urban hospital. Toward the end of his shift, Tim hurries to complete paperwork, ignoring the patients' call buttons buzzing around him. Other nurses leave their documentation to respond to the patients' needs. While Tim always leaves on time, the other nurses work overtime to complete their duties. Although they do not confront Tim, they vent their anger among themselves. When one of the nurses finally tells him how much the others resent his behavior, he informs her that he is a single parent, caring for two preschool-age children. If he does not pick the children up at the day care center at the appointed time, he is charged a penalty for each minute he is late. He cannot afford to be late. Torn between his parental role of needing to get his children on time and his professional role of being a team player and attending to client care and documentation, Tim may be experiencing personal conflict of an interrole nature. This conflict is causing internal stress for him and creating an interpersonal conflict between Tim and the other nurses.

**INTERPERSONAL CONFLICT**   Conflict develops at the interpersonal level when two or more individuals exhibit conflicting values or beliefs (Dove, 1998). For example, interpersonal conflicts frequently occur between nursing home staff members and residents' family members (Nelson & Cox, 2003; Pillemer, Hegeman, Albright, & Henderson, 1998). Nursing homes are structured organizations with rules and regulations. Sometimes they appear to provide impersonal client care. Family members, however, may provide more personal, albeit infrequent, care. Discrepancies about what is best for the client may arise. While staff members focus on the technical aspects of care, families may perceive that the emotional components are lacking and that their experiences are undervalued. Similarly, staff members might feel unappreciated by families. Because many nursing home residents, especially those with cognitive impairments, are unable to provide accurate information about their experiences, well-intentioned families may misinterpret what they see. Interpersonal conflict may ensue. If time restrictions further limit communication between staff and families, minor interpersonal conflicts can escalate into larger problems (Pillemer et al., 1998).

**INTRAGROUP CONFLICT**   Intragroup conflict exists when members within a group disagree with each other as to what course of action should be taken (Dove, 1998). Consider the Minelli family. For more than 10 years, Mr. Minelli has been caring for his wife at home. As her Alzheimer's disease has progressed, she has started to wander and is becoming combative. Mr. Minelli is seeking advice from his children. Of the six adult children in the family, three of them work in health care. Only the youngest daughter lives nearby.

The local daughter is the mother of five young children and has a husband who frequently travels for business. Experiencing interrole conflict between her roles as a mother, wife, and daughter, she cares for her nuclear family, while cleaning her parents' house and doing their laundry and shopping. Exhausted and frustrated, she suggested to her father that he consider placing her mother in a nursing home. The oldest son, who is a pediatrician, disagrees and has offered to pay for daytime respite care. The oldest daughter, who is a nurse, agrees with her younger sister. She believes her mother would receive excellent care in a long-term facility and that her father would be relieved of the burden. The youngest son, who is a pharmacist, thinks that everyone should "chip in" to build an apartment for the parents at his sister's house, making it easier for her to assist them. His sister's husband does not support this idea.

This family is experiencing intragroup conflict, and it is tearing them apart. Mr. Minelli wants to do whatever is best for his wife, but he does not know what that is. He loves his children and does not want to hurt their feelings, yet he is unable to make a decision. Siblings have heated arguments over the telephone and by e-mail correspondence. Alliances and counteralliances have developed. If the conflict remains unresolved, the family may be further torn apart. The Minelli family may need a neutral party, such as a social worker, to mediate the situation.

**INTERGROUP CONFLICT**    Intergroup conflict arises between two or more groups of people, departments, or organizations that have conflicting beliefs or needs (Dove, 1998). Consider Carmen Garcia, a 94-year-old woman recovering from a motor vehicle accident in which she sustained multiple fractures and internal injuries. She was in both the intensive care and medical/surgical units for several weeks and is now ready to be discharged from the acute care hospital. The health care team recommended that she go to a transitional care unit, where she will receive nursing care and therapy to increase her strength and endurance. In contrast, Mrs. Garcia and her family want her to go home. Her children and grandchildren believe that their cultural values oblige them to care for her at home, out of respect for her position in the family and their love.

Members of the health care team are quite concerned about the family's ability to care for Mrs. Garcia at home because she is weak and cannot bear weight on her casted right leg. She also has a fracture of her left humerus. Hospital staff members fear that either she will be further injured at home or that a family member will get hurt trying to help her.

The meeting between the two groups was confrontational. Even though a social worker attempted to mediate the situation, members of both groups refused to change their positions. Christmas was fast approaching, and both Mrs. Garcia and her family believed that this would be her last one at home. They wanted to spend it together in a family environment, not in the cafeteria of a health facility. The family ultimately brought Mrs. Garcia home, discharged against medical advice.

## Sources of Conflict

Conflicts include content, psychological, and procedural components (Moore, 1996). *Content issues* are related to specific factors, such as time and money. In the managed health care environment, a primary care physician may be in conflict with an insurance provider over how long a client may be able to stay in an acute care hospital following surgery. A physical therapist and a parent may be in conflict over the appropriate care of a child.

I visited my client and her family today. It was time to discuss the possibility of ordering a wheelchair for Brenda. Her mother became extremely insistent that Brenda's stroller was just fine for getting her around and that the use of a wheelchair would make her appear much more disabled. By using a trial wheelchair and some accessories I had available, I was able to demonstrate to Brenda's mother that Brenda could be significantly more functional and less disabled if her posture was improved. To my surprise, the demonstration proved convincing!

*—From the journal of Ron Johansen, physical therapist student*

By reframing the above situation, Ron was able to suggest an alternate perspective. The wheelchair became a symbol of independence rather than disability.

*Psychological elements* of conflict are multidimensional and include trust, respect, and the desire for inclusion (Moore, 1996). Involving clients, families, and appropriate care providers in decision making, introducing change slowly, and encouraging feedback can help reduce conflict (Davidhizar, Giger, & Poole, 1997). Using active listening techniques can also improve communication and diminish conflict. Listening to concerns and ideas attentively, eliminating unnecessary interruptions, and ensuring confidentiality will help cultivate a sense of trust. Providing adequate information and showing respect for everyone increases the probability that all involved will be able to manage conflict without the need for outside interventions (Purtilo & Haddad, 2007).

*Procedural components* of conflict involve policies, the chain of command, and decision-making responsibility. When policies are unclear, individuals may interpret them differently, resulting in conflicting views as to the appropriate course of action. Because content, psychological, and procedural components are interrelated, a conflict cannot be completely resolved until all three elements in this "satisfaction triangle" have been addressed (Moore, 1996).

Conflict can emanate from many sources. As discussed earlier, differing personal beliefs, goals, interests, and values may lead to conflict. Possible incompatibilities, based on temperaments, race, religion, culture, or other biases, may also result in conflict. Members of different cultures view conflict in different ways, a factor that must be taken into consideration when dealing with both clients and colleagues (Nibler & Harris, 2003; Xu & Davidhizar, 2004).

There is much ambiguity in health care. Individuals interpret available information in different ways, depending on their backgrounds and life experiences. Clients may be uncertain about options and potential outcomes. Decisions are complex, because many individuals are involved at different levels, which can result in competition for power, prestige, and status.

Lack of communication and unclear expectations are also sources of conflict. For example, in health care settings, clients may receive conflicting information from different staff members. Consider Nancy, a new mother who is having difficulty breast-feeding. Nurses on each of three successive shifts have offered her different and conflicting strategies. She is frustrated, confused, and anxious.

E-mail communication may also be a source of conflict. E-mail interactions lack both the verbal and nonverbal cues of face-to-face communication, leaving room for misinterpretation. In addition, people may be tempted to respond instantaneously to e-mail messages, rather than taking the time to consider what they are going to say. To prevent unnecessary conflict, it is important to follow-up on e-mail messages with telephone calls and face-to-face meetings to clarify questions or concerns (Umiker, 1997; Zweibel & Goldstein, 2001).

Life circumstances may also create conflict (Northouse & Northouse, 1998). For example, in contemporary society, family members often live long distances from each other, creating a geographic barrier when adult children attempt to assist parents with medical problems. Older adults sometimes fail to ask pertinent questions of their health care providers and, therefore, clients may not receive the services they need. Consider Ramona, a medical assistant working in southern California. Her elderly parents were both ill and living on the east coast. Ramona's mother had heart problems and required dialysis treatments twice a week. Her father had difficulty walking after having bilateral total hip replacements. In addition, he had a long history of smoking and emphysema.

Ramona became very frustrated when her attempts to contact her parents' primary care physician by e-mail were unsuccessful. She believed that the physician was not doing everything he could to help her parents. She made arrangements to fly home to accompany them to their next appointment. After Ramona described how much difficulty her parents were having, the physician immediately recommended a homemaker to assist with routine housekeeping and a company to provide meals. The doctor apologized profusely, stating that he was unaware of the difficulties Ramona's parents were having at home. In the end, enhanced communication made it possible for appropriate resources to be put into place.

Lack of advance directives from a legally incompetent client may be another source of conflict. Questions may exist about what is the "right" or "best" thing to do. Health care providers and clients' medical care surrogates do not always agree about the most appropriate care for a client who is unable to express his or her own wishes. Alpers and Lo (1999) describe a client who no longer had decision-making capabilities and had not left a clear advance directive. The family claimed that the client believed in the sanctity of life. Despite no hope for recovery, family members wanted the health care providers to prolong his life as long as possible. The health care professionals thought that the client was enduring unnecessary pain and suffering while life support systems kept him alive. Although his wife agreed with the health care team in principle, she would not go against the wishes of her children. This case illustrates the stress that family surrogates may experience and the need to provide them with the support and information required to help them make wise decisions.

## Strategies to Manage Conflict

Four elements affect the outcome of conflict: the issues at hand, cooperation among involved parties, the power bases of the participants, and the effectiveness of their communication skills (Miller, 1998). When conflict concerns relatively minor issues, cooperation and resolution may be fast and easy. At other times, conflict is related to substantive issues, where individuals or groups interpret facts differently, have opposing goals, or disagree on acceptable methods. When conflicting parties disagree on principles, cooperation may be nonexistent and resolution more difficult to achieve.

Although many health care professionals consider clinical skills as being most important for competent practice, they sometimes fail to recognize that communication and the ability to manage conflict successfully are of primary importance in ensuring effective health care outcomes (Pettrey, 2003). This is especially true in today's health care environment where there is an emphasis on interdisciplinary care. There is a tendency for individuals to "band together" in the "us" against "them" mentality described in Chapter 2. This can result in intragroup and intergroup conflict. Teams that work together to openly discuss differences and solve problems are much more effective than those that set up competitive goals (Alper, Tjosvold, & Law, 1998).

The ability to communicate effectively greatly assists people and groups in resolving conflicts. It is imperative to focus on the pertinent issues and avoid blaming and name-calling. When participants lose focus, the number of issues involved tends to expand, and the emphasis shifts toward winning rather than compromising. People begin to attack each other rather than the issues. Power tactics, including coercion and deception, are often employed.

Unfortunately, in today's society, violent behavior is becoming more prevalent. This may occur in the inpatient, outpatient, or home care settings and may involve coworkers, clients, or clients' family members. Organizations need to update staff members so they have the necessary skills to manage violent conflict in the workplace while continuing to deliver quality patient care. Educational programs are also needed to help providers recognize the warning signs of violence and understand the appropriate use of de-escalation and other interpersonal skills to contain and manage such situations (Young & Turner, 2009).

Thomas and Kilmann (1974) identified five styles of managing conflict—*avoidance, accommodation, competition, compromise,* and *collaboration*—that continue to be studied today (Lipcamon & Mainwaring, 2004). Most authors agree that no one single strategy is best. Rather, each situation needs to be evaluated to determine which strategy would be the most effective (Eason & Brown, 1999; Henrikson, 1998; Northouse & Northouse, 1998; Umiker, 1997). Although we have the ability to utilize each of the strategies in a given situation, each of us has our own preferred style of managing conflict. Understanding the strengths and weaknesses of each strategy and learning to identify our own as well as our colleagues' and clients' preferred styles will help us become better communicators and more effective health care providers. The following section describes the strengths and liabilities of each of these styles of managing conflict.

**AVOIDANCE**    Avoidance is an unassertive and uncooperative conflict management strategy in which individuals simply ignore or evade the fact that a conflict exists (Eason & Brown, 1999; Northouse & Northouse, 1998; Umiker, 1997). People who are passive and uncomfortable addressing conflict frequently use this style. Avoidance can be counterproductive, often prolonging, rather than resolving, issues and increasing stress levels. Consider a staff therapist who works in a large medical center. As clients are referred to the department, their names are posted on the bulletin board, and therapists select them. Most of the staff members add clients to their caseloads as the names become available, but one therapist purposely avoids "difficult" clients, leaving colleagues to care for those who have more complicated needs. Other staff members recognize this but do not address the situation with him. As a result, nothing changes—the problem continues, the rest of the staff remains frustrated, and staff morale decreases.

There are times when avoidance is a positive and necessary strategy. If individuals are angry, avoidance allows for a cooling-off period. It provides people with time to gain composure and gather additional information prior to addressing the issues. If a problem is perceived to be trivial, people may prefer to ignore it rather than deal with it. In addition, some problems resolve themselves over time. In those cases, it may not be worth the time and energy needed to confront them. When a problem is out of a provider's control, he or she may want to avoid becoming involved. In health care, minor conflicts might need to be set aside to ensure effective client care.

**ACCOMMODATION**    Accommodation is an unassertive but cooperative approach to conflict management. A person neglects his or her own needs to meet the needs of others. Those who seek constant approval frequently use this strategy (Eason & Brown, 1999; Henrikson, 1998; Northouse & Northouse, 1998; Umiker, 1997). Although this approach may appear to promote harmony and solve conflicts quickly, it may also be superficial and temporary. People who constantly accommodate may feel angry and frustrated because they failed to seize the opportunity to express their own thoughts, opinions, and feelings. For example, Shelley, a respiratory therapist, initially volunteered to work on major holidays so that her colleagues, whose extended families live out of state, could have the time off. What began as "team player behavior" became expected by the staff. Now, harboring feelings of frustration, she would like to have a holiday off but continues to accommodate colleagues' expectations. A better resolution may have emerged if Shelley had expressed her feelings, and the group had taken the time to consider alternative solutions.

Accommodation is an appropriate strategy to use when one realizes that the other party is right or when there is little chance of "winning." It can also be used when one party has little interest in the situation or when the outcome does not particularly affect him or her. In health care settings, accommodation may sometimes be useful to promote harmony and maintain good interpersonal relationships among staff members or interdisciplinary teams.

**COMPETITION**    Competition is an aggressive, uncompromising approach to managing conflict. It is power driven and frequently used by assertive individuals interested in pursuing their own goals, even at the expense of others (Eason & Brown, 1999; Henrikson, 1998; Northouse & Northouse, 1998; Umiker, 1997). Think of a situation in which a student proposes an alternative evidence-based treatment approach rather than one an experienced practitioner has been using for many years. The supervisor refuses to consider the students' proposal or listen to the rationale, insisting that it be done her way. This style may result in quick, short-term agreements. However, the results are based upon an "I win, you lose" strategy, which may be counterproductive over time and negatively affect client outcomes.

**COMPROMISE**    Compromise is a strategy midway between competition and accommodation. It includes an element of assertiveness, as well as a component of cooperation (Eason & Brown, 1999; Henrikson, 1998; Northouse & Northouse, 1998; Umiker, 1997). People who compromise use a "give-and-take" strategy. They are concerned with their own needs, as well as the needs and concerns of others, and realize that neither side can win completely. Although both parties may agree to the final outcome, neither side is perfectly satisfied with the results. Whereas this method may result in faster resolution of problems, more innovative and satisfying results may be achieved if the parties continue to negotiate.

Compromise can be an effective means of settling conflict. Consider Melissa, a 15-year-old girl with juvenile rheumatoid arthritis. Her medication made her drowsy and impaired her ability to think clearly, affecting her schoolwork. Her physician compromised and prescribed another medication that was not as effective but had fewer side effects.

**COLLABORATION**    Collaboration involves both assertiveness and cooperation. It is a problem-solving approach in which all parties want to fully address the concerns of everyone. It is designed to promote a "win–win" solution, with everyone committed to the final outcome. Participants believe that the achievement of mutual goals is more important than individual objectives (Eason & Brown, 1999; Henrikson, 1998; Northouse & Northouse, 1998; Umiker, 1997). Imagine a situation in which a manager enlists input from the entire staff to address how they might change the hours and staffing patterns of their operation. Although most authors agree that this is the preferred approach to managing conflict, it is the most difficult and often the most time consuming to achieve and, therefore, may not be appropriate in all situations.

People need to explore differences, identify commonalities, and work together to develop problem-solving strategies and initiate solutions acceptable to all involved. This requires everyone's dedication and hard work. As a result of the time and energy expended, innovative, cost-effective solutions usually result. Because both sides "win," everyone tends to feel satisfied. This helps build stronger relationships, promote trust, improve morale, decrease stress, and set the stage for more positive conflict resolution in the future.

It is important to note that the five styles of managing conflict just discussed may be used to varying degrees or in combination with one another, depending on the circumstances in each situation. A good communicator expresses his or her own viewpoints, listens carefully to the opinions of others, and works collaboratively to develop cooperative problem-solving strategies that lead to solutions acceptable to all parties (Miller, 1998; Umiker, 1997).

**MEDIATION**   Sometimes, individuals or groups may be unable to resolve conflict, and it escalates. Members of each side may try to convert otherwise neutral parties to their points of view. Stress levels increase while productivity decreases. At such junctures, mediation may be required (Fraser, 2001). A neutral third party is invited to facilitate the process. The mediator begins by developing a rapport with the parties in conflict. Once the conflict has been defined, alternative solutions are generated, with each possible solution considered until an agreement can be reached (Fraser, 2001; Rotarius & Liberman, 2000).

To be successful, individuals cannot blame one another. They must carefully listen to and understand all issues in the disagreement. For mediation to be successful, everyone has to agree from the outset to accept and implement the final decision, even if they do not agree with it.

## THE CLIENT INTERVIEW

The first section of this chapter described the components and importance of communication. This section provides information and suggestions for putting communication skills into practice. Client-interview models and the explanatory model of care are described. Skilled health care providers can efficiently and effectively develop a client-centered plan of care when they take the time to utilize effective communication techniques and listen to their client's stories during the interview process.

I don't think that I did a very good job with my client evaluation today. It was the first time I did one on my own, so of course, I was kind of nervous. Before I got started, my supervisor and I went over the chart, the diagnosis, and the kinds of symptoms to look for. Last night, I made a careful list to make sure that I didn't leave anything out.

Somehow, even though I asked all the right questions, I did not feel like things went very well. As I read down the list of questions, she answered briefly, using just a few words each time. She seemed sort of bored and did not offer any extra information. Although there was enough data to get started on the treatment, I didn't feel like I knew much about her or what she would like to get out of our sessions. Worse still, I am not sure how to motivate her to follow through on the home exercises.

—*From the journal of Jackie Marsh, occupational therapy student*

It has been said that there are three T's in TreaTmenT. The first "T" represents the *theory* that provides the scientific and philosophical basis for what we do. The second "T" stands for *technique*, which informs us what to do and how to do it—the so-called "tools of the trade." The final "T" is for *therapeutic* alliance, which allows us to apply our theories and techniques in a collaborative way with our clients to promote effective outcomes.

Developing relationships with clients is the most essential skill that we bring to the treatment setting. It is the foundation on which we build trust, understand each client's needs, and develop individualized treatment plans (Haidet & Paterniti, 2003; Smith & Hoppe, 1991). We begin to forge these alliances as soon as we meet and greet each new client. In this chapter, we discussed the importance of communication skills, and in Chapter 6, we will discuss collaborative treatment planning as a tool to support motivation and adherence. These skills provide the basis for all interactions within the health care setting and are an essential component of the client interview.

"The client interview is at the core of clinical interaction and the clinician's most important and intimate professional activity" (Kern et al., 2005, p. 65). In essence, the clinical interview is where the science of medicine joins the art of client care (Coulehan & Block, 2001; Epstein, 1999). The nature of the ideal interview is dynamic rather than static and it consists of more than just reviewing a checklist of symptoms to trigger information about clients' perceptions of their complaints. A good interviewer establishes a climate of safety in which clients feel they can discuss personal and psychosocial factors that contribute to the impact and meaning of various somatic symptoms. This information is crucial to effective client interventions. In this section, we describe the elements of a good client interview and explain how to perform one successfully.

## Types of Interviews

**THE BIOMEDICAL MODEL INTERVIEW**    The biomedical model of health care is founded on the premise that anatomy, physiology, pathology and other biological forces are responsible for health and illness, function and dysfunction. Therefore, the biomedical client interview was designed to identify disease or dysfunction and to determine an appropriate medical intervention (Donnelly, 1996); or, to phrase it more casually, it was concerned only with the "two Fs"—to find it and fix it (Tongue, Epps, & Forese, 2005).

Using the traditional biomedical model, health professionals have been taught to start the client interview by taking a history. They are instructed to ask open-ended questions that elicit client concerns and complaints. This is followed by the use of close-ended questions to gather specific diagnostic information. The intent is to allow the client to describe what has prompted the need for the visit and to provide increasingly specific information to determine a diagnosis and plan of care. However, this often does not proceed optimally. Studies have shown that, on average, practitioners who utilize this interviewing style interrupt clients after less than 20 seconds! Following this interruption, the provider takes control of the interview, and the client rarely has an opportunity to redirect it toward his or her concerns (Beckwith & Frankel, 1984; Lipkin, Frankel, Beckman, Charon, & Fein,1995). "The biomedical approach to medicine all too often overrides concern about patients' psychological and social experiences of illness" (Garden, 2008, p. 122).

Studies examining the biomedical interview model show that significant diagnostic information is never communicated by the client to the provider (Haidet & Paterniti, 2003; Smith & Hoppe,

1991). In part, this happens because the interviewer assumes that the first problem mentioned by the client is the most important one, and the focus quickly narrows to that issue. However, this is often not the primary problem or even the real reason that caused the client to seek medical attention (Roter & Hall, 1992). When this approach is taken, the care that is provided does not rise to the standard of evidence-based practice. Focusing only on symptoms or problems that the provider identifies as important generates biased and incomplete information, leading to inaccurate diagnoses and plans of care (Lipkin et al., 1995; Smith & Hoppe, 1991).

The biomedical interview is also designed to include social issues, sometimes known as a social history. This is where psychosocial information is usually requested. However, because the collection of information is typically provider driven within this model, questions are directed away from personal factors toward biomedical concerns (Smith & Hoppe, 1991). This lack of attention or acknowledgment of client concerns is prevalent, even in such emotionally laden settings as cancer care (Stacey, Henderson, MacArthur, & Dohan, 2009).

Consider the case of Mr. Mansur, who left an appointment with his orthopedist feeling very confused and upset. He went to the doctor because he was having pain in his knees that made walking difficult. The doctor conducted a very thorough exam, and in the process, determined that Mr. Mansur also had severe carpal tunnel syndrome. She spent the remainder of the visit discussing the importance of having surgical correction of his carpal tunnel syndrome. Because the physician judged the client's carpal tunnel syndrome to be a more serious problem than his knee pain, she lost sight of the reason why Mr. Mansur had sought medical advice and assistance in the first place. The client left the office determined to change health care professionals because this one did not understand his needs.

**THE CLIENT-CENTERED INTERVIEW**    "True patient-centered care places increased emphasis on the therapeutic encounter between the patient and the provider" (Tripicchio, Bykerk, & Wegner, 2009, p. 55). It abolishes the power differential that can exist in the client–provider relationship and creates an equal and collaborative partnership. Each client is viewed as the expert on his or her health and is given the opportunity to be heard and respected (Roter & Hall, 1992). This paradigm necessitates shared decision making, which considers the clients' beliefs and concerns as highly as those of the care provider (Tongue et al., 2005). Thus, there is shared knowledge, control, and decision making. The client-centered interview produces significantly better results as seen by improved outcomes, including trust, adherence, and empowerment, as well as client and provider satisfaction (Garden, 2008; Haidet & Paterniti, 2003; Kleinman, Eisenberg, & Good, 1978; Platt & Platt, 2003; Smith & Hoppe, 1991; Tongue et al., 2005).

A cornerstone of client-centered care is hearing clients' stories and learning what their symptoms and discomforts mean to them (Roter & Hall, 1992). Key questions that need to be answered include these: "Who is this person?" "What does she want from our encounter?" and "How does the client perceive or understand his health?" (Coulehan et al., 2001; Epstein, 1999). A provider who facilitates client storytelling will learn information about the client, as well as the problem that motivated him or her to come to the appointment. This approach enables the provider to obtain a more accurate medical history and provides a solid foundation, allowing the client and provider to develop a more effective relationship (Platt et al., 2001). Client-centered interviewing allows clients to set the direction of the exchange. It is the responsibility of the health provider to follow up on the client's lead by asking clarifying questions and offering reflections and information. A sample of questions providers might ask during the interview is found in Boxes 5–1 and 5–2.

---

**BOX 5–1   Sample Open-Ended Questions**

- Tell me about yourself.
- I'd like to know about you as a person.
- What brings you here today?
- Tell me more about that.
- How are things going for you?
- Is anything bothering you?
- How does that affect you?
- How do you feel about that?
- What do you think is going on?

- What are your concerns?
- What are your expectations?
- What do you think can be changed?
- What are your thoughts about your treatment plan?
- How can I help you?
- Is there anything else bothering you?
- Is there anything else that you would like to tell me?

---

As discussed in Chapter 4, it is important to assess whether the client has mental or spiritual distress along with physical changes or pain (Donnelly, 1996). Stress is prevalent in today's world and affects each of us differently, depending on an individual's available levels of support and his or her resilience in managing these issues. The client-centered model of care allows us to elicit information about the challenges our clients are facing, as well as the strategies and supports they find helpful. We can ask simple questions as described in Box 5–2 to obtain information. When we know what underlying factors may be contributing to the client's distress, we can collaborate to strengthen their support systems or help them find new resources if needed.

A problem that is frequently noted by health care providers is that clients bring up questions just as the care provider is leaving the room. Often, these are very important issues and may even be the primary reasons the client made the appointment. By providing clients time and comfort in which to express all their concerns, the client-centered interview makes it possible to avoid "doorknob" questions. Statements such as "Is there anything more you can tell me?" or "Is there anything else you would like me to know?" will allow this information to surface at an appropriate time and be included in the diagnostic process.

**EXPLANATORY MODEL OF CARE**   Arthur Kleinman is a psychiatrist and anthropologist who has done ground-breaking work on the interface between culture and medical care. In his approach to care, client interviews generate mini-ethnographies that help to explain how clients perceive their own problems. He calls the belief system that each person uses to understand his or her health and medical issues the *explanatory model*. It is important to keep in mind that health providers also have explanatory models that may substantially differ from or even conflict with

---

**BOX 5–2   Sample Psychosocial Questions (Social History)**

- Tell me about your living situation.
- What is your job like?
- Tell me about your family.
- What kinds of stress do you feel?
- What do you do to manage your stress?
- Who helps you with that?
- How does that affect your health?

- What are your social supports?
- What are you feeling?
- How far did you go in school? Do you ever have trouble understanding the things people tell you or give you to read? (health literacy)

---

the client's model (Kleinman et al., 1978). The importance of understanding the explanatory models of both the health care provider and the client is widely accepted as an important component of client-centered interviews (Coulehan & Block, 2001; Coulehan et al., 2001; Donnelly, 1996; Haidet & Paterniti, 2003; Platt et al., 2001; Smith & Hoppe, 1991; Stacey et al., 2009). What is most challenging about this paradigm is the need for providers to remain nonjudgmental and to respect the client's model as highly as the biomedical factors when designing a plan of care.

Each client is unique and has his or her own story to tell. Medical concerns do not occur in a vacuum, but as a component of everything the client is experiencing, as well as the cultural context and beliefs that shape the client's expectations. It is important to get the whole story. In other words, we can do a good physical exam, but can still miss important information if we do not incorporate the meaning of the problem to the client. Further, we may not be able to provide clients with care they will be willing to agree to if we do not ask what is acceptable to them. Eliciting each client's "explanation" provides the information needed to uncover clients' belief systems and understanding of their circumstances. This approach ties in nicely with the health belief model of behavior change that will be discussed in Chapter 6.

Effective implementation of Kleinman's explanatory model requires that clients be guided through the process of providing this information. In turn, the provider helps the client to understand his or her explanatory model of health care and to place client concerns within that context. Together, client and provider can develop a collaborative plan of action to address client concerns by utilizing the client's own resources and those available through the health care system. The most important step in this process is for providers to present themselves as client allies, ready to negotiate therapeutic plans that make sense to both the health care professional and the client. The latter is the most important aspect of this model, because it helps develop client trust and adherence (Kleinman, 1988; Kleinman et al., 1978).

Using the explanatory model requires breaking down the power differential that traditionally has existed between clients and providers. Eliciting clients' explanatory models of their medical conditions requires skills that are new to some health care providers. Examples of questions that may be helpful are included in Box 5–3. One should be flexible when asking questions and use words or phrases that seem most appropriate for each individual. The key questions to ask are

---

### BOX 5–3  Questions to Elicit Clients' Explanatory Models

- Tell me what brings you here today? What do you call your problem?
- What do you think has caused your problem?
- Why do you think it started when it did?
- Tell me your ideas about how the problem will change over time.
- What do you think your sickness does to you? How does it work?
- How severe is your illness? How long will it last?
- Tell me about the difficulties that your problem causes for you.
- How has this problem affected your life?
- What do you think is the best plan of care for you?
- What do you think is the best thing I can do for you?
- What kind of treatment do you think you should receive?
- What worries you most about your illness?
- Tell me what you are most afraid of.

---

*Sources:* Kleinman (1988), Kleinman et al. (1978), and Johnson, Hardt, & Kleinman (1995).

these: "What do you think is wrong?" "What caused it?" and "What do you want me to do?" (Kleinman, 1988, p. 239). This will allow the health care provider to understand the meaning the client has attached to his or her condition, as well as open the opportunity for a dialogue on how to proceed with treatment.

**INVITE, LISTEN, SUMMARIZE**    Boyle and associates (2005) have developed a simple system that guides practitioners in performing a client-centered interview. They call this strategy *invite, listen, and summarize*. It provides a helpful mnemonic device to help interviewers recall the necessary steps. At the beginning of the interview, health professionals briefly identify themselves and make a remark such as "You and I have never met before, and I would like to know something about you as a person before we begin our examination." This allows the clinician to see the client as a person first and to understand his or her story. It also provides a powerful message to clients: that the clinician wants to know them as people and is interested in their opinions. Other phrases that can be used to *invite* the client to provide important information include "Tell me a little about yourself" or "Tell me what brings you here today" (Boyle et al., 2005, p. 30).

Professionals actively *listen* to the client's story and use appropriate communication skills to show that they are engaged. As clinicians listen, they process and reflect on what they are hearing, while providing cues to the client to continue. During this stage, they request more information or provide confirmation that they are listening, by using statements such as "Tell me more," "Anything else you can tell me?" "What do you think about this?" "How do you feel about that?" (Boyle et al., 2005, p. 30). The clinician does not interrupt the flow of information or take control of the interview to pursue areas that might be important for diagnosis or treatment.

At this point, clinicians *summarize* what they have heard, using statements such as "You have been having chest pain for several weeks that does not seem related to exercise; did I hear that correctly?" "It sounds like there is a lot going on in your family, and I would like to know a little more about that" or "In the past, you have not been satisfied with your medical care because it did not fit with what you believe to be the best route to follow." This process of summarizing ensures that the client has been correctly heard and understood, which is important to all involved parties.

Once you have heard the client's story and elicited the symptoms, impact on life, and his or her understanding of the problem, you can move on to more close-ended questions and perform tests to narrow the diagnosis and treatment options. This is also the time to present your understanding and knowledge of the client's difficulties. You can describe how the symptoms reflect or affect physical or emotional functioning and what kinds of interventions you believe are most effective. There is often more than one solution to the client's difficulties, and you can present several viable options, while explaining which ones you feel will be most effective. Finally, the provider must be willing to negotiate with clients about the best course of treatment.

## In the Beginning

Entire books have been written on how to perform a good client interview. It is beyond the scope of this chapter to cover all potential encounters in different practice settings. However, this section provides basic information for organizing, structuring, and conducting the interview.

Planning for the client interview begins before the client even arrives in the office or clinic. It is assumed that the clinician will be knowledgeable, professional, and have well-developed communication skills. Before actually beginning the interview, it is important to prepare the room, the area, and yourself. Remember that it is not just the provider who interacts with the client but the office staff, receptionist, aides, students, and others, such as food service staff and cleaning personnel.

In any setting, the entire staff must help make the visit successful. It is important to realize that clients may be feeling a number of unpleasant emotions, including nervousness, embarrassment, worry, or anxiety. By providing a welcoming and respectful environment, clients will feel reassured that they are in good hands. For example, clients should be received into an area that ensures private interactions with friendly receptionists and that waiting areas are neat, clean, and pleasant. It is important to consider the furnishings and decorations that are used. Because many clients come from cultures other than Anglo American, artwork or other decorations that represent other cultures may help to indicate that this facility is welcoming to all.

The interview space should be private, quiet, and nondistracting, preferably with a door that closes. Clients can be distracted by a bustling clinic with ringing telephones, people walking in and out of the area, and perhaps an open clinic space where clients can see or hear each other. This will impair the client's ability to focus on the interview and provide answers with the depth and clarity that is needed. For this reason, it is also a good idea to separate clients from those who accompanied them to the appointment so that they can freely answer all questions and disclose their concerns. This, of course, would not be appropriate if clients need to have someone help provide a detailed medical history for them or to assist with communication due to hearing loss, literacy issues, and or other communication concerns. In addition, during an initial assessment, a client may need to be examined more fully than in later treatments, so concerns about physical privacy may exist.

Many students are anxious or uncertain about how to best communicate with clients. This is both understandable and positive. It indicates that students recognize and care about the psychosocial needs of their clients and understand the role of client–provider interactions. It is reassuring to know that while words are important, the caring, attentive, nonjudgmental attitude of the provider also speaks volumes. In the next section, we will emphasize that what you say is not nearly as important as how well you listen. Truly hearing the client is one of the most crucial skills we can bring to the encounter.

## Asking and Listening

As stated earlier, the successful client interview depends on skillful communication techniques. It permits us to hear each client's story, while gathering information about both the diagnosis and the type of care that will be acceptable to him or her. It also requires proficiency at organizing the structure and flow of the interview, pacing the questions and response times, using both open-ended and close-ended questions, and, of course, listening carefully to hear what the client is telling us. Perhaps the most essential skill in the client interview is silence, which allows the client time to tell us everything that we need to know (Smith & Hoppe, 1991). Research has confirmed that if the client is allowed to speak uninterrupted at the beginning of the interview, he or she is able to relay 80 percent of all relevant information in 2 to 3 minutes (Beckwith & Frankel, 1984; Lipkin et al., 1995; Tongue et al., 2005). One foundational belief of the client-centered interview is that the client has all the information the health care provider needs. Therefore, you must learn to listen attentively and wait for the client to give you that information (Shepard, 2007; Smith & Hoppe, 1991). It is very important to hear the clients' whole story if you are going to be asking them to incorporate changes, such as new medications, diet, or activity levels, into their lifestyles.

The interview typically begins with a simple greeting and an introduction, if the client is new to the provider: "Hello, my name is Jan, and I am going to be your nurse today." The introduction can quickly establish the relationship between the client and provider. A general rule is that the way providers introduce themselves should match the terms in which the client is addressed. If providers use formal terms for themselves, then the client must also be addressed using formal language, such as Mr., Mrs., Ms., or Dr. Some uncertainty exists about whether it is better to use formal or informal names, but the typical suggestion is that usage start out on a formal level and progress to an informal level as the relationship develops (Lipkin et al., 1995). Another way to handle this is to ask clients what they would like to be called.

In a busy health practice, confusion can arise over the roles of the many types of providers the client may encounter. It is not only rude, but very disconcerting, to interact with professionals who have not identified their roles on the team. Are you the nurse, the social worker, the doctor, or the medical technician? It is also helpful to briefly describe your role and what you will be doing, even if it is something as basic as taking vital signs.

After the initial greeting, the provider can make a remark about a neutral subject, such as the weather or the traffic. Avoid starting by casually asking, "How are you doing today?" because clients may reflexively answer "Fine," when in fact, they are not fine at all (Tongue et al., 2005). Once the client and provider are comfortably settled, the provider can ask an open-ended question, such as "Tell me how you are doing" or "Tell me what brought you here today." Remember that it is important to be patient and listen without interrupting; if we allow clients a few minutes to speak, they will tell us almost everything we need to know. Rather than being silent or immobile, we should nod, smile, and make statements such as "MmHm," "I see," "Tell me more about that," and "What was that like for you?"

Johnson, Hardt, and Kleinman (1995) suggest several skills that are necessary as part of the conversation to elicit the client's explanatory model. During this conversational portion of the interview, providers need to give their full attention to the client and be nonjudgmental about the information that is provided. This takes practice, because it involves not only words but body language. The questions provided in Box 5–1 are examples of the kind of information you will need to acquire and can be used as a guide. Remember to be flexible and authentic in your interview so that you are not stiff or stilted. Use words or phrases that are comfortable to you and the clients and be sensitive about how many questions to ask. You may need to interpret the reason for client reluctance to answer certain questions: Are they embarrassed by the question? Do they understand what you are trying to ask? Demonstrating interest and openness to what the client is and is not saying will generally provide sufficient information to reveal client concerns.

A mistake many providers make is asking too many questions, especially those that require only a yes/no or one-word answer. For example, rather than asking "How many servings of fruits and vegetables do you eat on a typical day?" "Do you have more pain in the morning or the evening?" or "Is your pain sharp, dull, or throbbing?" you can say "Tell me about your diet" or "Describe your pain to me." This can be followed up by asking the client to tell you more or by restating what you have heard and asking if you have correctly understood. It is important to ask how the condition affects the client, what he or she has done to try to deal with the problem, and what preferences, if any, the client has for care. Remember, before leaving this portion of the interview, it is important to ask if clients have anything else they think is important for you to know about their health or well-being.

Finally, health literacy is a factor that must be considered in all client interviews. It is particularly relevant when the client is a non-native English speaker and has limited English proficiency. For the purposes of a client-centered interview, the provider should avoid making any assumptions about literacy and should find a way for clients to demonstrate their understanding of information provided in medical encounters (Coulehan & Block, 2001). One technique is to ask clients to explain or describe in their own words what they have just heard you say. We can also ask if they have different words to explain the same thing.

## Summary

This chapter described the importance of communication and its relevance to health care. It is imperative to develop a rapport with a client in order to provide quality care. We reviewed the components of communication, which include being present in the moment, practicing mindfulness, using and appropriately interpreting verbal and nonverbal communication, the importance of active listening and understanding what the client is saying, and the use of client-sensitive language.

Appropriate and inappropriate humor in communication was described. Used effectively, humor can decrease tension and assist health care professionals in developing relationships with clients. Used inappropriately, humor can damage relationships, negatively effect adherence to treatment programs, and damage outcomes. Barriers to effective communication, such as role uncertainty, sensory overload, voice and word choice, physical appearance, and gender and cross-cultural differences were discussed.

This chapter also defined and presented an overview of conflict. Sources of conflict were identified, and elements of conflict resolution were explored. The advantages and disadvantages of common approaches to managing conflict were discussed. Methods of alternative conflict resolution were introduced.

Performing a good client interview is one of the most essential functions of the health provider. It allows us to develop relationships with clients, listen and hear their stories, and learn about how health concerns affect their lives. By using the concept of client-centered care, we are able to convey our willingness to understand and respond empathetically to those concerns. This is also the most effective and efficient way to obtain important diagnostic information. Students and novice health care professionals are often concerned about saying and doing the right thing. Rest assured that the practices of active listening, reflecting, and asking follow-up questions will provide you with the foundation needed to establish an effective plan of care that integrates client concerns with evidence based practice.

## Reflective Questions

1. a. What do you do to demonstrate that you are listening?
   b. How will you know if a client has heard what you intended to say?
   c. What can you do if you think a client received the wrong message?
2. Clients are not always able to express what they are thinking or feeling and cannot always generate questions related to something that is bothering them. What feelings may a client feel uncomfortable expressing?
3. What are some factors that might interfere with your ability to listen effectively to clients and members of the health care team?

4. Several concepts in this chapter may be new or unfamiliar to the reader, especially the concept of client-centered care. What do you see as the value of this approach to your profession?
5. We have described how to elicit a client's explanatory model of illness. Consider settings in which you have worked or hope to work in the future and develop a list of questions or guiding points that will help you integrate this approach to care.

## Case Study

Margaret James is a woman in her mid-50s who has come to your clinic because she has not been feeling well. She is overweight, sedentary, and loves to cook for her family. She presents with hypertension and is at high risk for type 2 diabetes. You are the first member of the health care team who will interview her for the purpose of developing an effective plan of care. Given her lifestyle, this is likely to be a very complicated matter that will involve a lot of interventions.

1. What factors or concerns will you address before you actually meet Mrs. James?

2. Using a client-centered model of care, describe how you would start your interview and your first few statements or questions to her.

3. How will you encourage her to provide you with the information you need? What questions might you ask?

4. a. Would you need to explore her explanatory model? Why or why not?

   b. If she seems reluctant to follow up on your concerns about her health, what might you say or do next?

## References

Alper, S., Tjosvold, D., & Law, K. S. (1998). Interdependence and controversy in group decision-making: Antecedents to effective self-managing teams. *Organizational Behavior and Human Decision Process, 74*(1), 33–52.

Alpers, A., & Lo, B. (1999). Avoiding family feuds: Responding to surrogate demands for life-sustaining interventions. *Journal of Law, Medicine and Ethics, 27*(1), 74–88.

Ang, M. (2002). Advanced communication skills: Conflict management and persuasion. *Academic Medicine, 77*(11), 1166.

Attewell, A. (1998). Florence Nightingale's relevance to nurses. *Journal of Holistic Nursing, 16*(2), 281–291.

Barringer, B., & Glod, C. A. (1998). Therapeutic relationship and effective communication. In C. A. Glod (Ed.), *Contemporary psychiatric-mental health nursing: The brain–behavior connection* (pp. 47–61). Philadelphia, PA: F. A. Davis.

Beach, M. C., & Inui, T. (2006). Relationship-centered care research network. Relationship-centered care. A constructive reframing. *Journal of General Internal Medicine, 21*, S3–S8.

Beckwith, F., & Frankel, R. (1984). The effect of physician behavior on the collection of data. *Annals of Internal Medicine, 101*(6), 692–696.

Bonvicini, K. A., Perlin, M. J., Bylund, C. L., Carroll, G., Rouse, R. A., & Goldstein, M. G. (2008). Impact of communication training on physician expression of empathy in patient encounters. *Patient Education and Counseling, 75*, 3–10.

Boyle, D., Dwinnell, B., & Platt, F. (2005). Invite, listen and summarize: A patient-centered communication technique. *Academic Medicine, 80*(1), 29–32.

Cann, A., Zapata, C. L., & Davis, H. B. (2009). Positive and negative styles of humor in communication: Evidence for the importance of considering both styles. *Communication Quarterly, 57*(4), 452–468.

Carney, B. T., West, P., Neily, J., Mills, P. D., & Bagian, J. P. (2010). Differences in nurse and surgeon perceptions of teamwork: Implications for use of a briefing checklist in the OR. *Association of Perioperative Registered Nurses, 91*(6), 722–729.

Charon, R. (2001). Narrative medicine: A model for empathy, reflection, profession, and trust. *Journal of the American Medical Association, 286*(15), 1897–1902.

Coombs, M. (2003). Power and conflict in intensive care clinical decision-making. *Intensive Critical Care Nursing, 19*(3), 125–135.

Coulehan, J. L., & Block, M. R. (2001). *The medical interview: Mastering skills for clinical practice.* Philadelphia, PA: F. A. Davis.

Coulehan, J. L., Platt, F. W., Egener, B., Frankel, R., Lin, C. T., Lown, B., & Salazar, W. (2001). "Let me see if I have this right . . ." Words that help build empathy. *Annals of Internal Medicine. 135*, 221–227.

Davidhizar, R. E., Giger, J. N., & Poole, V. (1997). When change is a must. *Health Care Supervisor, 16*(2), 193–196.

Davis, C. M. (2006). *Patient practitioner interaction: An experiential manual for developing the art of health care* (4th ed.). Thorofare, NJ: Slack.

Davis, M. A. (2009). A perspective on cultivating clinical empathy. *Complementary Therapies in Clinical Practice, 15,* 76–79.

Donnelly, W. J. (1996). Taking suffering seriously: A new role for the medical case history. *Academic Medicine, 71*(7), 730–737.

Dove, M. A. (1998). Conflict: Process and resolution. *Nursing Management, 29*(4), 430–432.

Eason, F. R., & Brown, S. T. (1999). Conflict management: Assessing educational needs. *Journal for Nurses in Staff Development, 15*(3), 92–96.

Ekman, P. (1999). Facial expressions. In T. Dalgleish & M. Power (Eds.), *Handbook of cognition and emotion* (pp. 45–60). New York, NY: John Wiley & Sons.

Epstein, R. M. (1999). Mindful practice. *Journal of the American Medical Association, 282*(9), 833–839.

Epstein, R. M., & Street, R. L. (2007). *Patient-centered communication in cancer care. Promoting healing and reducing suffering* (NIH Publication No. 07-6225). Bethesda, MD: National Cancer Institute.

Fox, F. E., Rodham, K. J., Harris, M. F., Taylor, G. J., Sutton, J., Scott, J., & Robinson, B. (2009). Experiencing "the other side." A study of empathy and empowerment in general practitioners who have been patients. *Qualitative Health Research, 19*(11), 1580–1588.

Fraser, J. J. (2001). Technical report: Alternative dispute resolution in medical malpractice. *Pediatrics, 107*(3), 602–612.

Garden, R. (2008). Expanding clinical empathy: An activist perspective. *Journal of Internal Medicine, 24*(1), 122–125.

Greenfield, B. H., Anderson, A., Cox, B., & Tanner, M. C. (2008). Meaning of caring to 7 novice physical therapists during their first year of clinical practice. *Physical Therapy, 88*(10), 1154–1166.

Haidet, P., & Paterniti, D. A. (2003). "Building" a history rather than "taking" one: A perspective on information sharing during the medical interview. *Archives of Internal Medicine, 163*(10) 1134–1140.

Halstead, L. S. (2001). The power of compassion and caring in rehabilitation healing. *Archives of Physical Medicine Rehabilitation, 82,* 149–154.

Hassed, C. (2001). How humour keeps you well. *Australian Family Physician, 1,* 25–28.

Hayes, J., & Cox, C. (1999). The experience of therapeutic touch from a nursing perspective. *British Journal of Nursing, 8*(18), 1249–1254.

Henkin, A. B., Dee, J. R., & Beatus, J. (2000). Social communication skills of physical therapist students: An initial characterization. *Journal of Physical Therapy Education, 14*(2), 32–38.

Henrikson, M. (1998). Managing through conflict. Harnessing the energy and power of change. *Association of Women's Health, Obstetric and Neonatal Nurses (AWHONN) Lifelines, 2*(4), 53–54.

Herdtner, S. (2000). Using therapeutic touch in nursing practice. *Orthopaedic Nursing, 19*(5), 77–82.

Hutchinson, T. A. (2005). Coming home to mindfulness in medicine. *Canadian Medical Association Journal, 173*(4), 391–392.

Jadad, A. R., & Delamothe, T. (2004). What next for electronic communication and health care? *British Medical Journal, 328,* 1143–1144.

James, T. & Cinelli, B. (2003). Exploring gender-based communication styles. *Journal of School Health, 73*(1), 41–42.

Jensen, G., Gwyer, J., Shepard, K., & Hack, L. (2000). Expert practice in physical therapy. *Physical Therapy, 80*(1), 28–52.

Johnson, T. M., Hardt, E. R., & Kleinman, A. (1995). Cultural factors in the medical interview. In M. Lipkin, S. M. Putnam, & S. M. A. Lazare (Eds.), *The medical interview: Clinical care, education and research* (pp. 153–162). New York, NY: Springer-Verlag.

Kabat-Zinn, J. (1994). *Wherever you go, there you are.* New York, NY: Hyperion.

Kearney, M. K., Weininger, R. B., Vachon, R. L. S., Harrison, R. L., & Mount, B. M. (2009). Self-care of physicians caring for patients at the end of life. *Journal of the American Medical Association, 302*(11), 1155–1164.

Kern, D. E., Branch, Jr., W. T., Jackson, J. L., Brady, D. W., Feldman, M. D., Levinson, W., & Lipkin, M. (2005). Teaching the psychosocial aspects of care in the clinical setting: Practical recommendations. *Academic Medicine, 80*(1), 8–20.

Kleinman, A. (1988). *The illness narratives.* New York, NY: Basic Books.

Kleinman, A., Eisenberg, L., & Good, B. (1978). Culture, illness and care. *Annals of Internal Medicine, 88,* 251–258.

Kummervold, P. E., Trondsen, M., Andreassen, H., Gammon, D., & Hjortdahl, P. (2004). Patient–physician interaction over the Internet. *Tidsskr Nor Laegeforen, 124*(20), 2633–2636.

Levinson, W., Roter, D., Mullooly, J., Dull, V., & Frankel, R. (1997). Physician–patient communication: The relationship with malpractice claims among primary care physicians and surgeons. *Journal of the American Medical Association, 277,* 533–559.

Lieberman, S. (2010). *Differences in male and female communication styles.* Retrieved from http://www.simmalieberman.com/articles/maleandfemale.html

Lipcamon, J. D., & Mainwaring, B. A. (2004). Conflict resolution in healthcare management. *Radiology Management, 26*(3), 48–51.

Lipkin, M., Frankel, R. M., Beckman H. B., Charon, R., & Fein, O. (1995). Performing the medical interview. In M. Lipkin, S. M. Putnam, & S. M. A. Lazare (Eds.), *The medical interview: Clinical care, education and research* (pp. 65–82). New York, NY: Springer-Verlag.

Loscalzo, M. (1999). In coping with cancer, gender matters. *Journal of the National Cancer Institute, 91*(20), 1712–1714.

Martin, S. T. (1999). Language shapes thought. *PT—Magazine of Physical Therapy, 7*(6), 44–45.

McCray, A. T. (2005). Promoting health literacy. *Journal of the Medical Information Association, 12*, 152–163.

Mead, N., & Bower, P. (2002). Patient-centered consultations and outcomes in primary care: A review of the literature. *Patient Education and Counseling, 48*, 51–61.

Mentgen, J. L. (2001). Healing touch. *Holistic Nursing Care, 36*(1), 143–157.

Miller, B. J. (1998). The art of managing conflict. *Journal of Christian Nursing, 15*(1), 14–17.

Misra-Hebert, A., D. (2003). Physician cultural competence: Cross-cultural communication improves care. *Cleveland Clinic Journal of Medicine, 70*(4), 289–303.

Monroe, C. K. (2009). The effects of therapeutic touch on pain. *Journal of Holistic Nursing, 27*(2), 85–92.

Moore, C. (1996). *The mediation process* (2nd ed.). San Francisco, CA: Jossey-Bass.

Nelson, H. W., & Cox, D. M. (2003). The causes and consequences of conflict and violence in nursing homes: Working toward a collaborative work culture. *Health Care Management, 22*(4), 349–360.

Nibler, R., & Harris, K. L. (2003). The effects of culture and cohesiveness on intragroup conflict and effectiveness. *Journal of Social Psychology, 143*(5), 613–631.

Northouse, L. L., & Northouse, P. G. (1998). *Health communications: Strategies for health professionals* (3rd ed.). Stamford, CT: Appleton & Lange.

O'Day, B. L., Killeen, M., & Iezzoni, L. I. (2004). Improving health care experiences of persons who are blind or have low vision: Suggestions from focus groups. *American Journal of Medical Quality, 19*(5), 193–200.

Pettrey, L. (2003, February). Who let the dogs out? Managing conflict with courage and skill. *Critical Care Nurse*, pp. S21–S24.

Pillemer, K., Hegeman, C. R., Albright, B., & Henderson, C. (1998). Building bridges between families and nursing home staff: The partners in caregiving program. *The Gerontologist, 38*(4), 499–503.

Platt, F. W., Gaspar, D. L., Coulehan, J. L., Fox, L., Adler, A. J., Weston, W. W., . . . Steward, M. (2001). "Tell me about yourself": The patient-centered interview. *Annals of Internal Medicine, 134*(11), 1079–1085.

Platt, F., & Platt, C. (2003). Two collaborating artists produce a work of art. *Archives of Internal Medicine, 163*(10), 1131–1132.

Purtilo, R., & Haddad, A. (2007). *Health professional and patient interaction* (7th ed.). Philadelphia, PA: W. B. Saunders.

Raica, D. A. (2009). Effect of action-oriented communication training on nurses' communication self-efficacy. *Medical Surgical Nursing, 18*(6), 343–360.

Rakel, D. P., Hoeft, T. J., Barrett, B. P., Chewning, B.A., Craig, B. M., & Niu, M. (2009). Practitioner empathy and the duration of the common cold. *Family Medicine, 41*(7), 494–501.

Rotarius, T., & Liberman, A. (2000). Health care alliances and alternative dispute resolution: Managing trust and conflict. *Health Care Manager, 18*(3), 25–31.

Roter, D., & Hall, J. (1992). *Doctors talking with patients: Patients talking with doctors.* Westport, CT: Auburn Books.

Routasalo, P. (1999). Physical touch in nursing studies: A literature review. *Journal of Advanced Nursing, 30*(4), 843–850.

Saha, S., Beach, M. C., & Cooper, L. A. (2008). Patient centeredness, cultural competence, and healthcare quality. *Journal of the National Medical Association, 100*(11), 1275–1285.

Schacher, C. L., Stalker, C.A., & Teram, E. (1999). Toward sensitive practice issues for physical therapists working with survivors of childhood sexual abuse. *Physical Therapy, 79*(3), 248–261.

Schmitt, N. (1990). Patients' perception of laughter in a rehabilitation hospital. *Rehabilitation Nursing, 15*(3), 143–146.

Schneider, J., Kaplan, S. H., Greenfield, S., Li, W., & Wilson, I. B. (2004). Better physician–patient relationships are associated with higher reported adherence to antiretroviral therapy in patients with HIV infection. *Journal of General Internal Medicine, 19*(11), 1096–1103.

Schon, D. (1983) *The reflective practitioner: How professionals think in action.* San Francisco, CA: Jossey Bass.

Schouten, B. C., & Meeuwesen, L. (2006). Cultural differences in medical communication: A review of the literature. *Patient Education and Counseling, 64*, 21–34.

Shepard, K. (2007). Are you waving or drowning? *Physical Therapy, 87*(11), 1543–1554.

Simon, V. & Pedersen, H. (2005). Communicating with men at work: Bridging the gap with male co-workers and employees. Retrieved from http://www.itstime.com/mar2005.htm

Smith, R. C., & Hoppe, R. B. (1991). The patient's story: Integrating the patient- and physician-centered approaches to interviewing. *Annals of Internal Medicine, 115,* 470–477.

Stacey, C. L., Henderson, S., MacArthur, K. R., & Dohan, D. (2009). Demanding patient or demanding encounter? A case study of cancer. *Social Science and Medicine, 69,* 729–737.

Stiefel, F., Barth, J., Bensing, J., Fallowfield, L., Jost, L., Razavi, D., & Kiss, A. (2010). Communication skills training in oncology: A position paper based on a consensus meeting among European experts in 2009. *Annals of Oncology, 21,* 204–207.

Studdert, D. M., Mello, M. M., Burns, J. P., Puopolo, A. L., Galper, B. Z., Truog, R. D., & Brennan, T. A. (2003). Conflict in the care of patients with prolonged stay in the ICU: Types, sources, and predictors. *Intensive Care Medicine, 29*(9), 1489–1497.

Sutcliffe, K. M., Lewton, E., & Rosenthal, M. M. (2004). Communication failures: An insidious contributor to medical mishaps. *Academic Medicine, 79*(2), 186–194.

Taylor, R. R., Wook Lee, S., Kielhofner, G., & Ketkar, M. (2009). Therapeutic use of self: A Nationwide survey of practitioners' attitudes and experiences. *The American Journal of Occupational Therapy, 63*(2), 198–207.

Teal, C. R., & Street, R. L. (2009). Critical elements of culturally competent communication in the medical encounter: A review and model. *Social Science and Medicine, 68,* 533–543.

Thomas, K., & Kilmann, R. (1974). *Thomas Kilmann conflict mode instrument.* Tuxedo, NY: Xicom.

Thompson, V. L., Cavazos-Rehg, P. A., Jupka, K., Caito, N., Gratzke, J., Tate, K. Y., . . . Kreuter, M. W. (2007). Evidential preferences: Cultural appropriateness strategies in health communication. *Health Education Research, 23*(3), 549–559.

Tongue, J. R., Epps, H. R., & Forese, L. L. (2005). Communication skills for patient-centered care: Research-based, easily learned techniques for medical interviews that benefit orthopedic surgeons and their patients. *Journal of Bone and Joint Surgery, 87*(3), 652–658.

Tripicchio, B., Bykerk, K., &Wegner, J. (2009). Increasing patient participation: The effect of training physical and occupational therapists to involve geriatric patients in the concerns-clarification and goal-setting process. *Journal of Physical Therapy Education, 23*(1), 55–61.

Umbreit, A. W. (2000). Healing touch: Applications in the acute care setting. *American Association of Critical Care Nursing Clinical Issues, 11*(1), 105–119.

Umiker, W. (1997). Collaborative conflict resolution. *Health Care Supervisor, 15*(3), 70–75.

Vanderhoff, M. (2005). Patient education and health literacy. *PT–Magazine of Physical Therapy, 13*(9), 42–46.

Wainwright, S. F., Shepard, K. F., Harman, L. B., & Stephens, J. (2010). Physical therapist clinicians: A comparison of how reflection is used to inform the clinical-decision-making process. *Physical Therapy, 90*(1), 75–88.

Wanzer, M., Booth-Butterfield, M., & Booth-Butterfield, S. (2005). If we didn't use humor, we'd cry: Humorous coping communication in health care settings. *Journal of Health Communication, 10,* 105–125.

Williams, K., Kemper, S., & Hummert, M. L. (2004). Enhancing communication with older adults: Overcoming elderspeak. *Journal of Gerontological Nursing, 30*(10), 17–25.

Woltersdorf, M. (1998). Body language. *PT–Magazine of Physical Therapy, 6*(9), 112.

Xu, Y., & Davidhizar, R. (2004). Conflict management styles of Asian and Asian American nurses: Implications for the nurse manager. *Health Care Management, 23*(1), 46–53.

Young, A., & Turner, J. (2009). Developing inter-professional training for conflict resolution—A scoping audit and training pilot. *Mental Health Review Journal, 14*(1), 4–11.

Zweibel, E. B., & Goldstein, R. (2001). Conflict resolution at the University of Ottawa faculty of medicine: The pelican and the sign of the triangle. *Academic Medicine, 76*(4), 337–344.

# Motivation, Adherence, and Collaborative Treatment Planning

I'm finding that when I begin each treatment by asking the clients how things are going and how they're handling everything, I see an enormous improvement in therapy results.

Just today, I listened carefully while Mr. Jorgensen revealed how much pain he was having and how that affected his ability to walk and do other important activities. Because I was fully attentive and listened with my whole heart and soul, I was able to understand his psychosocial needs and found the words to encourage him to persevere. Although he was reluctant to ambulate further because of his pain, he responded to me and doubled the distance that he walked.

*—From the journal of Denise Motley, nursing student*

As clinicians, we ask clients to adhere to many things, such as monitoring blood glucose levels, taking prescribed medications, using orthoses, and doing exercises. The more motivated and willing clients are to be actively involved in their therapeutic intervention, the more adherent they will be and the better their outcomes. Most clients are highly motivated to get well. However, many of us have had the experience of working with clients who feel sorry for themselves, feel the world is against them, and want to spend the rest of their lives moping around or staying in bed. In addition, some clients are unwilling to make changes. Why do clients with the same diagnosis, age, gender, and socioeconomic status act so differently?

Motivation is a two-part multifactorial phenomenon. The client first has to possess a desire to achieve a goal and then commit to an action to accomplish it. If the clinicians singularly set the goals, the clients may not be adherent because the goals are not their own, a considerable barrier to motivation. In addition, clients may feel they face too many barriers to be adherent, such as lack of transportation, time, finances, pain, fatigue, family conflicts, and differences in health beliefs and culture.

Motivation and adherence are critical elements in rehabilitation and are frequently used as outcome measures. Adhering to a treatment regimen is one variable of a positive outcome (Brewer, 1999), and motivation seems to increase the degree of adherence (Brewer, van Raalte, & Cornelius, 2000). In studies of home exercise programs that complement clinic-based physical therapy, 60 to 76 percent of clients did not completely comply with therapeutic regimens (Sluijs, Kok, & van der Zee, 1993; Taylor & May, 1996).

Many factors affect therapeutic adherence. Some are motivators that enhance it; others are barriers that thwart adherence (King et al., 2002; Resnick & Spellbring, 2000). This chapter discusses theoretical concepts that influence motivation and adherence, describes collaborative relationships, identifies common barriers to collaborative treatment planning, and explores strategies that health care practitioners can use to enhance client motivation and adherence.

The phenomenon presented here as adherence is known in some fields as compliance. Studies generally define adherence as the degree to which clients follow a treatment regimen (Rand, 1993; World Health Organization [WHO], 2003). The treatment program could be in a clinic or at home and might include activities such as a diet, exercise plan, or other lifestyle changes. In fact, the WHO (2003) uses a model of five dimensions of adherence: patient-related factors, social/economic factors, therapy-related factors, condition-related factors, and health system-related factors.

Some studies use clinic attendance or self-reports to assess adherence. In others, the clinician evaluates the degree to which clients adhere with specific programs. The Sport Injury Rehabilitation Adherence Scale (SIRAS) (Bassett & Prapavessis, 2007) is an example. This 5-point scale measures three items: intensity of exercises, extent that recommendations and directions are followed, and receptiveness to changes in the program. Another example uses a multivariate approach, integrating several kinds of measurements. The 4-item subscale from the Situation Motivational Scale (Guay, Vallerand, & Blanchard, 2000) was used to examine clients' beliefs about the intrinsic and extrinsic benefits of a physical therapy program by asking them "Why are you starting physical therapy?"

The importance of motivation and adherence in improving outcomes has been well documented in the literature. For example, adults with osteoarthritis who adhered to a community-based aquatic exercise program showed improvements in physical function and quality of life and well-being (Belza, Topolski, Kinne, Patrick, & Ramsey, 2002). Long-term independent adherence by clients with chronic low back pain, after supervised rehabilitation ended, resulted in significant improvements in many parameters, including scales of perception of disability and pain (Hartigan, Rainville, Sobel, & Hipona, 2000).

Now that you've read about how motivation and adherence benefit the client, consider how nonadherence might influence you as a practitioner. Think about how you might feel or react when a client does not adhere to your therapeutic regimen. Think about how frequent nonadherence, over time, could influence what you prescribe for future clients. Could you see yourself ever "giving up" on some clients or prescribing a different program based on how you "read" them?

Physical therapists during their first year of clinical practice defined the "difficult patient" as one who is not open to therapy, is opposed to therapy, or lacking in motivation (Greenfield, Anderson, Cox, & Tanner, 2008). Sometimes, therapists blame their clients, which affects both parties. As one novice therapist said, "I shut off a little bit . . . if you don't care about yourself, then why should I care about you" (Greenfield et al., 2008, p. 1159)? This inexperienced therapist's attitude was judgmental and unethical, failing to respect the dignity and autonomy of the client to make his or her own choices. If we listen to clients, we can better assess how ready, willing, and able they are to make changes, to understand actual or perceived obstacles, and to help them become successful.

von Korff and coworkers (1997) identified important principles regarding increasing motivation and adherence for us to consider when working with clients. First, *illness management skills are learned, and behavior is self-directed.* Most clients grow and develop without concerns related to illness or disability. Until a need arises, these illness management skills cannot be practiced. Clients who have survived previous hardships will adapt to illness or disability more readily. Those who have not will benefit from additional counseling and education. However, until clients value the information as necessary for their own health, independent management is not likely to occur. Patience and individualized education are needed with those learning these skills for the first time.

Second, *motivation and self-confidence are important determinants of behavior.* As we will discuss, clients must be motivated to make changes in their health behaviors. They also must believe that they are capable of achieving success. It is critical to identify what is most important in their lives, what they enjoy doing, and what they find easy to do. Goals established with these elements in mind are more likely to be motivating and achievable. For example, if the goal is to quit smoking, it might be motivating to focus the client's attention on a child or spouse who would be left alone should he or she die from lung disease.

Finally, *the process of monitoring and responding to changes, symptoms, emotions, and functions improves adaptation to illness.* Learning to adapt to an illness or disability requires the acquisition of many new skills. The process of monitoring and responding to changes related to the illness or disability provides a natural and incremental method for learning to deal with all that is entailed. Consider the life of Sebastian, a 22-year-old man who sustained a cervical 7 spinal cord injury approximately 14 months ago. His initial recovery was hampered by the involvement of his well-meaning, but overprotective, mother. Over time, family counseling has helped both Sebastian and his mother understand the importance of separation. Recently, he has assumed full responsibility for managing his new life.

Education and persuasion can be used to help motivate clients, but strategies to overcome barriers toward progress must be continually refined. Rewards, such as recognition and praise, may be helpful in encouraging the maintenance of positive changes, but the recognition and praise have to be authentic. Health care professionals need to be more than "cheerleaders" who praise clients for the slightest changes. The client must feel praiseworthy for this to be effective.

## FACTORS AFFECTING MOTIVATION AND ADHERENCE

### Locus of Control

Psychologists and other health care providers have long been interested in determining why individuals behave the way they do. Why do some people practice "wellness" behaviors, eating a balanced diet and exercising regularly, while others smoke and overindulge in food and alcohol, even though they know it is detrimental to their health? Why do some clients with chronic pain manage well, while others develop maladaptive behaviors?

One of the early researchers to study behavior was Julian Rotter. He described a theory that he called "locus of control," which is based on life experiences and influenced by one's culture and family. According to Rotter's seminal 1966 work, people develop preconceived expectations about what will happen to them in the future. Those who believe they can influence what will happen to them are described as having an internal locus of control. They tend to be self-motivated and follow suggested treatment protocols because they believe they can make a difference in their lives. Other individuals have an external locus of control, believing that what happens to them is a result of outside influences or events. They may be less adherent to treatment protocols because they believe that their efforts will not make a difference.

Many studies have examined the relationship between locus of control and health-related behaviors. Hussey and Gilliland (1989) report that individuals with an internal locus of control are more health oriented and more likely to follow suggested health care plans than those whose locus of control is external. In reviewing the nursing literature, Oberle (1991) found that some studies support the Hussey-Gilliland findings, whereas others contradict them. This may be due to the fact that locus of control is a dynamic concept with many points on its continuum. It can range from strongly internal to strongly external. In addition, the measures of locus of control assess tendencies that can vary and even change (Wallston, 1992).

Clients with chronic pain who have a strong internal locus of control are better able to deal with their pain than those with a strong external locus of control (Toomey, Mann, Abashian, & Thompson-Pope, 1991). However, because of its dynamic nature, locus of control can shift. Evidence of this was generated when clients with chronic pain were treated in multidisciplinary pain management clinics and were able to increase their internal locus of control and, as a result, better manage their pain (Coughlin, Bandura, Fleischer, & Guck, 2000).

Clients' beliefs in the benefits and effects of treatment strongly affect adherence. Engstrom and Oberg (2005) found that clients with chronic pain who had lower expectations of therapy did not fully adhere to treatment recommendations and, as a result, experienced more pain, more disability, and deficient overall health. To facilitate treatment adherence habits, clinicians need to explore the client's beliefs about the benefits of the proposed therapy. The good news for clients and health care providers is that locus of control is a fluid concept. Even clients with a strong external locus of control can learn to take control of their situations. Note, however, that although health care providers need to understand the importance of locus of control, we must recognize that other factors also influence motivation and adherence.

## Self-Efficacy

Why do some clients improve, while others, with similar problems, do not? This happens for many reasons, and one of them is the client's own perception of his or her reality. Sometimes, there is a gap between what clients can actually do and what they think they can do. This can be particularly true if clients have not been able to do for a long duration what they had previously been able to do. This becomes their new reality and can hamper improvements. As clinicians, you can help change perceptions and emphasize clients' assets to facilitate a more realistic self-perception of what they should be able to achieve.

This phenomenon of a client's perception of reality is known as self-efficacy (Burton, Shapiro, & German, 1999; Conn, 1998), which was first introduced by Bandura (1977). It is a sense of competence and ability that is related to how successful people believe they can be in accomplishing a task. The idea that people believe that they are able to control their actions and behavior can affect their rehabilitation (Jensen & Lorish, 2005; Schenkman, Hall, Kumar, & Kohrt, 2008; Woodard & Berry, 2001).

Some people avoid a task if they do not believe they can adequately participate or complete it. In contrast, those who believe they will ultimately succeed continue their efforts, even if they are having difficulty. People judge their own abilities, which, in turn, affects their behavior, level of motivation, and adherence to health care regimens. This self-judgment can also determine how long someone persists with a difficult task. It is important to note that these personal judgments are not always accurate.

When people misjudge their abilities, they may become angry and frustrated and lose their focus on the task. They believe things are more difficult than they really are. However, people with a strong sense of self-efficacy may see a difficult situation as more of a challenge, causing them to try even harder (Bandura, 1997). This may partly explain why clients may react differently to the same circumstances.

Individuals with a strong sense of self-efficacy are better able to cope following a disability or illness (Maciejewski, Prigerson, & Mazure, 2000; Robinson-Smith, Johnston, & Allen, 2000). For instance, women who survived breast cancer and participated in a strength/weight training program for 6 months demonstrated a high degree of self-efficacy and adhered to their exercise programs (Ott et al., 2004). In a study of people with chronic low back pain before and 2 years following treatment, 80 percent exercised regularly because they believed that their actions could be successful. In fact, they did show improvements in flexibility, strength, pain levels, and disability scores (Mailloux, Finno, & Rainville, 2006).

A corollary of self-efficacy and a key motivator for adherence is outcome expectation. Adults in a retirement community who adhered to a walking program reported that they did so because they believed they were able to participate (self-efficacy) and that their actions would result in specific health benefits (outcome expectation) (Resnick & Spellbring, 2000). Fortunately, like locus of control, self-efficacy is a dynamic concept. People can improve their sense of efficacy by observing others accomplishing tasks and by learning to successfully complete tasks themselves (Bandura, 1997; Resnick, Palmer, Jenkins, & Spellbring, 2000). This is important information for health care professionals. We can assist our clients by introducing them to clients with similar diagnoses who have functionally integrated their illness or disability into their lives. Experienced survivors can serve as role models for those who have recently been diagnosed or injured. In addition, we can assist our clients by establishing reasonable short-term goals. Clients develop a sense of accomplishment, improve their sense of self-efficacy, and become motivated to comply with future treatments as they successfully achieve goals.

## Self-Esteem

Like locus of control and self-efficacy, self-esteem affects motivation. Self-esteem describes how individuals feel about themselves. Do they accurately assess their self-worth in comparison to others? Do they have pride in their abilities? A person with strong self-esteem is more likely to feel in control of his or her life and be more motivated to be an active participant in health care than a person with low self-esteem (Turner, 1999).

Many factors affect self-esteem. What may appear to be insignificant to us might be extremely important to a client. People in a rehabilitation setting or skilled nursing facility may feel better if they are able to wear their own clothing rather than hospital attire. A woman who uses a wheelchair may feel better about herself if a hairdresser is available to cut, color, and style her hair. Someone with burns might improve his self-esteem if he learns to apply cosmetics to mask his injuries. It may also help to have personal items nearby to remind clients of their homes and families. A simple compliment from a health care provider can also help boost a client's self-esteem.

Self-esteem is often negatively impacted by alterations in body image. For example, children who had amputations of limbs to treat primary malignant bone tumors reported significantly lower levels of self-esteem than their counterparts who could be treated with surgical limb-sparing procedures (Marchese et al., 2007). Similarly, low self-esteem, anxiety, difficulty with social relationships, changes in body image, and depression are seen in clients with craniofacial conditions, facial injuries, facial cancer, and conditions to surgically correct face and jaw problems (DeSousa, 2008). One symptom of depression (see Chapter 13) is low self-esteem. The lowered self-esteem can affect a client's motivation to participate in treatment.

## Social Determinants of Health

In addition to locus of control, self-efficacy, and self-esteem, a number of social determinants play a significant role in determining a client's motivation and treatment adherence. Factors such as race/ethnicity, literacy, education, income, and place of residence can influence lifestyle decisions about whether clients do things like exercise, take their medications, and eat healthy diets. Behavior change occurs where our clients live—at home, work, and school—but some communities fail to offer the infrastructure needed to modify lifestyle (Woolf, 2008). For instance, if a plan entails healthier nutrition, is there a store with fresh fruit nearby? Can clients or members of their support system get there? Is the food affordable (Woolf, 2008, 2009)?

Adherence to medical regimens, whether they involve medication, diets, exercise programs, or stress management, requires that clients be both willing and able to make the desired changes. Often a client faces barriers to change that are difficult for health care providers to detect. In Chapter 3, we discussed cultural issues that affect health care. However, it is important to mention here that a culturally sensitive and knowledgeable provider will communicate with clients in ways that respect their beliefs and values when making recommendations. For example, it is important to consider the role of the family and community in decision making and support, the desire to use alternative medicine, and the amount of trust the client places in the providers' advice (White et al., 2007). When clients are comfortable with medical recommendations, they are more likely to be adherent. The information needed is most likely to be elicited and negotiated in a skillful client interview (see Chapter 5).

**COMMUNITY RESOURCES**    Intensive counseling is often required to change poor habits, for example, addictions to substances such as alcohol or cigarettes. This takes a considerable amount of time and usually occurs outside of medical encounters in programs available at community locations, such as the YMCA or Weight Watchers®. Unfortunately, clinicians generally lack adequate knowledge of existing programs outside of formal medical environments to make referrals. When such information is available, however, lack of ability to pay for nonmedical programs and lack of transportation can be deterrents. It is crucial for health providers to avoid underestimating the difficulty of changing behavior and adhering to treatment programs. We must not assume that providing information and support will always be sufficient (Woolf, 2008).

**SOCIAL SUPPORT**    The presence of social support, which shows people that they are loved, cared about, and valued, can enhance well-being. Clients who are supported are more optimistic, experience less depression and anxiety, have higher self-esteem and a better quality of life, and adhere more to treatment interventions (Platt et al., 2001; Symister & Friend, 2003). Social support leads to a winning combination: The more supported people feel, the more satisfied they are with their care, resulting in greater adherence (Bylund & Makoul, 2002). Lack of social support has been associated with low levels of motivation and may lead to nonadherence; therefore, it is beneficial to consider social support mechanisms when developing plans of care.

Another principle of von Korff and coworkers (1997) regarding motivation and adherence is that *social factors influence health behaviors*. The social environments at home, work, and in the health care system can support or impede health behaviors. Changes in these environments may be necessary to promote optimal health. Consider Jon, a college sophomore who has been diagnosed with hepatitis C. His liver biopsy shows early signs of cirrhosis. He lives near campus with a group of friends who host "keg" parties nearly every weekend night. Because he finds it impossible to avoid drinking in this environment, his health care provider might help him to see that moving into a new setting would be a healthy choice, though it would come at the expense of cutting ties with close friends.

It is important for health providers to determine clients' histories and what they bring to their current circumstances. People with illness or injury may find that they are unable to perform many of their activities of daily living. Frustration, anger, and lack of motivation may follow. A social support system can make it easier for clients to function. For example, people may be able to keep medical appointments if they have transportation. Members of a social support system may encourage a client to adhere to treatment plans, such as reminding a client to take medication, eat healthy meals, and exercise. This support can motivate a client to remain hopeful and adherent, even in difficult times.

Clients who live with a spouse or another adult have somewhat greater adherence to medical treatment than adults who live alone (DiMatteo, 2004a). A study of caregivers for clients discharged from an outpatient geriatric assessment center found that those caregivers who agreed with health provider recommendations had greater adherence to treatment protocols and were more likely to help clients reach the goals (Bogardus et al., 2004). In a broader sense, when caregivers and health providers work together and caregivers believe in the efficacy of recommendations, clients are the winners.

The stress that caregivers experience can significantly impact adherence. One study involving children with disabilities showed that as family stress increased, children's adherence to home exercises decreased, resulting in a loss of functional skills (Rone-Adams, Stern, & Walker, 2004). Health care professionals can help reduce family stress by recommending appropriate resources for assistance, such as stress management programs, caregiver support groups, and respite care.

If clients do not have support systems in place, they can be referred to appropriate community resources. For example, Meals-on-Wheels can provide nourishment. Transportation may be provided by local town governments. A home health aide might assist with activities of daily living. Health care providers are responsible for knowing about the programs and resources that are available in their clients' community, so they can inform them about these services.

Information can empower clients, providing they have the resources needed to act on the information learned. With the information and resources required to make health behavior changes, clients are able to gain control over what they are experiencing and, therefore, may be in a better position to adhere to a recommended therapeutic regimen. Empowerment is a strong motivator. It helps to strengthen relationships between clients and health care professionals, building trust and reducing anxiety so that goals can be achieved. A sense of empowerment strengthens confidence and self-efficacy, which may also result in participatory decision making and self-management (Heisler, Bouknight, Hayward, Smith, & Kerr, 2002).

In addition to locus of control, self-efficacy, self-esteem, and social determinants, other factors that affect a client's motivation and ability to participate with health care include coping styles. In one study of people with cystic fibrosis, their coping style influenced how adherent they were to treatments, such as physical therapy, enzymes, and vitamins (Abbott, Dodd, Gee, & Webb, 2001).

Motivation and adherence go hand in hand. In a study investigating why children do not take their asthma medication (that is to say, lack of adherence to the treatment regimen), the children gave reasons of lack of motivation, difficulty remembering to do so, and social barriers. This occurs even in the face of the perceived consequences of nonadherence, such as feeling sick and not being able to participate in peer activities (Penza-Clyve, Mansell, & McQuaid, 2004).

## BARRIERS TO ADHERENCE

Just as there are motivators that increase therapeutic adherence, there are also barriers that decrease it. These barriers may predict inadequate adherence with a therapeutic regimen and, as a result, negatively impact achievement of goals. Health professionals need to address barriers before expecting people to change their behavior. We have already discussed many barriers, such as lack of finances, transportation, interest, and social support. In addition, the impact of an illness can affect one's ability to adhere to treatment regimens. This lack of ability is manifested as pain, fatigue, and feeling overwhelmed. There are also psychosocial barriers that can influence self-assessment of function, such as secondary gain; secondary loss; emotional distress (i.e., anger, anxiety, depression); psychopathology; somatization, symptom magnification, and malingering; and comprehension and mental status (Gatchel, 2004).

Traditionally, health care practitioners believed that education about the value and importance of exercise and other healthy behaviors, in and of itself, would be ample motivation for clients to alter their actions. We now understand, however, that changing human behavior is a far more complicated process. Identifying barriers is a by-product of good communication. Once you identify barriers, you can work to mitigate them.

## ROLE OF HEALTH CARE PROVIDERS IN PROMOTING MOTIVATION AND ADHERENCE

Mrs. Menendez is at home recuperating from total hip replacement surgery. She fractured her hip when she fell on the ice in front of her home. Recently discharged from the hospital, she will receive services from the Visiting Nurses Association.

My supervisor and I visited Mrs. Menendez to evaluate her home to eliminate falling hazards. I was appalled! She had numerous scatter rugs throughout her home. I suggested she remove them immediately so that she wouldn't trip on them. She refused. The rugs had belonged to her mother, and she enjoys having them in her home; they make her feel comfortable and connected to her family. In addition, she has a 20-pound Boston Terrier, who has a habit of jumping on people. I was concerned that he would knock her over. I really thought she should put him in a kennel while she recuperated. She said, "No way! I love my dog and missed him when I was in the hospital." She likes to have him sit on her lap in the evening because he helps her "relax and calm down."

Her husband is another problem. While I was trying to encourage Mrs. Menendez to do things for herself, he wanted to wait on her "hand and foot." He didn't want her to move from her comfortable chair in the living room. I tried to explain that she needed to walk to become stronger, to improve her balance, and increase her endurance. He didn't want to listen to me. He was afraid that she might fall again, and he didn't want to "lose her." They've been married for over 50 years. What was I to do?

*—From the journal of Samantha Marino, physical therapist student*

The interaction between Samantha and the Menendez family illustrates the importance of the health provider in motivating clients to comply with care. Health providers need to recognize clients' values and priorities and incorporate them into a care plan to establish reasonable and effective outcomes. Flexibility is also an important component of the interaction. For example,

Mrs. Menendez might have considered removing the scatter rugs, if she knew she could replace them once she was more stable on her feet. Samantha could suggest that the dog be put into a closed room while Mrs. Menendez is walking and be present when she is seated. In addition, Samantha could also work with Mr. Menendez to establish goals to increase his wife's strength and endurance. With these strategies, she would include him as a valued team member. Perhaps he could record his wife's daily progress. Samantha needs to understand and respect that Mr. Menendez, the dog, and the scatter rugs are all part of Mrs. Menendez's frame of reference. Samantha could utilize these resources to motivate her client to comply with treatments.

## STRATEGIES TO ENHANCE MOTIVATION AND ADHERENCE

### Modifying Health Behaviors

Various approaches to changing or modifying health behaviors are documented in the medical literature. Treatment interventions based on behavior theory seem most likely to have positive outcomes, particularly when clients and providers work together toward shared goals (Hirano, Laurent, & Lorig, 1994; Lorish & Gale, 1999, 2002; Meyer & Mark, 1995; von Korff et al., 1997). Multiple factors need to be addressed to improve adherence, such as those associated with the individualized behavioral, cognitive, emotional, and technical needs of the client (DiMatteo, 2004b; Haynes, McKibbon, & Kanani, 1996; Herborg, Haugbolle, Sorensen, Rossing, & Dam, 2008; McDonald, Garg, & Haynes, 2002; Pampallona, Bollini, Tibaldi, Kupelnick, & Munizza, 2002; Schroeder, Fahey, & Ebrahim, 2004; Weingarten et al., 2002).

Therapeutic interventions can be developed that foster motivation and adherence by modifying health behaviors. To effectively promote motivation and adherence, health care professionals need to understand basic theories of behavior and change. Several models have been designed to change health behaviors, and there are too many to include in this chapter. We will provide information here about four models that are frequently utilized and illustrate how they can be applied: the health belief model, the transtheoretical model for health behavior change, the five A's behavioral intervention protocol, and motivational interviewing.

**HEALTH BELIEF MODEL**    The *health belief model*, developed by Hochbaum, Leventhal, Kegeles, and Rosenstock, utilizes psychological theories of decision making to determine what actions individuals might choose when presented with various health care choices (Rosenstock, 1966). This model is based on the earlier seminal work of Lewin and colleagues (1944), who believed that health behaviors and choices are influenced by the value people place on a potential outcome and their belief that a certain course of action would result in that desired outcome.

Wallston (1992) suggests that health-related behavior also depends on the value that people place on their health. People who perceive that they can control their illness may place a higher value on health and comply with treatments in order to improve. In contrast, those who believe they have no control over their illness may place less emphasis on their health. They may be nonadherent with treatment, believing that their actions will not positively influence their health. These perceptions and beliefs, either positive or negative or accurate or not, can influence therapeutic outcomes. So, too, can expectations and apprehensions of being able to participate and reap benefits from treatment (Jensen & Lorish, 2005; Schenkman et al., 2008; Woodard & Berry, 2001). Clients tend to adhere to treatment interventions and have higher attendance levels if they believe that the treatments are meaningful to them (Campbell et al., 2001; Taylor & May, 1996).

The health belief model is intricately entwined with people's perceptions of their health status. As such, it is based on subjective beliefs, as opposed to objective measurements. According to the health belief model, in order for people to change behavior, they must be ready to make a change. This readiness is based on their health beliefs and includes an understanding of what causes the problem. If clients believe that health is given by a higher power, then they will also believe that they have no ability to make a change in their status. Some clients believe that they are capable of making the change but also believe that the barriers that have to be overcome are not worth it. For instance, if we ask the "cook in the family" to change his or her diet, this can affect the way he or she cooks for the whole family. If that client believes the family will be highly resistant to this change, he or she may be reluctant to make the change because of the conflict it is likely to create.

Clients must also believe that the value of making the change is stronger than the consequences of not making the change. Hypertension typically has no noticeable symptoms and is rarely detected by the client. Therefore, asking a client to take a medication that causes side effects will not be valuable if the client sees no benefit in controlling blood pressure. Health beliefs can also affect clients' sense of self-efficacy and whether or not they believe that they have the ability to be successful in achieving their goal.

To help motivate clients to make the changes we suggest, clients' beliefs must align with our view that Western medicine provides appropriate solutions. In Chapter 3, we discussed some common health beliefs of various cultures. It is important to elicit these beliefs so that they can be discussed and form the basis for a truly collaborative plan of care to which the client is willing to adhere.

**TRANSTHEORETICAL MODEL FOR HEALTH BEHAVIOR CHANGE** The *transtheoretical model for health behavior change* focuses on motivation. Although this is a heavily utilized and often discussed model, few guidelines are available for applying it. In addition, evidence of efficacy in the short term is greater than that which exists for long-term behavioral change (Adams & White, 2005). "There is abundant evidence that other external and social factors, such as age, gender, and socioeconomic position, influence exercise behavior, motivation to participate in physical activity, and stage of activity" (Adams & White, 2005, p. 239).

Change in health behavior is a process that takes time. The transtheoretical model for health behavior change, also called the stages of change model (Prochaska, DiClimente, & Norcross, 1992; Prochaska, Redding, & Evers, 2002; Prochaska & Velicer 1997), recognizes that change does not happen easily and that people move through various stages of readiness to change. Identifying the signs of these stages will help us tailor our interventions to current needs. Further, even when progress toward change occurs, clients are likely to relapse into earlier stages. In fact, relapse appears to be a necessary element in the process and must be addressed so clients can begin anew. As described in Table 6–1, clients are likely to pass through six nonlinear stages on their way to change, including the following:

- *Pre-contemplation* An abundance of clients are in this stage when we first encounter them and have no plans to begin to make a change. During pre-contemplation, clients are not expecting to make any changes within the next 6 months. At this stage, people may be uninformed as to the consequences of their behaviors or may have given up, having been unsuccessful at earlier attempts to change. These clients tend to refuse to discuss or consider consequences of their actions. Although they may be perceived and labeled as unmotivated, they may just not be *ready* to change. Providing them with additional information regarding the positive aspects of change can help them progress to the next stage, known as contemplation.

| **Table 6–1** Transtheoretical Model for Health Behavior Change/Stages of Change Model | | |
|---|---|---|
| Pre-contemplation | No thought of change | "I'm not changing my diet; why should I?" |
| Contemplation | Considering change | "I'm not changing my diet now but may begin at some point." |
| Preparation | Preparing to change | "I will make changes in the next year." |
| Action | Implementing change | "I've been exercising for 30 minutes, three times a week, for the past few months." |
| Maintenance | Maintaining change | "I've been exercising for 30 minutes, three times a week, for over 6 months now." |
| Termination | Change is integrated | "I test my blood sugar four times a day, like clockwork." |

- *Contemplation*   In the contemplation stage, clients are aware of the need to change and are considering doing so within the next 6 months. They have "done their homework" and have learned the pros and cons of their situation. However, these clients can sometimes feel overwhelmed with information and become stuck in this stage for months. They are not ready for action, but encouraging them, providing additional resources, and reducing their barriers to change may help them move to the next stage, known as preparation.
- *Preparation*   During the preparation stage, people plan to take action in the near future. They know what they need to do and have a plan as to how they will achieve their goals. In addition, they recognize that the positive aspects of change outweigh the negative elements. They are prepared and tend to quickly move to the action stage where observable changes can be measured.
- *Action*   Health professionals perceive clients in the action stage as highly motivated. When clients adhere to home programs, lose weight, and join gyms or health clubs, the health providers feel a sense of satisfaction for having helped them achieve their goals.
- *Maintenance*   Once people achieve their goals, they progress to the maintenance stage and can remain there for 6 months to 5 years. During this period, they continue to develop self-confidence and are less tempted to relapse to their former behavior. However, clients often do relapse and may return to any of the earlier stages.
- *Termination*   The final stage, termination, occurs when clients have reached their goals, incorporated positive lifestyle changes, and are confident that they will not return to their "old ways."

Health care professionals who understand where clients are in the process of change can better provide appropriate support and help them move forward. Attempting to force a person who is in the pre-contemplation stage to the action phase can be frustrating for both the client and the health provider and will usually result in only short-term success and a high dropout or relapse rate.

**FIVE A'S BEHAVIORAL INTERVENTION PROTOCOL**   Lorish and Gale (2002) built on the theoretical components of the models discussed above and developed the *five A's behavioral intervention protocol*. The five steps are easy to follow, take little time to complete, and have been shown to be more successful in promoting client motivation and adherence than information and advice alone. This model is also closely aligned with the transtheoretical model and motivational interviewing.

The five A's model provides a structure and format for interacting with clients capable of developing a collaboration that will support them to make behavioral changes to improve health. The first A is to *address the issue.* We need to make sure that we have the clients' attention and that we are also fully attentive. We name the problem and present the need for intervention. Second, we *assess the clients.* In this step, we determine where they are in the stages of change, as well as identifying any barriers preventing them from engaging in more healthful behaviors. We can ask the clients what they would like to change and how prepared they are to implement changes. It will be helpful to determine any previous attempts to change behavior. Third, we *advise the clients.* This is where we include the traditional medical role of providing information and educating the clients about their illness and the reasons why changes are needed. We can help the clients understand the benefits of change and the consequences of not changing. Fourth, we *assist the clients* to make change. This is where we negotiate an agreeable plan of care. Finally, we *arrange for follow-up.* Behavior change is a long and difficult journey, and one appointment will typically not result in change. Schedule another appointment to review progress, address barriers, and renegotiate the protocol.

In order for clients to change, they must be knowledgeable about their situation, motivated to change, and have the resources to make it happen. The five A's address all of these issues and involve a dialogue between the health care provider and the clients to reduce barriers and negotiate positive behavioral changes.

Numerous other behavioral techniques have been found to improve health management among clients who have chronic illnesses (Beresford et al., 1992; Ignacio-Garcia & Gonzalez-Santos, 1995; Woodard & Berry, 2001). These include the following: collaborative goal setting; assessing readiness for new behaviors in small, manageable steps; providing personalized education, observation, and feedback; self-monitoring of changes and symptoms; and counseling in techniques to obtain appropriate social support. Health care providers must design structured behavioral interventions that incorporate these behavior techniques to facilitate clients' independence in using important health management skills.

**MOTIVATIONAL INTERVIEWING**    Motivational interviewing is predicated on the belief that clients are responsible for their own actions and health and, consequently, for changing their health behaviors. It epitomizes client autonomy and self-determination. Because self-efficacy and outcome expectations shape actions, motivational interviewing can be a valuable strategy to enhance motivation and adherence. Initially used with the treatment of addictions and alcohol use, it is a client-centered, directive counseling approach first developed by Miller (1983) and later expanded by Miller and Rollnick (1995). It is now used in medical, public health, and other health promotion arenas (Britt, Hudson, & Blampied, 2004; Resnicow et al., 2002) for promoting physical activity in clients with chronic heart failure (Brodie & Inoue, 2005), promoting public health (Shinitzky & Kub, 2001), changing behavior in clients with chronic obstructive pulmonary disease (Rollnick, Miller, Butler, & Aloia, 2008), and weight reduction in women with type 2 diabetes (West, DiLillo, Bursac, Gore, & Greene, 2007).

An evidence-based, directive, client-centered counseling approach, motivational interviewing helps a client's intrinsic motivation to change by delving into ambivalence and working to end it (Levensky, Forcehimes, O'Donohue, & Beitz, 2007); that is to say, it help clients adhere to treatment recommendations. Building on the transtheoretical model for health behavior change (Prochaska et al., 1992, 2002; Prochaska & Velicer 1997), motivational interviewing follows four key counseling principles (Levensky et al., 2007; Miller & Rollnick, 2002):

- *Express empathy*    The health care provider communicates an understanding of what clients are experiencing and accepts their ambivalence. "Readiness to change" comes from within the client and can ebb and flow. Clients are helped to overcome their "ambivalence or lack of resolve" to change.

- *Develop a discrepancy*   The provider helps clients become aware of the discrepancies between their present unhealthy behaviors and the goals and values that they would be striving to achieve. The responsibility to self-determine and reach a commitment to change rests with the client.
- *Roll with resistance*   Because motivation to change ultimately comes from the client rather than the provider, the health provider does not directly interfere with any client resistance. Coercion, persuasion, and confrontation are counterproductive and contradictory to the core concepts of motivational interviewing.
- *Support self-efficacy*   The health provider supports and communicates the belief that clients are able to effect change. A partnership exists between the client and clinician rather than a paternalistic relationship (Miller & Rollnick, 1995).

Important skills for motivational interviewing include reflective listening, asking open-ended questions, affirming, and summarizing (see Chapter 5). Because the premise is to help clients become aware of their problems, for example, nonadherence, and what consequences can ensue from lack of following the recommended course of behavior, we ask key questions to elicit inherent motivation rather than provide the information. Four important questions to ask are listed in Box 6–1.

Patient education looks different with motivational interviewing because it uses an ask–tell–ask approach. For example, "Tell me what you already know about diabetes and how it is treated" (*ask* the question). Ask for permission to provide more information as needed (*tell* the information). For instance, "It sounds like you know that drinking is not good for your liver. I have some specific information that I would like to share with you. Is that all right?" *Ask* what the client thinks about the new information you provided.

As an "interpersonal style," clinicians facilitate alternate thinking, a new picture with better results, which can help motivate the client to change behavior and instill commitment to that change. To do that, they work with clients to negotiate a plan of action. With information you have already elicited from the clients, you can then ask questions, such as "Are there things that you think you could change, even if they are small things?" "Can you think of one thing that you are able to change?" "What else would you be willing to change?" "What might you be willing to change later if this change is successful?" "What do you need to help you change?" Health professionals affirm and support all facets of the conversation to change.

## Goal Setting

"Goal-setting has long been regarded as a cornerstone of effective rehabilitation" (Lawler, Dowswell, Hearn, Forster, & Young, 1999, p. 402) and is important in treatment success. Goals need to be negotiated between clients and providers, participating as equals, and clients' needs, not those of health providers, should be the focus. Goals that are important in clients' lives tend

---

### BOX 6–1   Key Questions to Elicit Motivation

- What is the best thing that can happen to you if you do not change?
- What is the worst thing that can happen to you if you do not change?
- What is the best thing that can happen to you if you do change?
- What is the worst thing that can happen to you if you do change?

to be functional, meaningful, and motivating (Randall & McEwen, 2000; von Korff et al., 1997). Because the goals have relevancy in their lives, clients tend to be more committed to them. When clients are involved in establishing goals, they become partners in their care (Playford et al., 2000; Skinner, 2004).

Ideally, the client not only sets short-term and long-term goals but also enters into a contract to reach these goals by adhering to healthy behaviors (Bodenheimer, Lorig, Homan, & Grumbach, 2002). Clients are most successful in achieving treatment outcomes when their goals are specific, challenging, and achievable, and they have the opportunity to successfully practice the skills (Bandura, 1977, 1997; Locke, Shaw, Saari, & Latham, 1981). Therefore, we must be careful to agree on goals that are neither too high nor too low. If a goal is set too high, clients will be unable to achieve success. If a goal is too low, clients may achieve success but will lack a sense of accomplishment. In either case, this may lead to frustration and nonadherence.

Clinicians should review the goals with the client and mutually revise them as needed. This is also a good opportunity to discuss concerns and barriers and explore strategies to mitigate them (Schenkman et al., 2008). Clients' involvement should be active enough that they realize their collaborative role. This means that if clients are asked to identify their goals for treatment, responses should mirror the goals recorded in their health care records. Incorporating clients' goals into the plan of care requires active listening to ensure that we fully understand what clients are conveying. Their ideas then need to be developed into attainable and measurable goals that not only meet the criteria for standards of professional documentation but also maximize the chance of health insurance reimbursement (Chinman et al., 1999).

Once goals have been established, it can be helpful for clients to write out their goals in their own words. They may record them in a journal or calendar so that they can regularly review them. You can help clients establish realistic time frames for completing these goals. It is important to note, though, that goals do not always indicate forward progress. Some goals may be to maintain function or to slow the rate of decline that occurs with some long-term illnesses (Cott & Finch, 1991). In addition, having clients sign personal contracts stating they will adhere to treatment plans has been shown to improve motivation and adherence (Jones & Kovalcik, 1988).

Health care professionals and clients need to recognize that most people will not adhere to treatment programs 100 percent of the time. For example, clients occasionally forget to take medications or follow dietary recommendations. These minor lapses are considered normal. According to Barsa del Alcazar (1998), clients who are "moderately adherent" are demonstrating adaptive behavior. This is especially true of clients who are undergoing long-term treatments, such as dialysis. Health care professionals need to recognize and accept this adaptive behavior because it allows clients to continue to have control of their own lives. They can also help clients' family members understand this behavior so they will continue to be supportive, rather than critical, of the behavior of their loved ones.

Following illness or injury, clients' goals frequently include returning immediately to their previous state of health. Health care professionals need to discuss prognosis and anticipated time frames for recovery. Educating clients about the importance of short-term goals and their relationship to long-term goals is critical (Adams & White, 2005; Bradley, Bogardus, Tinetti, & Inouye, 1999). Health practitioners need to provide sufficient education so that clients can make constructive, informed decisions (Daily Mock, 2001). They also need to integrate the clients' viewpoints and work from a perspective that realistically conforms to the clients' perspective (Herborg et al., 2008 ).

Long-term goals are sometimes more important to patients than short-term goals. In a study of patients with osteoarthritis, long-term instead of short-term goals, as well as being

actively involved in the process, were strongly associated with long-term adherence to the therapeutic intervention (Veenhof et al., 2006). When clients understand and appreciate the link
between short- and long-term goals, they may be more motivated to adhere to programs. In
addition, early and continued involvement in goal setting promotes active participation, and
clients take responsibility for their own care.

Clients expect clinicians to know what questions to ask to retrieve important information
regarding concerns, goals, resources, treatment ideas, and outcomes. Although this may occur in
long-term care, professionals working in fast-paced environments may have only one opportunity to ask clients to identify their goals. Asking one question about goals during the initial examination, however, is not enough. In addition, clients may rely on health care professionals to share
established goals with other members of the team. This may not happen. Even clients who are ill
enough to require care in an intensive care unit may move from that setting to transitional care
and, finally, to outpatient or home care, sometimes after only a few days in each setting. Transfers
of service are likely to be accompanied by a complete change in the members of the health care
team, with little or no continuity other than what is provided by written reports. Ideally, these reports should relay all details that are important to consider.

## Education and Empowerment

Client education is an important component of health care (Jensen, Gwyer, Shepard, & Hack,
2000; Mostrom & Shepard, 1999; Vanderhoff, 2005). Studies have shown that educated clients
practice wellness behaviors and, if ill or injured, remain motivated and adhere to treatment programs (Sluijs, 1991). Client education needs to be culturally sensitive (see Chapter 3) and utilize
the components of effective communication (see Chapter 5). Ask clients if they will be able to
adhere to the program that you have both agreed on. If not, ask why and make appropriate
modifications. Attempt to eliminate any barriers that might interfere with adherence.

According to an early study by Treichler (1967), classroom students remember only 10 percent of what they read, but the retention increases as they are more engaged in this experience,
climbing to 80 percent of what they personally experience and 90 percent of what they teach to
others. In the clinical setting, clients and families are also learners. Providing clients with written
directions, pictures, and time to discuss instructions and ask questions will help them remember
prescribed treatment programs. All treatment adjuncts need to be clear and easy to understand,
customized to meet the needs of the clients, and relevant to them. To be beneficial, clinicians need
to review any form of documentation and share feedback.

Various educational approaches have been found useful, including treatment booklets with
clear graphics; videotapes, DVDs, iPods®, iPhones®, and YouTube; informational conversations
with clinicians, and equipment (i.e., for exercise) and adjunct equipment (i.e., inhalers or oxygen) (Bassett & Prapavessis, 2007; Moore, von Korff, Cherkin, Saunders, & Lorig, 2000; Stelzner,
Rodriguez, Krapfl, Jordan, &Schenkman, 2003; Sweeney, Taylor, & Calin, 2002).

Have clients repeat directions or demonstrate tasks to ensure they understand. In addition,
according to Treichler's model, giving clients the opportunity to teach their program to significant others, under your guidance, may aid in their retention.

Sluijs (1991) noted that the more information clients are given at one time, the more likely
they are to forget. They will forget even more if they are worried, concerned, or in pain when they
receive information. When possible, try to mitigate anxiety and discomfort at the outset. Yet, how
often do we overload clients with information during our first encounter? Ideally, provide clients
with basic information during the initial meeting, emphasizing the most important components

of the instruction. More complex information can be given at a later time. During subsequent sessions, determine whether clients correctly remember instructions. If a client has only one treatment session, however, you should communicate only the most essential information. Encourage clients to contact you with questions or concerns and provide your telephone number and e-mail address.

People have different teaching and learning styles. Most people tend to teach the way they prefer to learn (Brock & Allen, 2000; Mostrom & Shepard, 1999). However, this may not always be effective. Our teaching approach may not match the client's learning style. Some individuals prefer to hear only the facts, whereas others prefer a more personable approach. Allow time for clients to tell you how they feel and to ask questions. This strategy may instill comfort and prepare clients to absorb the information you are prepared to communicate. Whereas some people learn best by watching a demonstration and listening to instructions, others prefer trying things immediately. Recognizing and making adjustments for individual learning styles can make health care professionals more effective teachers and clinicians (Lawrence, 1997; Vanderhoff, 2005).

Today, a great deal of information on health care is available. Clients can open a newspaper, watch television, or listen to the radio to hear about the latest medical research. In addition, more people have access to the Internet, at home or through local libraries and schools. Clients need to be educated on how to evaluate all sources of information because some are unreliable (Vanderhoff, 2005). As health care professionals, we need to be well informed so that we can answer questions appropriately and ensure that clients receive accurate information. Motivation and adherence can be enhanced if clients are well educated regarding their diagnosis and prognosis.

## Feedback and Follow-Up

Positive feedback has been shown to improve self-esteem, enhance individuals' perceptions of their own competency, and improve motivation and adherence (Goudas, Minardou, & Kotis, 2000; Mulvaney, 2009). Health care professionals track clients' progress in medical records, but do we adequately share this information with clients? Understanding the progress they have made can give clients a sense of control and motivate them to continue (Lawler et al., 1999). It is important to give feedback in a timely manner. Positive feedback may be provided whenever clients follow through with program guidelines or make progress toward their goals. For example, clients with multiple myeloma and bone lesions who received encouragement and support were able to adhere to an aerobic and strengthening exercise program, in spite of the discomfort they experienced while they were receiving high-dose chemotherapy and stem cell transplantation (Coleman, Hall-Barrow, Coon, & Stewart, 2003). Other forms of feedback are also useful. Clients with heart failure who had already completed a supervised exercise program had greater adherence to exercise when they received graphic feedback and used goal setting and guidance (Duncan & Pozehl, 2002).

Clients can give themselves positive self-feedback. For example, they may track their own progress in journals or calendars. Reviewing this information can be a motivator. Consider Mrs. Thompson, who was trying to lose weight and increase her endurance following cardiac surgery. She had been in a cardiac rehabilitation program for several months and had become discouraged. As a result, she started "forgetting" about her exercise and walking program and no longer made time to adhere to other aspects of her treatment plan. Her exercise physiologist suggested she review the progress she had recorded in her journal. Reading the entries, Mrs. Thompson was surprised at how far she had come. Identifying her accomplishments enhanced her self-esteem and motivated her to return to her program with renewed energy.

Feedback to clients depends on consistent follow-up, can enhance adherence (Hall, 1999), and can take many forms, such as telephone calls, e-mails, group attendance, and personal counseling. In addition, scheduled assessment visits with clinicians may be helpful to review information, discuss how the client is progressing, and identify any barriers that have arisen. Follow-up contact is an opportunity to bolster sagging adherence, identify challenges early, and modify programs as necessary. Just as introducing the concept of adherence and setting mutual goals at the outset of a therapeutic program are key elements, supervised training with follow-up checks and feedback are continuing critical ingredients.

Health care practitioners need to encourage, support, educate, communicate, and build sustaining therapeutic alliances with clients. Having information, and being able to use it, and being involved in partnerships increases the clients' self-efficacy, which, in turn, may result in greater adherence to their therapeutic intervention. This is why the last of the five A's behavioral intervention protocol is to *arrange for follow-up*.

## Peer Support Groups

Peer group participation has been shown to help people clarify values, improve self-esteem, increase knowledge, develop coping strategies, maintain healthy lifestyle habits, and reduce or eliminate addictions (Bernard, 1991). In fact, groups are so beneficial and popular, it seems as though they exist for almost any problem, condition, or diagnosis. Interacting with others who have gone through or are going through similar experiences may assist clients in understanding their own limitations or impairments and give them greater confidence in their ability to succeed (Resnick et al., 2000; Turner, 1999). Support groups also benefit family members who are learning to live with an individual who has been diagnosed with an illness or who has sustained an injury. Groups offer social support and provide a forum for sharing stories and strategies for success. Clients with ankylosing spondylitis who were in a self-help group exercised more frequently, strengthened their own locus of control, utilized external support more freely, and continued to improve outcome measurements over time (Barlow, Macey, & Struthers, 1993).

Peer support groups can be especially effective in promoting positive health and wellness behaviors. For example, Turner (1999) described peer-led initiatives as a social support system for adolescents. Teens often feel more comfortable talking to one another rather than discussing their concerns with adults. Turner cautions, however, that when teen peer groups are developed, peer leaders need extensive training in listening and basic counseling skills in order to be effective. He emphasizes the need for adequate training, adult support, and the availability of appropriate referral resources. There must also be a trained adult available whom they can contact immediately if the need arises. Developing effective peer support programs can be quite time consuming, but the results are worth the effort.

Health care professionals direct some peer support groups, but group members direct others, as in the teen group noted above. Such programs can be a positive adjunct to professional health care services. However, when developing these programs, health care providers must remember that peer leaders have the same concerns and problems as group members. Therefore, it is important to provide professional social support mechanisms for all peer leaders if their problems begin to overwhelm them (Sherman, Sanders, & Yearde, 1998).

Information regarding peer group meetings is often available from local newspapers, hospitals, libraries, or churches. National resources, such as the Muscular Dystrophy Association and the United Cerebral Palsy Association, can be found on the Internet. Practitioners may consider developing peer support groups at their own facilities if none are available in the community.

## Functional Programs

Following illness or injury, many clients are concerned with their ability to be independent. Studies have shown that clients are more motivated to adhere to treatment programs that are related to functionality (Brody, 2005). In addition, clients are more likely to comply with programs that cause the least disruption in their lifestyles. Finding ways to fit treatment plans into a client's normal routine helps ensure long-term adherence (Brody, 2005).

Keep programs realistic and avoid complex instructions. Provide variety and choice when possible to prevent clients from becoming disinterested. Develop functional programs based on daily routines. For example, if a client needs to follow a complicated medication schedule, suggest the client purchase a weekly medication dispenser. Guide the client to identify the best time each week to fill the dispenser and establish a realistic strategy for remembering to take the medication on time. If the medication needs to be taken with food, he or she may want to leave the dispenser on the table where meals are eaten.

Be sure that home programs are functional in nature. Consider Mrs. Farrari, who slipped in the supermarket and fractured her shoulder. The therapist first suggested a nonfunctional exercise program. Mrs. Farrari stated the exercises were "boring" and did not interest her. After careful questioning about her home environment, where she lived alone, the therapist suggested that Mrs. Farrari move frequently used items to higher shelves. The client relocated teacups and glasses in the kitchen cabinets and towels and facecloths in the bathroom closet. As a result, as her day progressed, so did her accomplishments of her treatment goals. While a more structured exercise program might have accelerated her progress, she would not have made any progress if she did not adhere to the therapeutic program.

It is especially beneficial for families with children who have disabilities to integrate home exercise programs with a functional routine, such as bathing, dressing, and playing. It is incumbent upon the health provider to collaborate with caregivers to simplify activities so that stress is minimized, and limited time and energy are used most effectively (Rone-Adams et al., 2004).

## Primary and Secondary Control-Enhancing Strategies

Some clients start out motivated but lose their impetus over time. This is especially true for clients dealing with a chronic impairment or terminal illness. No matter how hard they work, their condition is not likely to significantly change or improve. Maintaining motivation can also be difficult for elderly people. Even healthy people experience decreased hearing acuity and loss of muscle tone, strength, flexibility, and memory as they age. They cannot participate in activities the way they could when they were younger.

How can we help these clients sustain their motivation to adhere to programs and achieve therapeutic outcomes? Studies have shown that a two-step approach, involving primary and secondary control-enhancing strategies, can be very effective (Chipperfield & Perry, 2006; Wrosch, Heckhausen, & Lachman, 2000). These strategies allow clients to feel in control of their lives, maintain their self-esteem, and remain motivated.

Primary control-enhancing strategies allow people to accomplish desired goals in new ways by modifying the environment. Consider Mrs. McKenzie, who loved to walk to the corner store to get her daily newspaper. As her rheumatoid arthritis progressed, she purchased a motorized scooter that allowed her to continue her routine. When primary control-enhancing strategies no longer achieve the goals, secondary strategies can be utilized to retain a form of personal control. Clients who use secondary control-enhancing strategies modify their internal environment by altering their expectations and reframing what is important. As her condition worsened,

Mrs. McKenzie found that she could not control the scooter and began to have her newspaper delivered to her home. Both types of strategies require the client to be cognitively flexible and to be able to adjust to changing circumstances. This can be difficult and require the support of both health care professionals and the social network.

### Creative Strategies to Support Motivation and Adherence

In addition to goal setting, other techniques that promote adherence and healthy behaviors include individualized action plans (Moore et al., 2000) and contracts with built-in incentives for goal achievement. Peer support with spouses and exercise partners has helped with smoking cessation, improving eating habits, and exercise/walking (Prochaska & Velicer, 1997). Reminders, such as laminated cue cards and exercise clothes, if applicable, can be placed in strategic locations in the client's environment (Bassett & Prapavessis, 2007; Sweeney et al., 2002).

The use of technology also fosters motivation and adherence. Clients with chronic stroke who participated in a program of physical therapy plus robotic devices showed high scores on the Intrinsic Motivation Inventory, sustained their interest, and received specific feedback (Colombo et al., 2007). Virtual reality systems, such as the Nintendo Wii™ system, are being used in many health care settings, including private practices, extended care facilities, and hospital-based rehabilitation units (Coyne, 2008). In addition, Dance Dance Revolution® is being used for aerobic conditioning and airway clearance for patients with cystic fibrosis (Coyne, 2008).

## COLLABORATION

I had a terrible experience in the clinic today. I was working in the gym with Mrs. Swanson, a woman who had her left leg amputated above the knee because of complications related to her diabetes. Just as she was finishing her exercises, one of the medical residents came by. Apparently, Mrs. Swanson agreed to participate in a study that was designed to examine how well clinicians at our hospital collaborate with patients on establishing goals and treatment plans. I asked for permission to sit in on the interview. What a mistake! This is how the interview went:

*Interviewer:*   Who decides what you are going to do in physical therapy?

*Mrs. Swanson:*   Well, Suzy does, of course! She's so smart. I don't know how I would have gotten this far without everything she has taught me.

*Interviewer:*   Do you ever suggest to Suzy that you would like to try a different exercise or work on something specific that you need to be able to do at home?

*Mrs. Swanson:*   Oh, no. She really knows just what I need to learn. After all the schooling she's had, how would I know anything more?

At first, I felt touched and kind of proud, but as the interview continued, I became embarrassed. The questioning continued about Mrs. Swanson's home situation. She mentioned how sad she was that she probably wouldn't be able to participate in her weekly line dancing class now that she was missing a leg. She started sobbing and talking about how she would be no good to anyone any more. I really thought that I had done a good job of incorporating her goals into my treatment plan. Today, I realized I had not.

*—From the journal of Suzanne Ballis, physical therapist student*

We have discussed the importance of establishing therapeutic partnerships with our clients that are based on genuine concern and mutual respect and trust. A healthy client–provider relationship involves understanding clients' perspectives and leads to explicitly shared expectations for outcomes. Collaborative goal setting is an important step toward empowering clients to take responsibility for their own recovery. Providing opportunities to make real choices in treatment goals and planning stimulates clients to utilize their own skills and resources to achieve positive outcomes. In addition, client satisfaction is positively associated with the degree of client involvement in the collaborative design and implementation of health care plans (Daily Mock, 2001; Green et al., 2008).

This is true even when the collaboration involves end-of-life care. A hematologist-oncologist said: "A patient may relapse and die of his disease. But, in the effort that he and I both put into this as partners in fighting his disease, there's a great solace. . . . I hope to do my very best in helping him die with ease" (Kearney, Weininger, Vachon, Harrison, & Mount, 2009, p. 1158).

Health practitioners agree that plans of care should be client centered and established and managed in collaboration with clients and all of their care providers (Baker, Marshak, Rice, & Zimmerman, 2001; Randall & McEwen, 2000). In early intervention, for instance, transdisciplinary teams consist of the child's parents, along with professionals from a variety of disciplines (King et al., 2009; Rapport, McWilliams, & Smith, 2004). Ideas and expertise are shared among team members to evaluate and meet the needs of the child being served. Once the collaborative plan has been established, team members train each other to provide hands-on interventions. For example, a special education teacher may train the child's parents in behavioral techniques to obtain their child's attention and cooperation. An occupational therapist may instruct a special educator in the principles of positioning to facilitate the child's involvement in classroom activities that require upright sitting. Professional members of the team assume a consultative role, providing assistance to bring about changes in the care plan as needed. Active family involvement is central to the process, and this helps to ensure that a holistic approach is maintained.

Consider the case of Lisa Marie, a 2-year-old girl with a diagnosis of cerebral palsy. She has been treated by the same physical therapist (PT), occupational therapist (OT), and speech/language pathologist (SLP) since she came home from the neonatal intensive care unit. The individualized family service plan (IFSP) was coordinated by a case manager and involved Lisa Marie's parents and all health care professionals who would be involved in her care. Although only one member of the health care team can visit each month, collaborative planning occurs, involving all team members, especially the family. Occasional tension does exist between the practitioners and Lisa Marie's parents regarding what is "right" for her care, but this tension forces periodic reexamination of the goals and the progress being made.

Because family involvement is essential, team members have established bonds with Lisa Marie, her parents, and two older siblings. All family members have learned how they can help facilitate Lisa Marie's development. Her parents use effective handling skills, which were taught by the PT and OT. Her brother, Eric, helps position her in the seating system she uses for eating meals and participating in family activities. The SLP taught Eric to position Lisa Marie in a way that minimizes the risk of aspiration when she is eating. Lindsay, Lisa Marie's sister, plays videogames with her, prerequisites for power-mobility training, which Lisa will begin once she makes the transition to her new school-based program next year.

Lisa Marie will soon be 3 years old, and the therapists have been helping prepare everyone for the transition to a public preschool program in the fall. She will be entering an innovative program, in which children with special needs are integrated with neighborhood children who have no identified special needs. Each of Lisa Marie's therapists has participated in the development of her individualized education plan (IEP). In addition to submitting written reports of all aspects of Lisa Marie's life, they also participated in a team meeting with the family and school-based personnel. Her services must be linked to educational goals, so part of the work of both teams of professionals has been to help the family understand which services would be "appropriate."

## BARRIERS TO COLLABORATION

Chinman and colleagues (1999) conducted a needs assessment in a large mental health clinic to determine the levels of interest and willingness of both clients and providers to participate in collaborative treatment planning. They identified the most significant barriers to collaboration as clients' disabilities, nonadherence, and clients' lack of interest in collaboration. Conversely, clients perceived the main barriers as providers' lack of time, uncertainty that treatment goals would be helpful, and inadequate knowledge about how to collaborate in treatment planning. The researchers suggested two additional reasons why some practitioners fail to provide this opportunity. First, they must relinquish some power in the relationship if they are going to empower clients. Second, they feel that *they* know what is best for their clients. For collaborative treatment planning to be successful, practitioners need to provide clients with opportunities for participation and may need to educate them in the actual techniques of collaborative planning.

Another potential barrier to collaboration is failure to take clients' premorbid lifestyle and history into account, except in a very superficial way. Clients may feel "stripped" of their previous identity. Their former lifestyle may seem somewhat irrelevant in light of significantly altered physical or cognitive function. On the other hand, when important aspects of the premorbid lifestyle are considered, motivating factors can be identified and used to develop an effective treatment plan.

Consider the case of Jenny, whose story of successful recovery from traumatic brain injury was summarized by Price-Lackey and Cashman (1996). Hers was actually a story of self-recovery. When the therapists involved in her rehabilitation failed to capture and incorporate Jenny's life history, she became frustrated, discharged herself from her residential treatment program, and struggled to develop her own, eventually successful program. Had the therapists fully examined Jenny's history, they would have discovered that she had always been remarkably independent and self-disciplined. She sought out progressively greater challenges and worked diligently until she mastered them. Throughout her life, Jenny reframed adverse situations (see Chapter 8), enabling her to view potentially negative experiences as opportunities for change and growth and strive for completion in the face of adversity. She eventually incorporated these skills into her self-directed therapy, which she described as a long and lonely process. Counseling that emphasized cognitive restructuring would have been extremely helpful to Jenny in the early stages of recovery, but failure to identify this important aspect of her history prevented this from happening.

Clients conceptualize their needs in terms of the functional abilities and resources needed to help them return to their premorbid lifestyles. Therefore, providers need to conceptualize clients in terms of more than diagnoses and symptoms that must be matched with appropriate treatment options. Coordination and integration of both perspectives through effective collaboration are beneficial.

## STRATEGIES FOR IMPROVING COLLABORATION

Asking clients to identify the biggest problems they are facing in managing their illness may provide the basis for improved collaboration. Consider the following example:

> I tried something new with my patients this month. About one week prior to each client's appointment, I sent out a brief questionnaire. Clients were asked to answer a few basic, open-ended questions before coming in for their visits. The questions addressed concerns or problems they might be experiencing with their health or lifestyle. I was amazed at the results. I had expected the majority would respond, but every one of my clients did! The other expectation I had was that this simple reflection would help focus our sessions. It did, but other benefits occurred, too. Patients reported feeling more relaxed during the visit because they knew all their concerns would be addressed. One of my clients suggested that I add a section to record my answers to concerns discussed during the visit. They'll be given a copy of this to take home.
>
> *—From the journal of Cathy Smith-Peterson, nurse practitioner student*

In addition to asking clients to identify questions or problems, it may be helpful to ask them other pointed questions at various intervals in the treatment process. For example, they could be asked to define their own role in maintaining and improving their health, how they perceive the role of the health care professional, and how they define concepts, such as help, therapy, rehabilitation, goals, and outcomes. This type of discussion not only provides baseline information about client beliefs, it can also provide an opportunity to clarify any confusion the client may be experiencing (von Korff et al., 1997).

As discussed earlier, client education is an essential element of health care. In addition to information about a specific illness or disability, some clients may have to learn how to be more active participants in goal setting and taking charge of their health. This might require instruction in helpful concepts and terminology (Daily Mock, 2001). By modeling the process of evaluation and task analysis and communicating in terms that clients can easily understand, health providers can help their clients learn how to independently solve functional problems. For example, if a client tends to identify problems in broad-based terms such as "I want to be able to provide for my family," you may need to help him or her reframe the problem in terms of specific functions. This will facilitate achievement of the ultimate goal of every health plan—independent health care management.

It is important for providers to identify clients' health beliefs, values, and practices because these can be key determinants of motivation and behavior. For example, if a client believes that herbal supplements offer more benefit than the insulin that has been prescribed as a treatment for diabetes, a change in this belief must be encouraged before a successful outcome can be achieved.

Forms designed to guide treatment planning tend to include information required by payers but may be relatively void of prompts to record client beliefs, strengths, resources, hopes, dreams, and practical needs. Including this information on these forms can enhance collaborative care by providing data of value to the entire health care team.

## Summary

This chapter discussed the theoretical concepts related to motivation and adherence, including locus of control, self-efficacy, self-esteem, and the role of important social determinants of health. Strategies to enhance motivation and adherence involved understanding the importance of shared goal setting; developing realistic and functional goals and treatment plans that are relevant, meaningful, and mutually valued by both the clients and the health provider; ensuring that clients understand instructions; developing and adjusting educational programs to meet clients' learning styles; and providing clients with positive feedback. In addition, methods to help clients adjust goals to effectively deal with chronic illness and impairments were presented. Barriers to motivation were discussed, and principles of behavior theory, which may be helpful in modifying health behaviors, were reviewed.

The concept of collaboration was discussed from both client and provider perspectives, and common barriers to collaborative planning were identified. When working with clients, we need to remember that many feel a loss of control as a result of illness or injury. We can empower them by facilitating a move toward independent management of their care. Even if complete independence of a task is not possible, many people are able to direct aides, nurses, therapists, and others to assist in a way that is comfortable for the clients. Regaining control of even small tasks can provide motivation to adhere to established programs so that long-range goals can be realized.

## Reflective Questions

1. Think about a person you know who lacks motivation and has difficulty following through with most things.
   a. What factors do you believe contribute to his or her lack of motivation?
   b. Describe three strategies that might help the person become or stay motivated.
2. a. When do you feel challenged?
   b. What motivates you to keep trying?
   c. What barriers interfere with your motivation?
3. What are some important attitudes and beliefs that you can use to elicit clients' motivation?
4. Think about a health care encounter experienced by you, a friend, or family member that was not client centered. .
   a. How might collaboration have improved the experience?
   b. How might the outcome have been different?
5. How will you respond if a client disagrees with your recommendations?

## Case Study

Russell Lewis is a 14-year-old boy who sustained multiple trauma in a motor vehicle accident. He is quite depressed and refuses to cooperate with treatments. His parents, grandparents, and younger sister are very concerned about his prognosis and make sure that someone is always with him, the grandparents all day and the parents and sister during the evening following work and school. Although the physician informed them that Russell may never walk again, they believe that he will. They are very active in their local church, and the entire congregation is praying for Russell's speedy recovery.

1. Consider the earlier discussion about locus of control.
   a. Where might Russell be at this point in time on the continuum from internal to external locus of control?
   b. What factors form your rationale?
   c. Given the dynamic nature of locus of control and self-efficacy, as well as the specifics of this case, what kinds of interventions might help shift Russell's locus of control in a more positive direction?

**2.** Bandura and others found that clients are most successful in achieving treatment outcomes when goals are specific, challenging, and achievable, and they are afforded the opportunity to practice specific skills.

   a. Develop at least three goals for Russell that meet these criteria.

   b. How will you include Russell in establishing these goals?

**3.** a. What do you think might motivate Russell?

   b. What are some possible barriers to his adherence?

   c. What barriers exist for successful collaboration between Russell and the health care team?

   d. What strategies can you develop to overcome these barriers?

**4.** a. What behavioral techniques could be used with Russell to improve his health care?

   b. What principles support your response?

# References

Abbott, J., Dodd, M., Gee, L., & Webb, K. (2001). Ways of coping with cystic fibrosis: Implications for treatment adherence. *Disability and Rehabilitation, 23*(8), 315–324.

Adams, J., & White, M. (2005). Why don't stage-based activity promotion interventions work? *Health Education Research, 20*(2), 237–243.

Baker, S. M., Marshak, H. H., Rice, G. T., & Zimmerman, G. J. (2001). Patient participation in physical therapy goal setting. *Physical Therapy, 81*(5), 1118–1126.

Bandura, A. (1977). Self-efficacy: Toward a unifying theory of behavioral change. *Psychological Review, 84*(2), 191–215.

Bandura, A. (1997). *Self-efficacy: The exercise of control.* New York, NY: W. H. Freeman.

Barlow, J. H., Macey, S. J., & Struthers, G. R. (1993). Health locus of control, self-help and treatment adherence in relation to ankylosing spondylitis patients. *Patient Education & Counseling, 20*(2–3), 153–166.

Barsa del Alcazar, C. (1998). Spectrum of adherence among hemodialysis patients. *Journal of Nephrology Social Work, 18*, 53–65.

Bassett, S. F., & Prapavessis, H. (2007). Home-based physical therapy intervention with adherence-enhancing strategies versus clinic-based management for patients with ankle sprains. *Physical Therapy, 87*(9), 1132–1143.

Belza, B., Topolski, T., Kinne, S., Patrick, D. L., & Ramsey, S. D. (2002). Does adherence make a difference? Results from a community-based aquatic exercise program. *Nursing Research, 51*(5), 285–291.

Beresford, S. A., Farmer, E. M., Feingold, L., Graves, K. L., Sumner, S. K., & Baker, R. M. (1992). Evaluation of a self-help dietary intervention in a primary care setting. *American Journal of Public Health, 82*, 79–84.

Bernard, B. (1991). The case for peers. *The Peer Facilitator Quarterly, 8*, 20–27.

Bodenheimer, T., Lorig, K., Holman H., & Grumbach, K. (2002). Patient self-management of chronic disease in primary care. *Journal of the American Medical Association, 288*(19), 2469–2475.

Bogardus, S. T., Bradley, E. H., Williams, C. S., Maciejewski, P. K., Gallo, W. T., & Inouye, S. K. (2004). Achieving goals in geriatric assessment: Role of caregiver agreement and adherence to recommendations. *Journal of the American Geriatric Society, 52*(1), 99–105.

Bradley, E., Bogardus, Jr., S., Tinetti, M., & Inouye, S. (1999). Goal-setting in clinical medicine. *Social Science and Medicine, 49*, 267–278.

Brewer, B. W. (1999). Adherence to sport injury rehabilitation regimens. In S. J. Bull, (Ed.), *Adherence issues in sport and exercise.* (pp. 145–168). New York, NY: John Wiley & Sons.

Brewer, B. W., van Raalte, J. L., & Cornelius, A. E. (2000). Psychological factors, rehabilitation adherence, and rehabilitation outcome after anterior cruciate ligament reconstruction. *Rehabilitation Psychology, 45*, 20–37.

Britt E., Hudson, S. M., & Blampied, N. M. (2004). Motivational interviewing in health settings: A review. *Patient Education and Counseling, 53*(2), 147–155.

Brock, S., & Allen, J. (2000). Working with type in health care: Same words, different meanings? *Journal of Psychological Type, 53*, 4–10.

Brodie, D. A., & Inoue, A. (2005). Motivational interviewing to promote physical activity for people with chronic heart failure. *Journal of Advanced Nursing, 50*(5), 518–527.

Brody, L. (2005). Principles of self-management and exercise instruction. In C. M. Hall & L. T. Brody (Eds.), *Therapeutic exercise: Moving toward function* (pp. 35–46). Philadelphia, PA: Lippincott Williams & Wilkins.

Burton, L. C., Shapiro, S. B., & German, P. S. (1999). Determinants of physical activity initiation and maintenance among community-dwelling older persons. *Preventive Medicine, 29,* 422–430.

Bylund, C., & Makoul, G. (2002). Empathic communication and gender in the physician–patient encounter. *Patient Education and Counseling, 48,* 207–216.

Campbell, R., Evans, M., Tucker, M., Quilty, B., Dieppe, P., & Donovan, J. L. (2001). Why don't patients do their exercises? Understanding non-compliance with physiotherapy in patients with osteoarthritis of the knee. *Journal of Epidemiology and Community Health, 55,* 132–138.

Chinman, M. J., Allende, M., Weingarten, R., Steiner, J., Tworkowski, S., & Davidson, L. (1999). On the road to collaborative treatment planning: Consumer and provider perspectives. *Journal of Behavioral Health Services and Research, 26*(2), 211–218.

Chipperfield, J. G., & Perry, R. P. (2006). Primary and secondary control-enhancing strategies in later life: Predicting hospital outcomes in men and women. *Health Psychology, 25*(2), 226–236.

Coleman, E. A., Hall-Barrow, J., Coon, S., & Stewart, C. B. (2003). Facilitating exercise adherence for patients with multiple myeloma. *Clinical Journal of Oncology Nursing, 7*(5), 529–534,540.

Colombo, R., Pisano, F., Mazzone, A., Delconte, C., Micera, S., Carrozza, M. C., . . . Minuco, G. (2007). Design strategies to improve patient motivation during robot-aided rehabilitation. *Journal of Neuroengineering and Rehabilitation, 19*(4), 3.

Conn, V. S. (1998). Older adults and exercise: Path analysis of self-efficacy related constructs. *Nursing Research, 47,* 180–189.

Cott, C., & Finch, E. (1991). Goal-setting in physical therapy practice. *Physiotherapy Canada, 43*(1), 19–22.

Coughlin, A. M., Bandura, A. S., Fleischer, T. D., & Guck, T. P. (2000). Multidisciplinary treatment of chronic pain patients: Its efficacy in changing patient locus of control. *Archives of Physical Medicine and Rehabilitation, 81,* 739–740.

Coyne C. (2008). Video "games" in the clinic: PTs report early results. *PT–Magazine of Physical Therapy,, 16*(5), 22–28.

Daily Mock, K. (2001). Effective clinician–patient communication. *Physician's News Digest.* Retrieved from http://www.physiciansnews.com/law/201.html

DeSousa, A. (2008). Psychological issues in oral and maxillofacial reconstructive surgery. *British Journal of Oral and Maxillofacial Surgery, 46*(8), 661–664.

DiMatteo, M. R. (2004a). Social support and patient adherence to medical treatment: A meta-analysis. *Health Psychology, 23*(2), 207–218.

DiMatteo, M. R. (2004b). Variations in patients' adherence to medical recommendations: A quantitative review of 50 years of research. *Medical Care, 42*(3), 200–209.

Duncan, K. A., & Pozehl, B. (2002). Staying on course: The effects of an adherence facilitation intervention on home exercise participation. *Progress in Cardiovascular Nursing, 17*(2), 59–65, 71.

Engstrom, L. O., & Oberg, B. (2005). Patient adherence in an individualized rehabilitation programme: A clinical follow-up. *Scandinavian Journal of Public Health, 33*(1), 11–18.

Gatchel, R. J. (2004). Psychosocial factors that can influence the self-assessment of function. *Journal of Occupational Rehabilitation, 14*(3), 197–206.

Goudas, M., Minardou, K., & Kotis, J. (2000). Feedback regarding goal achievement and intrinsic motivation. *Perceptual and Motor Skills, 90,* 810–812.

Green, C. A., Polen, M. R., Janoff, S. L., Castleton, D. K., Wisdom, J. P., Vuckovic, N., . . . Oken, S. L. (2008). Understanding how clinician–patient relationships and relational continuity of care affect recovery from serious mental illness: STARS study results. *Psychiatric Rehabilitation Journal, 32*(1), 9–22.

Greenfield, B. H., Anderson, A., Cox, B., & Tanner, M. C. (2008). Meaning of caring to 7 novice physical therapists during their first year of clinical practice. *Physical Therapy, 88*(10), 1154–1166.

Guay, F., Vallerand, R. J., & Blanchard, C. (2000). On the assessment of situational intrinsic and extrinsic motivation: The Situational Motivational Scale (SIMS). *Motivation and Emotion, 24,* 175–213.

Hall, L. K. (1999). Health and disease management: Expanding the cardiac and pulmonary rehabilitation model. *Clinical Exercise Physiology, 1*(1), 42–46.

Hartigan, C., Rainville, J., Sobel, J., & Hipona, M. (2000). Long-term exercise adherence after intensive rehabilitation for chronic low back pain. *Medicine & Science in Sports & Exercise, 32*(3), 551–555.

Haynes, R. B., McKibbon, K. A., & Kanani, R. (1996). Systematic review of randomised trials of interventions to assist patients to follow prescriptions for medication. *Lancet, 348*(10), 383–386.

Heisler, M., Bouknight, R. R., Hayward, R. A., Smith, D. M., & Kerr, E. A. (2002). The relative importance of physician communication, participatory decision-making and patient understanding in diabetes self-management. *Journal of General Internal Medicine, 17*(4), 243–252.

Herborg, H., Haugbolle, L. S., Sorensen, L., Rossing, C., & Dam, P. (2008). Developing a generic, individualised adherence programme for chronic medication users. *Pharmacy Practice, 6*(3), 148–157.

Hirano, P. C., Laurent, D. D., & Lorig, K. (1994). Arthritis patient education studies, 1987–1991: A review of the literature. *Patient Education Counseling, 24,* 9–54.

Hussey, L. C., & Gilliland, K. (1989). Compliance, low literacy, and locus of control. *Nursing Clinics of North America, 24,* 605–611.

Ignacio-Garcia, J. M., & Gonzalez-Santos, P. (1995). Asthma self-management education program by home monitoring of peak expiratory flow. *American Journal of Respiratory and Critical Care Medicine, 151*(2), 353–359.

Jensen, G. M., Gwyer, J., Shepard, K. F., & Hack, L. M. (2000). Expert practice in physical therapy. *Physical Therapy, 80*(1), 28–43.

Jensen, G. M., & Lorish, C. D. (2005). Promoting patient cooperation with exercise programs: Linking research, theory, and practice. *Arthritis Care & Research, 7*(4), 181–189.

Jones, J., & Kovalcik, E. (1988). Goal-setting: A method to help clients escape the negative effects of stress. *Stress Reduction, 83*(1), 257–261.

Kearney, M. K., Weininger, R. B., Vachon, M. L. S., Harrison, R. L., & Mount, B. M. (2009). Self-care of physicians caring for patients at the end of life. *Journal of the American Medical Association, 301*(11), 1155–1164.

King, G., Strachan, D., Tucker, M., Duwyn, B., Desserud, S., & Shillington, M. (2009). The application of a transdisciplinary model for early intervention services. *Infants & Young Children, 22*(3), 211–223.

King, M. B., Whipple, R. H., & Gruman, C. A., Judge, J. O., Schmidt, J. A., & Wolfson, L. I. (2002). The Performance Enhancement Project: Improving physical performance in older persons. *Archives of Physical Medicine and Rehabilitation, 83,* 1060–1069.

Lawler, J., Dowswell, G., Hearn, J., Forster, A., & Young, J. (1999). Recovering from stroke: A qualitative investigation of the role of goal-setting in late stroke recovery. *Journal of Advanced Nursing, 30*(2), 401–409.

Lawrence, G. (1997). *Looking at type and learning styles.* Gainesville, FL: Center for Applications of Psychological Type.

Levensky, E. R., Forcehimes, A., O'Donohue, W. T., & Beitz, K. (2007). Motivational interviewing: An evidenced-based approach to counseling helps patients follow treatment recommendations. *American Journal of Nursing, 107*(10), 50–58.

Lewin, K., Dembo, T., Festinger, L., & Sears, P. S. (1944). Level of aspiration. In J. M. Hunt (Ed.), *Personality and the behavior disorders: A handbook based on experimental and clinical research* (pp. 333–378). New York, NY: Ronald Press.

Locke, E. A., Shaw, K. N., Saari, L. M., & Latham, G. P. (1981). Goal-setting and task performance. *Psychological Bulletin, 90*(1), 125–152.

Lorish, C. D., & Gale, J. R. (1999). Facilitating behavior change: Strategies for education and practice. *Journal of Physical Therapy Education, 13*(3), 31–37.

Lorish, C. D., & Gale, J. R. (2002). Facilitating adherence to healthy lifestyle behavior changes in patients. In K. F. Shepard & G. M. Jensen (Eds.), *Handbook of teaching for physical therapists* (2nd ed., pp. 351–385). Boston, MA: Butterworth-Heinemann.

Maciejewski, P. K., Prigerson, H. G., & Mazure, C. (2000). Self-efficacy as a mediator between stressful life events and depressive symptoms. *British Journal of Psychiatry, 176,* 373–378.

Mailloux, J., Finno, M., & Rainville, J. (2006). Long-term exercise adherence in the elderly with chronic low back pain. *American Journal of Physical Medicine and Rehabilitation, 85*(2), 120–126.

Marchese, V., Rai, S., Carlson, C., Hinds, P., Spearing, E., Zhang, L., . . . Ginsberg, J. (2007). Assessing functional mobility in survivors of lower-extremity sarcoma: Reliability and validity of a new assessment tool. *Pediatric Blood Cancer, 49*(2), 183–189.

McDonald, H. P., Garg, A. X., & Haynes, R. B. (2002). Interventions to enhance patient adherence to medication prescriptions. *Journal of the American Medical Association, 288,* 2868–2879.

Meyer, T. J., & Mark, M. M. (1995). Effects of psychosocial interventions with adult cancer patients: A meta-analysis of randomized experiments. *Health Psychology, 14,* 101–108.

Miller, W. R. (1983). Motivational interviewing with problem drinkers. *Behavioural Psychotherapy, 11,* 147–172.

Miller, W. R., & Rollnick, S. (1995). What is motivational interviewing? *Behavioural and Cognitive Psychotherapy, 23,* 325–334.

Miller, W. R., & Rollnick, S. (2002). *Motivational interviewing: Preparing people for change* (2nd ed.). New York, NY: Guilford Press.

Moore, J. E., von Korff, M., Cherkin, D., Saunders, K., & Lorig, K. (2000). A randomized trial of a cognitive behavioral program for enhancing back pain self care in a primary care setting. *Pain, 88*(2), 145–153.

Mostrom, E., & Shepard, K. F. (1999). Teaching and learning about patient education in physical therapy professional preparation: Academic and clinical considerations. *Journal of Physical Therapy Education, 13*(3), 8–17.

Mulvaney, S. A. (2009). Improving patient problem-solving to reduce barriers to diabetes self-management. *Clinical Diabetes, 27*(3), 99–104.

Oberle, K. (1991). A decade of research in locus of control: What have we learned? *Journal of Advanced Nursing, 16,* 800–806.

Ott, C. D., Lindsey, A. M., Waltman, N. L., Gross, G. J., Twiss, J. J., Berg, K., . . . Henricksen, S. (2004). Facilitative strategies, psychological factors, and strength/weight training behaviors in breast cancer survivors who are at risk for osteoporosis. *Orthopedic Nursing, 23*(1), 45–52.

Pampallona, S., Bollini, P., Tibaldi, G., Kupelnick, B., & Munizza, C. (2002). Patient adherence in the treatment of depression. *British Journal of Psychiatry, 180,* 104–109.

Penza-Clyve, S. M., Mansell, C., & McQuaid, E. L. (2004). Why don't children take their asthma medications? A qualitative analysis of children's perspectives on adherence. *Journal of Asthma, 41*(2), 189–197.

Platt, F. W., Gaspar, D. L., Coulehan, J. L., Fox, L., Adler, A. J. , Weston, W. W., . . . Stewart, M. (2001). "Tell me about yourself": The patient-centered interview. *Annals of Internal Medicine, 134*(11), 1079–1085.

Playford, E. D., Dawson, L., Limbert, V., Smith, M., Ward, C. D., & Wells, R. (2000). Goal-setting in rehabilitation: Report of a workshop to explore professionals' perceptions of goal-setting. *Clinical Rehabilitation, 14*(5), 491–496.

Price-Lackey, P., & Cashman, J. (1996). Jenny's story: Reinventing oneself through occupation and narrative configuration. *American Journal of Occupational Therapy, 50*(4), 306–314.

Prochaska, J. O., DiClimente, C. C. & Norcross, J. C. (1992). In search of how people change. *American Psychologist, 47,* 1102–1104.

Prochaska, J. O., Redding, C. A., & Evers, K. E. (2002). The transtheoretical model and stages of change. In K. Glanz, B. Rimer, & Lewis F. M. (Eds.), *Health behavior and health education: Theory, research, and practice* (3rd ed., pp. 99–116). San Francisco, CA: Jossey Bass.

Prochaska, J. O., & Velicer, W. F. (1997). The transtheoretical model of health behavior change. *American Journal of Health Promotion, 12*(1), 38–48.

Rand, C. S. (1993). Measuring adherence with therapy for chronic diseases: Implications for the treatment of heterozygous familial hypercholesterolemia. *American Journal of Cardiology, 72,* 68D–74D.

Randall, K. E., & McEwen, I. R. (2000). Writing patient-centered functional goals. *Physical Therapy, 80*(12), 1197–1203.

Rapport, M. J., McWilliams, R. A., & Smith, B. J. (2004). Practices across disciplines in early intervention: The research base. *Infants & Young Children, 17*(1), 32–44.

Resnick, B., Palmer, M. H., Jenkins, L. S., & Spellbring, A. M. (2000). Path analysis of efficacy expectations and exercise behavior in older adults. *Journal of Advanced Nursing, 31*(6), 1309–1315.

Resnick, B., & Spellbring, A. M. (2000). Understanding what motivates older adults to exercise. *Journal of Gerontological Nursing, 26,* 34–42.

Resnicow, K., Dilorio, C., Soet, J. E., Borelli, B., Hecht, J., & Ernst, D. (2002). Motivational interviewing in health promotion: It sounds like something is changing. *Health Psychology, 21*(5), 444–451.

Robinson-Smith, G., Johnston, M. V., & Allen, J. (2000). Self-care, self-efficacy, quality of life and depression after stroke. *Archives of Physical Medicine and Rehabilitation, 81,* 460–464.

Rollnick, S., Miller, W. R., Butler, C. C., & Aloia, M. S. (2008). Motivational interviewing in health care: Helping patients change behavior. *Journal of Chronic Obstructive Pulmonary Disease, 5*(3), 203–205.

Rone-Adams, S. A., Stern, D. F., & Walker, V. (2004). Stress and compliance with a home exercise program among caregivers of children with disabilities. *Pediatric Physical Therapy, 16,* 140–148.

Rosenstock, I. M. (1966). Why people use health services. *Milbank Memorial Fund Quarterly, 44,* 94–127.

Rotter, J. B. (1966). Generalized expectancies for internal versus external control of reinforcement. *Psychological Monographs, General and Applied, 80,* 1–28.

Schenkman, M., Hall, D., Kumar, R., & Kohrt, W. M. (2008). Endurance exercise training to improve economy of movement of people with Parkinson disease: Three case reports. *Physical Therapy, 88*(1), 63–76.

Schroeder, K., Fahey, T., & Ebrahim, S. (2004). How can we improve adherence to blood pressure-lowering medication in ambulatory care? Systematic review of randomized controlled trials. *Archives of Internal Medicine, 164,* 722–732.

Sherman, B. R., Sanders, L. M., & Yearde, J. (1998). Role-modeling healthy behavior: Peer counseling for pregnant and post-partum women in recovery. *Women's Health Issues, 8*(4), 230–238.

Shinitzky, H. E., & Kub, J. (2001). The art of motivating behavior change: The use of motivational interviewing to promote health. *Public Health Nursing, 18*(3), 178–185.

Skinner, T. C. (2004). Psychological barriers. *European Journal of Endocrinology, 151*(Suppl. 2), T13–T17.

Sluijs, E. (1991). *Patient education in physical therapy.* Utrecht, Netherlands: Nederlands Institut voor Onderzoek Van de Eerstel I jnsgezondheidszorg NIVEL.

Sluijs, E. M., Kok, G. J., & van der Zee, J. (1993). Correlates of exercise compliance in physical therapy. *Physical Therapy, 73,* 771–782.

Stelzner, D. M., Rodriguez, J. W., Krapfl, B., Jordan, S. L., & Schenkman, M. L. (2003). *Instructor's adherence protocol: Instructor's guidelines for assisting participants.* Denver: Physical Therapy Program, University of Colorado at Denver and Health Sciences Center.

Sweeney, S., Taylor, G., & Calin, A. (2002). The effect of a home based exercise intervention package on outcome in ankylosing spondylitis: A randomized controlled trial. *Journal of Rheumatology, 29,* 763–766.

Symister, P., & Friend, R. (2003). The influence of social support and problematic support on optimism and depression in chronic illness: A prospective study evaluating self-esteem as a mediator. *Journal of Health Psychology, 22*(3), 123–129.

Taylor, A. H., & May, S. (1996).Threat and coping appraisal as determinants of compliance with sports injury rehabilitation: An application of protection motivation theory. *Journal of Sports Science, 14,* 471–482.

Toomey, T. C., Mann, J. D., Abashian, S., & Thompson-Pope, S. (1991). Relationship between perceived self-control of pain, pain description, and functioning. *Pain, 45,* 129–133.

Treichler, D. G. (1967). Are you missing the boat in training aids? In *Audiovisual communications.* New York, NY: United Business Publications.

Turner, G. (1999). Peer support and young people's health. *Journal of Adolescence, 22,* 567–572.

Vanderhoff, M. (2005). Patient education and health literacy. *PT–Magazine of Physical Therapy, 13*(9), 42–46.

Veenhof, C., van Hasselt, T. J., Koke, A. J., Dekker, J., Bijlsma, J. W., & van den Ende, C. H. (2006). Active involvement and long-term goals influence long-term adherence to behavioural graded activity in patients with osteoarthritis: A qualitative study. *Australian Journal of Physiotherapy, 52*(4), 273–278.

von Korff, M., Gruman, J., Schaefer, J., Curry, S. J., & Wagner, E. H. (1997). Collaborative management of chronic illness. *Annals of Internal Medicine, 127*(12), 1097–1102.

Wallston, K. A. (1992). Hocus-pocus, the focus isn't strictly on locus: Rotter's social learning theory modified for health. *Cognitive Therapy and Research, 16*(2), 182–199.

Weingarten, S. R., Henning, J. M., Badamgarav, E., Knught, K., Hasselblad, V., Gano, Jr., A., & Ofman, J. J. (2002). Interventions used in disease management programmes for patients with chronic illness—which ones work? Meta-analysis of published reports. *British Medical Journal, 325,* 925.

West, D. S., DiLillo, V., Bursac, Z., Gore, S. A., & Greene, P. G. (2007). Motivational interviewing improves weight loss in women with type 2 diabetes. *Diabetes Care, 30*(5), 1081–1087.

White III, A. A., Hill, J. A., Mackel, A. M., Rowley, D. L., Rickards, E. P., & Jenkins, B. (2007). The relevance of culturally competent care in orthopaedics to outcomes and health care disparities. *Journal of Bone and Joint Surgery, American Volume, 89*(6), 1379–1384.

Woodard, C. M., & Berry, M. J. (2001). Enhancing adherence to prescribed exercise: Structured behavioral interventions in clinical exercise programs. *Journal of Cardiopulmonary Rehabilitation, 21,* 201–209.

Woolf, S. H. (2008). The power of prevention and what it requires. *Journal of the American Medical Association, 299*(20), 2437–2439.

Woolf, S. H. (2009). Social policy as health policy. *Journal of the American Medical Association, 301*(11), 1166–1169.

World Health Organization. (2003). Adherence to long-term therapies: Evidence for action. In *Noncommunicable diseases and mental health adherence to long-term therapies project.* Geneva, Switzerland: Author.

Wrosch, C., Heckhausen, J., & Lachman, M. E. (2000). Primary and secondary control strategies for managing health and financial stress across adulthood. *Psychology and Aging, 15*(3), 387–399.

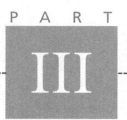

PART

III

# Loss/Grief, Coping, and Family

# Loss and Grief

My client Anita had a miscarriage, and it was an early miscarriage at that. I don't want to seem insensitive, but it's not like she lost an actual baby. You should have seen her. She was hysterical! On her follow-up appointment today, she was in the throes of grief. If anyone has a reason to grieve like that, it would be my other client Priscilla. I can't even imagine carrying a baby to term and then discovering that the umbilical cord had become wrapped around a foot. I still don't understand why the doctor kept her in the hospital for 12 hours, with a dead baby inside of her, before finally delivering it.
—*From the journal of Linda Whitehead, nursing student*

Who can say which loss is more valid? A response to a loss is influenced by how people perceive the loss and the meaning they attach to what is lost. Although reactions to loss are as unique as the people who experience it, the process of grieving is a universal and natural phenomenon. Linda Whitehead, the nursing student who wrote this journal entry, is only partially right. Stillbirth *and* miscarriage both initiate feelings of despair and confusion, just at the vulnerable moment when families are expecting happiness. Far more is lost than the loss of the awaited child. Perinatal loss results in the loss of dreams, self-esteem, the parental role, and the confidence in the ability to create and deliver a healthy baby (Weiss, Frischer, & Richman, 1989).

This chapter begins our discussion of the continuum of loss, grieving, and coping, which will be continued in the following chapter. It explores loss and grieving from the perspective of the "three D's"—disease, disability, and death—and recognizes loss, grieving, and coping as a process rather than finite stages.

## UNDERSTANDING LOSS

By the time we assume our professional roles, we have experienced many changes, which we often perceive as losses. To the adage that "the only constants in life are death and taxes," we can add loss. People experience "separations and departures from those we love, our conscious and unconscious losses of romantic dreams, impossible expectations, illusions of freedom and power, illusions of safety—and the loss of our own younger self, the self that thought it always would be unwrinkled and invulnerable and immortal" (Viorst, 1986, p. 2).

As health care professionals, we do not always understand the meaning and value that loss of health or function holds for both the client and those who provide personal support. We may not value the need for a client to have a support system. Do we focus on a "cure," thereby giving credence to what Siegal (1986) calls a "failure orientation?" He believes that many physicians focus on physiology and overlook the impact that the client's attitude has on the outcome of treatment and the quality of life. If we believe in the primacy of the medical model, do we overlook clients' needs and desires in our goal setting and treatment intervention?

Oncologists who self-described using principally a biomedical model felt more detached from patients, felt ineffective at not being able to improve their circumstances, and experienced a lack of support from colleagues (Jackson et al., 2008). They did not believe they could influence how clients and their families coped with impending death and, consequently, offered little information about treatment options. However, oncologists who incorporated a biomedical *and* a psychosocial model found that end-of-life care was gratifying, and they communicated more freely, accepting the progression.

Hospice clients in the terminal phase of their illnesses benefit from palliative care, not a "cure" mentality. They will not have the same therapeutic goals as clients with short-term, reversible problems. Comfort measures, rather than aggressive medical therapies, form the plan of care. Health professionals need to adjust their sights and goals accordingly to deal with individuals' losses.

Many insights in health care are afoot, but people's attitudes are still slow to change. In the 1960s, sociologist Coser (1963) reported that nurses were strongly influenced by the medical model's orientation toward cure. Nurses in a rehabilitative setting were professionally stimulated by the therapeutic goals of helping clients achieve positive outcomes and return home. Their work afforded them a measure of self-esteem and satisfaction. In contrast, nurses working with clients who were terminally ill or who had custodial needs did not derive professional gratification or self-esteem. Rather than being challenged by the different goals and needs, these nurses perceived their work as mechanical and routine. They did not experience the same degree of involvement with the clients. In *today's* health care arena, *some* things have changed. Contemporary studies recognize that the prospect of progressive debilitation and dependency on a caregiver add to the anguish of clients with advanced diseases who are facing death (Cheville, 2000). The health care team can work to mitigate these issues. Many of these same concerns also apply to losses other than death.

### Types of Loss

Illness takes its toll on the body. *Loss of health*, even in small degrees, can result in changes, such as those in the musculoskeletal, neurological, and pulmonary systems. Muscle strength, coordination, endurance, and balance may be partially or completely lost. Loss of bowel and bladder function diminishes personal control and may affect one's social activities. One loss often leads to additional losses. Clients with diabetes, for instance, may face the loss of extremities that would impact mobility and independence. Life partners of people with Alzheimer's disease have a loss of mutuality and the relationship they once knew (Garner, 1997), even before they face the loss of life.

Memory, cognitive, and intellectual losses and functional limitations may have a negative impact on social roles, self-esteem, and independence. For example, people who have had a cerebrovascular accident (stroke) may have difficulty going outside their homes, walking and communicating as they once did, and participating in the leisure activities that they enjoyed prior to the neurological insult. They may experience confusion and deteriorating memory. Activities of daily living, such as washing, bathing, and dressing, may pose additional problems. All of these changes can result in losses of freedom, social contact, and the once-valued roles they previously held (Pound, Gompertz, & Ebrahim, 1998).

The *loss of these social roles* is also a reflection of a *loss of autonomy*, which negatively influences personal decision making and control of one's life. Cancer, for example, can result in a loss of occupational identity, control, and "normalcy," which can lead to anxiety and depression (Peteet, 2000). There may also be concerns about the side effects and efficacy of treatment. Many clients are distressed by the possibility of uncontrolled pain. This is actually two blended issues, pain and loss of control. Fears are related to the loss of autonomy, as well as impending isolation (Breitbart, Chochinov, & Passik, 1998). Sometimes, it feels like there is little "choice" to be made between certain death and the acceptance of painful, debilitating cancer treatments. In addition, clients consider the "loss of the ability to do what one wants" a significant issue (Axelsson & Sjoden, 1998). These losses can be sufficiently distressing for the person to consider suicide or assisted suicide (Breitbart, 1990; Breitbart & Rosenfeld, 1999; Fairclough, 1998).

Although some losses are expected, predictable, and integral parts of life and growth, others are not. Losses may be *sudden*, like a child flying over a bicycle's handlebars, hitting the pavement, and sustaining a traumatic brain injury. Others are *gradual*, like the progressive loss of function, speech, and breathing of amyotrophic lateral sclerosis, commonly known as Lou Gehrig's disease, or ALS. Some losses are *anticipated* because the disease process is more predictable, such as in cystic fibrosis. Others are associated with *uncertainty*, as in the form of multiple sclerosis characterized by remissions and exacerbations.

Loss may be *total*, like the death of a loved one or the anticipated death of oneself. It may be *partial*, like a severely damaged rotator cuff in a pitcher's shoulder. Loss may also be *permanent*, like the paralysis resulting from a complete spinal cord injury, or *temporary*, like the paralysis often seen in the neurological syndrome Guillain-Barré.

*Age-related* changes in function represent another type of loss. Even a healthy older person experiences alterations in hearing, vision, and the musculoskeletal system. Osteoarthritis, for example, is a significant source of disability and functional limitation in older people (Burke & Flaherty, 1993). In older people with declining physical health, there can also be a loss of vitality, increased risk of disease, and fear of falling.

A person can lose *external objects*, such as one's home. A move to an assisted environment, when a person is no longer able to independently function in his or her home, is a loss. In addition to the physical loss of the home and all of the memories associated with it, this may also be a symbolic loss, representing loss of some aspect of oneself. Perhaps it is loss of personal *freedom and control, self-worth*, or *life role*, such as that of breadwinner or head of the household.

*Primary internal losses* can result in secondary external losses. For example, a person who is diagnosed with acquired immune deficiency syndrome (AIDS) may experience physical and/or mental deterioration (primary loss), which necessitates assistance from others. Even with legislation to protect people's rights, the person with AIDS may face many *secondary losses*, such as employment, residence, and insurance, as a result of the primary loss. Although new and effective treatments have helped some people return to the workforce, employment may no longer be possible for others. Loss of friends and family may occur. Social isolation may become a factor due to the stigma and discrimination that still surround this medical disease. People with other chronic conditions also face many of these same issues.

We see physical, psychological, symbolic, or a combination of these types of losses in clients with whom we work, secondary to their pathology and injuries. As a result of their losses, they may encounter additional losses in independence, body parts or function, and a sense of wholeness (Drench, 1995). These losses disrupt a person's present time frame and can have far-reaching effects, not only on the individual but also on their friends and family members. The losses also change the future that the person had envisioned.

*Chronic medical conditions* require long-term management (refer to Chapter 11). They tend to affect mental health, although the level of psychological distress varies with the type of condition and the individual person. Hearing and vision impairments, neurological, pulmonary, and cardiac diseases, and chronic pain conditions have strong correlations with psychological distress, perceptions of disability, and, to a lesser extent, with a sense of capability and competency (Ormel et al., 1997).

The sustained or relapsing aspects of chronic conditions can be wearing on an individual and may directly lead to depression. In addition, this depression can also be *indirectly* exacerbated by the effect that a chronic condition has on relationships, occupational changes, and emotional and economic status. Diminished self-esteem, personal control, and mastery can also indirectly fuel depression (Vilhjalmsson, 1998). For example, people with lymphedema experienced increased feelings of depression, with some reporting, " I have become withdrawn because I feel like a freak when I go outside" and "Lymphedema has ended the life I once had and has given me a sad life" (Maxeiner, Saga, Downer, & Arthur, 2009, p. 14).

Any type of psychological distress is influenced by the loss of resources associated with a chronic medical condition. In addition, the severity of the disability can also be a factor, with more severe conditions creating greater psychological distress. Finally, the psychological attributes of the client play a role in the degree of distress that is experienced. Those who are able to adopt effective long-term coping strategies generally experience less psychological distress. The idea of a condition or disease being chronic means that the people involved would have to make long-term adjustments.

A nurse told a client that his AIDS was now considered a chronic, rather than terminal, disease. She indicated that he could live with this for a long time instead of dying "within a month or two, like it had been in the early days of the disease. You can live with the idea of a chronic disease because it means you can live" (Drench, 1998, p. 137). Helping the client to understand the diagnosis and prognosis facilitates adaptation and coping.

Some chronic conditions can have positive manifestations. Following a stroke, a person faces unfamiliar restrictions and losses and may experience sorrow. Yet, hope for the strength to endure the situation can entwine with dreams of what may come. Perspective can change, and the person may appreciate life in a different light. Suddenly, the ordinary in life is not so "ordinary." In addition, nurturing relationships can be supportive and give the person a much-needed boost (Pilkington, 1999).

People with acquired hearing losses, which are common long-term conditions, may perceive a loss of control caused by insecurity in social encounters (Eriksson-Mangold & Carlsson, 1991). Yet, some people integrate the hearing loss into their lives, making the necessary lifestyle changes (Herth, 1998). This calls for modifying one's perspective on life and making some practical accommodations, such as minimizing distracting sounds and positioning oneself to read lips or hear to one's best advantage. However, not everyone is willing or able to make accommodations. Some people react with strong feelings of fear and sadness, which can produce a stress response.

Mrs. Williams is 60 years old. She's absolutely beside herself! I saw her today in the clinic, and she continued to complain about dizziness and ringing in her right ear. She says that she doesn't sleep well, has increasing headaches, and can't concentrate on her bridge game. She feels like she's not fun to be with any more, not even for herself. She feels like her quality of life is going down the tubes, and I feel so helpless. I wish there were some things I could do to support her.

*—From the journal of Robert Evans, audiology student*

Perceptions about loss of control, fear of serious illness, and anticipation of a severe episode of vertigo (dizziness) may be associated with an intensifying cycle of vertigo, anxiety, and restriction of activity (Yardley, 1994). The frequency of headaches is significantly related to the severity of the tinnitus (ringing in the ears), which strongly correlates to perceived attitudes (Erlandsson, Hallberg, & Axelsson, 1992). If the health professional can help Mrs. Williams alter her perceptions, perhaps the relationship between the audiological and psychological issues, dizziness, headaches, and tinnitus may be modified. A person's perceptions and feelings can often influence how he or she copes, grieves, and adjusts to a loss.

In some conditions, the precipitating loss is not chronic, but the resulting feelings may become long lasting. In an *acute loss*, low self-esteem and loss of personal control can become *chronic feelings*. These perceptions of inadequacy, which can include feeling anxious and depressed, are directly proportional to the intensity of stress, bereavement, and psychological suffering. If not addressed, they can last for years or even a lifetime. For example, 4 years after perinatal loss of a baby due to congenital abnormalities, parents can continue to experience these feelings (Hunfeld, Wladimiroff, & Passchier, 1997), a phenomenon known as *chronic sorrow*. This is not unusual, as we will discuss later.

In many situations where loss is involved, the impact on the client and family is uncertain and unclear. *Ambiguous loss* (Boss, 1999; Boss & Couden, 2002) is a phenomenon in which, for example, a person may exist physically but not cognitively, such as in dementia or in the terminal phase of life, and their life roles may dramatically fluctuate or completely change. The person can be there but not "really" there or not be the person he or she and others knew. In addition, people can be so preoccupied with pain or taking care of illness or disability that they are no longer engaged in employment or other life activities. Some physical pathologies have unclear prognoses, no cure, "mystery" diagnoses, or cause abilities and symptoms to vary.

This ambiguity impacts the client, family, and all relationships and can result in anxiety, depression, hopelessness, and loss of control, which can thwart grieving for and coping with losses. Decision making and day-to-day plans and activities are often in limbo. Boss and Couden (2002) include examples of the husband with "so much pain all the time that he is emotionally unreachable," the wife who is "no longer interested in sex" following a hysterectomy, and the parent who "no longer wants to talk to the children" once he or she has become terminally ill with cancer (p. 1352).

## LOSS FOR THE PERSONAL CAREGIVER

Health care providers should realize that the individual personally facing the illness or injury is not the only one experiencing loss. Often, clients' significant others—those we expect to administer medications, perform home care procedures, and enforce exercise regimens—are also grieving. Sadly, the needs of this group are often neglected.

Regardless of whether caregivers are siblings, sons or daughters, nieces or nephews, friends, or other relation, they, too, may endure this kind of personal loss and grief. Family and friends may also experience a loss of future dreams, such as retirement strategies, travel plans, and social lives. In addition, they tend to lose part of themselves in their role as caregiver, as they become enmeshed in attending to the needs of the other person (Loos & Bowd, 1997). White and Grenyer (1999) report that clients with end-stage renal disease experience feelings of anger, depression, and hopelessness, whereas their partners feel sadness, resentment, guilt, and loss.

Personal caregivers can face significant losses. Mothers whose children sustain traumatic brain injuries have to deal with grief over the loss of the child they knew, the effects on their own health, the short- and long-term impact on their family, and changing roles within the family, all while trying to cope with the losses the child has sustained and coordinating services (Clark, Stedmon, & Margison, 2008).

Sirki, Saarinen-Pihkala, and Hovi (2000) noted similar findings among family members who lost children after terminal care and those during active anticancer therapy. Parents report physical and mental problems with similar frequency, self-reported recovery times, and times for returning to work. Mothers need longer recovery times and greater intervals of time before returning to work than do fathers. Siblings of children who die during active anticancer therapy have more difficulties than brothers and sisters of children who die after terminal care. Their issues include fear, behavioral and social problems, and problems associated with school. The good news is in knowing that mothers, fathers, brothers, and sisters of children who die (from cancer) have the ability to move through the grieving process and recover. They are, however, forever changed.

Bobby threw his sister's stuffed bears against the walls and on the floor. He was yelling, "She wasn't supposed to die! All those months of throwing up. Going bald. Missing school. It seems like Mom and Dad spent years at the hospital with her, while the rest of us tried not to feel ignored. They said we should understand. It was temporary. She'd get better, and everything would be back to normal. The leukemia would be history. Well, it's not! Things will never be normal again." I let Bobby rant until he collapsed in my arms. We sat on the floor and wept together.

—*From the journal of Sanjay Patel, nursing student*

Grieving for loss, whether it is disability or death related, is a necessary and difficult process, one that can put people at a higher risk for their own illness, such as poorer perceived health, health-risk behaviors, anxiety, and depression symptoms (Beach, Schulz, Yee, & Jackson, 2000; Evans, Bishop, & Ousley, 1992; Smith et al., 2004). For instance, in one study, caregivers of people who had experienced a stroke 1 year earlier were more anxious than depressed but were still willing to provide care; coping strategies were ineffective (Smith et al., 2004).

Positive outcomes are possible (Folkman & Moskowitz, 2000). Men who provided care for people with AIDS and had greater degrees of social coping and positive affect had fewer physical symptoms than those with lower degrees of social coping and a negative affect; in contrast, those who had greater cognitive avoidance had the opposite consequence (Billings, Folkman, Acree, & Moskowitz, 2000). Relationships within the family are often a powerful source of support for those providing care to people with disabilities, regardless of the nature of the disability, and can strengthen over time (Evans et al., 1992). Loss and grief can also have positive outcomes for those whose family members and friends die, by giving them the "gifts" of a clearer appreciation for their own lives and the lesson to enjoy themselves (Lev & McCorkle, 1998). A psychiatric nurse said, "I see people every day who wish that they could go back in time and have moments to live over again or wish they could have done things differently" (Drench, 1998, p. 172). A developing sense of gratitude and a healthy perspective about life are often part of the legacy left behind.

Grief holds possibilities for empowering people to grow and mature, but again, it can be a double-edged sword. Psychiatrist Viktor Frankl (1984), who survived the concentration camps of Auschwitz and Dachau during World War II, asserts that despair can occur when people suffer and perceive no meaning in the experience. However, a painful and lingering experience *can* facilitate self-discovery of one's deepest beliefs and overturn negative experiences. He also asserts that grief does not cause pain; rather, it is grief without meaning that causes pain. Perhaps that is one of the motivators for those who have loved ones who are ill, have a disability, or have died to join or initiate activities or foundations, such as the many fund-raising walks supporting illnesses or the National Cristina Foundation, which provides donated computer technology to people with differing abilities. Created by Bruce McMahan, it was inspired by his daughter Cristina, who has cerebral palsy and had difficulty writing in school.

## LOSS FOR THE HEALTH CARE PROFESSIONAL

Mrs. Moriarty was a pale, shrinking form, lying in a sea of white sheets. We were working so hard to wean her off the ventilator, at first for only moments at a time. Finally, success! I felt strong and empowered. When she died, I was crushed. After work, I cried on the bus the whole way home.

—*From the journal of Dinah Rogers, respiratory therapy student*

Dinah's reflections illustrate that health care providers also experience loss. Oncology nurses, for example, who frequently confront different kinds of losses, have high levels of despair, social isolation, and somatization (Feldstein & Gemma, 1995). A nurse who works with patients in a long-term care setting speaks about the small losses often being more difficult than death itself:

When they die, it's hard, but it's not that hard. It's not as hard as having them lose control of their bladder and bowels. This is real sad. It's hard for us because we're talking to an otherwise competent client about Depends® saying, "Are you going out? Do you have enough diapers with you?" Or they'll be talking to you and say, "God, I had an accident," and sometimes you have to clean them up. It's the day-to-day stuff that's the hard part. By the time they get around to dying, it's almost easy. It's not easy, and it's sad, but the things you have to do to them while they're living are much harder than watching them die. (Drench, 1998, p. 97)

Confronting these many small losses along the continuum of loss, grief, and coping can lead to grief overload and take its toll.

Health professionals sometimes feel anxious or guilty that they are unable to respond to all clients' needs (Drench, 1992), especially in a health system where a premium is placed on cost effectiveness, budgeting of time, and volume of clients, all of which translate into reimbursement costs. Some retreat physically or emotionally, which clients can perceive as abandonment when their need is most significant, dashing all hope (Bruce, 2007). Care providers who work with clients over a long period of time, such as in a rehabilitation setting, skilled nursing facility, or hospice care, often develop relationships with the clients and deeply feel the losses. When clients with whom strong bonds are shared die, the losses can be acutely felt (Drench, 1998). Yet, ambivalence may exist. As sad as it feels to lose a client, health care providers occasionally feel a sense of relief when a struggle is over (Drench, 1992).

Health care providers encounter loss daily, from A to Z—from anterior cruciate ligament tears in athletes' knees to the "zoning out" of a client with mental deterioration. They need to handle the loss and reactions of clients and significant others, as well as of themselves. Part of their occupational core identity is that of a "helping" person. An effective helping relationship includes a certain level of sharing the clients' feelings of loss. Although their work may yield professional and personal satisfaction, health care providers may also perceive defeat and ineffectiveness as clients' losses amass (Drench, 1992).

Health care providers may also experience depression in response to dealing with clients' losses, treating a client who is terminally ill, and losing a client. We are educated and socialized to maintain a professional distance in order to minimize personal involvement. This is designed to help us make objective decisions regarding client care and prevent an unhealthy level of attachment. Although emotional detachment can be a protective insulator against loss and separation, it can also compromise compassion and sensitivity. A certain degree of therapeutic bonding makes the relationship more effective. The other side of this "therapeutic coin" is that a sense of loss is a by-product of that emotional bonding between professional and client.

In addition, new loss can reignite previous losses. Unresolved loss in the health care provider's personal history may also be triggered by a client's loss if the professional overidentifies with the client (Drench, 1992). These unresolved loss and mourning experiences can come back and jar us awake when we least expect it. We grieve for the client. We grieve for others we may have personally lost. We grieve for ourselves.

Hainsworth (1998) studied eight nurses, asking them to reflect on their experiences working with clients in acute care who had sustained catastrophic loss through severe brain injury. The nurses perceived their overall work experiences as negative, as they struggled to connect with clients and get support from colleagues and physicians. They experienced empathy but also felt vulnerable, futile, and abused by clients' families, who were struggling with their own dynamics. Although these acute care nurses sometimes felt ineffective and unsupported, they continued to seek professional satisfaction through their work. Overall, they wrestled with poor workplace experiences with patients who were neurologically devastated. In addition, health professionals working with people with AIDS report feelings of frustration, pervasive sadness, and anger, as well as gratification, challenges, and joy (Drench, 1998).

One loss is hard. Two is more difficult. Never-ending losses, especially with people with whom you work closely, can be devastating. These losses, with or without death, are very real to the health care provider and can contribute to or cause "singe-out," "rust-out," or in the extreme, burnout. They may experience burnout as a result of their relationship with the work milieu (Maslach, Schaufeli, & Leiter, 2001), or may develop compassion fatigue as a result of their relationship with the client, what Figley (1995) refers to as the "cost of caring" (p. 7). This, too, may result in burnout. When the demands and stress in the workplace become too great, the healer may become overwhelmed (Hall, 1997). House staff, medical oncologists, and nurses at Memorial Sloan-Kettering Cancer Center had greater emotional exhaustion and less empathy, that is, "depersonalization," than their counterparts in general medicine (Kash et al., 2000).

As health care professionals, we need to confront and understand our own responses to loss and openly acknowledge them. In doing so, we become more aware and sensitive to the needs of others, develop empathy for their losses from illness or injury, and clarify the impact of our clinical interventions.

## UNDERSTANDING GRIEF

Where there is loss, there is the universal human phenomenon of grief, a neuropsychobiological process that occurs in response to loss in every age group and culture. It is a painful process during which those who have a loss experience powerful and confusing emotions. Grief can affect all dimensions of a person—physical, emotional, cognitive, behavioral, and spiritual. To grieve effectively, people need to integrate the losses into their lives and come to terms with both the reality of the situation and the symbolic meaning of the loss. They must reframe their goals, priorities, and values to incorporate the person(s) they have become. Only then can they work to accommodate the loss into their existence.

### Types of Grief

In his seminal work on attachment and loss, British psychologist John Bowlby (1980) described the goal of mourning as accepting the reality of loss. The purpose of cultural traditions and rituals associated with death, such as wakes and funerals, is to help mourners face their losses. They create an acceptable opportunity for individuals to express feelings and receive comfort. They also "bring home the fact that a loss has in fact occurred" (p. 234). Yet, the process of grieving is also one of healing and recovery, helping people feel better. In today's fast-paced society of immediate gratification, people tend to underestimate the intensity of their distress, the problems that they face, and the length of time that the distress and problems will endure. In addition, Western culture can be death denying, with people minimizing the time, duration, and potency of the experience.

Grief is a natural phenomenon in response to loss and is part of the continuum of adjustment. Inherently, it is not pathological, although it may become so in extreme forms. Although the need to grieve is universal across cultures, the grieving process is influenced by religious and social mores. However, regardless of the manner in which someone grieves, there are typical psychological and physical reactions. Psychological signs include an initial shock and disbelief, followed by sorrow and often regret. Grief-related emotions, such as anger, guilt, despair, sadness, depression, denial, and fear, tend to be powerful, confusing, and overwhelming. Physical signs associated with a grief reaction include fatigue, sighing, hyperventilation, feelings of physical emptiness in the abdomen and chest, and a sense of a lump in the throat. Anorexia, insomnia, and disorientation may also be present. Cognitive signs are often present as well, including anxiety, confusion, and difficulty making decisions:

> I am new to this thing called widowhood.
> No one can tell you about grief, about its limitless boundaries, its unfathomable depths. No one can tell you about the crater that is created in the center of

your body, the one that nothing can fill. No matter how many times you hear the word *final*, it means nothing until final is actually final.

It has been just over four months since the day Bill died, and still I am paralyzed. I am a woman without a country, an alien who has dropped to earth from some other planet. I am in a capsule on the moon, bouncing from side to side, floating in space, but I cannot imagine emerging from the capsule to offer one small step for mankind. I keep thinking I will see a 224-point headline that reads DERANGED WIDOW FOUND SUSPENDED IN OUTER SPACE, and then realize that the headline refers to me. (Coughlin, 1993, p. 3)

Just as there are different types and reactions to loss, there are different types and responses to grief: anticipatory, acute, chronic, delayed, and suppressed grief. Grief has typically been considered to have two temporal phases. *Anticipatory grief* is experienced prior to the actual loss, and *"conventional" grief* occurs after the fact, following a loss. These two types of grief have similarities and differences. For instance, although anticipatory and conventional grief are similar in expression and duration among husbands and wives whose spouses die, anticipatory grief is associated with greater intensities of anger, loss of emotional control, and atypical grief responses (Gilliland & Fleming, 1998). Both anticipatory and conventional grief affect the survivors prior to and following a death. It is important to remember, though, that the client undergoing loss also grieves. Anticipatory grief includes preparing for losses that will occur as a result of surgery and disease progression, as well as death. This type of grief was significantly associated with caregiver burden in individuals who care for people with dementia, as they dealt with progressive decline of cognitive and physical capacities (Holley & Mast, 2009). Anticipatory grief may have signs similar to those of acute grief, but the timing is different.

Although widely accepted as a phenomenon in the literature, anticipatory grief can be a confusing concept. It is not always clearly distinguished from a "forewarning of loss" (Fulton, Madden, & Minichiello, 1996). In addition, it is not experienced in the same way by everyone. In a retrospective study of caregivers, five major processes of expected loss in palliative care were identified: "realization," "caretaking," "presence," "finding meaning," and "transitioning" (Clukey, 2008). Recommendations for health care practitioners to aid caregivers in anticipatory mourning were to:

• Appreciate how the roles and relationships in the family become altered, further stressing family dynamics.
• Be aware of the burdens placed on family caregivers and their necessity to get information, assistance, and support.
• Be forthcoming with knowledge and experience to prepare caregivers for what to expect.
• Be compassionate and caring.
• Control the client's pain and other symptoms.

Similar to the experience of caregivers, anticipatory grief in clients with advanced cancer involves facing many losses and, ultimately, death and being concerned with their role and relationship within the family (Cheng, Lo, Chan, Kwan, & Woo, 2010). Important information for health care providers is that comprehension of the anticipatory grief of clients who are terminally ill, personally and within the family system, may result in the need for more therapeutic interactions.

Conventional grief, which develops following a loss, can be acute, chronic, delayed, or suppressed. In contrast to anticipatory grief, *acute grief* begins following a recent or sudden loss. The loss could be the death of a loved one. It could be the loss of an important function, such as vision, or the loss of perfect health due to a chronic illness. It could be a devastating diagnosis that disrupts one's life. The severity of the grief tends to be directly proportional to the perceived void resulting from the loss. The person who is acutely grieving may experience profound sadness, anxiety, denial, anger, and depression. He or she may feel overwhelmed, confused, numb, helpless, and hopeless (Sullivan, 2003).

Grief can also become *chronic*. With chronic grief, a person enters a state of perpetual mourning. In some cultures, following the death of their husbands, widows dress completely in black for the rest of their lives. Although the attire does not necessarily indicate that their grief continues at the same intensity over time, it does serve as an outward symbol of their position in the community.

Symptoms of prolonged grief disorder, a stress response syndrome also known as complicated grief, are different from those of anxiety and depression, and can also forecast diminished functioning. This functional impairment, evidenced by lower quality of life and challenges with mental health (Boelen & Prigerson, 2007), is also aggravated by the avoidance of things associated with the loss (Shear et al., 2007). Models of prolonged grief disorder differ in duration, that is, 6 months post-loss (Prigerson et al., 1999; Prigerson & Jacobs, 2001) and 14 months (Horowitz et al., 2003). They have similar diagnostic criteria, though, with percentages of signs and symptoms, that cause significant impairment in social, occupational, and other fields of functioning. Prolonged or complicated grief disorder will be a new diagnostic category in the *Diagnostic and Statistical Manual of Mental Disorders, Fifth Edition*(DSM-V), to be published in 2012.

Grief may also be *delayed* or *absent*. Some people suppress their grief; however, it can be triggered at a later date. This may occur when the individual perceives that the time and environment are safe for grieving or when the grief can no longer be inhibited. Consider the woman who suppressed her grief at the time of each of her three miscarriages. Years later, when her daughter had a miscarriage, she was overcome with grief, not only for her awaited first grandchild, but also for her three previous losses. She said, "I honestly thought I was over it. I can now see that I never even dealt with what happened. I buried my babies inside, just as if I buried them in the ground."

## GRIEVING BEHAVIOR

Although many people may grieve the same information or event, not everyone grieves as intensely as others. There are typically primary and secondary mourners. Primary mourners are people who perceive that they have lost the most—the client, family, and close friends. Secondary mourners also despair, but there is less of a void in their lives. They are likely to be coworkers and less close friends.

Social worker Susan Berger (2009) identifies five types of grieving that describe how individuals react to a major loss and adjust to changed life circumstances: (1) *Nomads* have unresolved grief and may not grasp the effect that the loss has in their lives. (2) *Memorialists* create memorials, rituals, and tributes to honor the memory of their family/friends. (3) *Normalizers* welcome a sense of family and community. (4) *Activists* reach out to help others who are facing the same illness or circumstances that resulted in the death of people they loved. (5) *Seekers* embrace spiritual, philosophical, or religious beliefs to find comfort and meaning. Berger's contention is that a major loss impacts people's worldviews and alters their values, priorities, life meaning, perception of mortality, sense of time, and how they see themselves "fitting" in society.

Grief or sorrow (emotional suffering) caused by bereavement (having something taken away) have come to be used interchangeably. Like other life-span issues, bereavement behaviors as a response to loss are influenced by religious beliefs, age, cultural and community aspects, the personality of the grieving person, and the relationship between who is grieving and what is lost. Cultural healing rituals help mourners face death. These include practices such as photographic collages or collections at memorial services, candle lighting, charitable funds, condolence visits, specific prayers, stuffed animals and flowers left at the scene of accidents, and the AIDS quilt of memorial panels (initiated by the Names Project). However, there is a paucity of rituals associated with losses from a disability. The support at the onset of a disability or impairment often seems to evaporate over the long term. Consider the barrage of visitors, flowers, candy, and notes that accompany the person who is newly incapacitated from a spinal cord injury, head trauma, or diagnosis of cancer, for example; at some point, these people return to the fabric of their own lives and do not become a sustained source of support. Perhaps, in part, avoiding contact with the client and family is a way of avoiding one's own feelings of inadequacy.

In our fast-paced society, mourners are "allowed" only a few days of grief and are quickly encouraged to "get on with life." In contemporary, industrialized societies, the mourner is perhaps allotted 2 or 3 days away from the workplace. Mourning is considered morbid, and some people grow impatient with the time others need. Many people do not view grief as normal. Prolonged grief (timing is in the minds of the beholder), therefore, becomes pathological. The message is firm—if you need all this time and have all this pain, you are not adjusting well; you are somehow deficient. Consider the case of Dr. Jones who lost his 10-year-old son to cancer. When he returned to the office, his secretary said, "It's been a week; get over it." She clearly did not understand the depth of his grieving experience.

Some cultures see death as a transition rather than the kind of loss others perceive. In other societies, people minimize the loss they feel from a death, referring to the death experience in indirect terms, such as "returning to one's Maker," "entering the Kingdom," and "passing away" (or "passing on" or "passing over"). In our efforts to protect children, such as excluding them from the bedside of a dying person or a funeral, we rob them of the opportunity to say goodbye, gain closure, and understand the process of living and dying. We want to quickly replace the loss—a hamster, a mother—as though someone or something else could be substituted. This behavior is not reserved only for children. Sometimes during the grieving period, we hear, "You're young. You'll marry again." This mentality provides little comfort.

Some cultures have even abdicated many of the rituals that comforted and helped move people through the mourning process in the past. It is no longer common to see people wearing black armbands or dressing all in black for an extended period of time. Black wreaths and banners may be hung on public buildings for some losses but not typically on homes. Bodies are generally not laid out in the house; vigils are no longer the rule.

In a highly mobile society, people often live a distance from their extended family and friends. The built-in support that was once common in one's own neighborhood or town is rare today. Because so many of us do not live in insular communities, we do not grow up exposed to loss and death experiences. We often grieve alone, no longer blanketed by those around us. Clients and their families who are dealing with, for example, amputation, paralysis, or diminished capacity from cardiopulmonary problems, are also grieving their losses, but that is not always recognized nor is as high a value placed on this as a death.

The society in which one lives influences the outward behavior of a grieving person. Clear messages in mainstream American culture are "You have to be brave for the children," "Big boys don't cry," and "You're young; you can have another baby" (Cable, 1998, p. 63). Therefore, it is no surprise that the outward behavior of a grieving person can be deceiving. Whereas some people keen and wail, others remain in control. "Quiet" mourners may cry in private or not at all. Others stoically harbor their grief, but it can be prompted later by a memory, an association, or a subsequent loss. Sometimes the loss is met with ambivalence, with both grief and relief—grief over the loss and relief especially after a particularly prolonged, painful, or deteriorating death.

Behaviors associated with acute grief frequently include crying and agitation. There may be wringing of the hands, deep sighing, and general tension. This grief response usually happens immediately after the loss has occurred. The grieving person may become withdrawn, not eat, have difficulty sleeping or sleep more than usual, pace frenetically or sit lethargically, and lose interest in pleasurable things. He or she may express feeling numb, hopeless, helpless, and exhausted. It may seem that life no longer has any meaning. The world feels like an empty place. There is a loss of connection between the person in mourning and the rest of the world. They often wonder how others can go about "business as usual" while they are "dying inside." Mourners feel as though they are on the outside looking in.

If the mourning is in response to the loss of a person, there is often a tendency to place the person on a pedestal, idealizing the individual who has died. In contrast, some deaths, illnesses, or circumstances carry a stigma that compounds the complexities faced by the grieving people and often yields less compassion and support. People are sometimes blamed for their own happenstances, if their losses or deaths are perceived as resulting from poor lifestyle choices, such as substance abuse, AIDS, suicide, or foolish accidents (Cable, 1998). Similarly, clients can feel responsible for their problems and blame themselves, such as those with lung cancer who smoked. Sadly, personal and professional caregivers sometimes imply that this is true, resulting in a greater sense of isolation and loneliness (Wess, 2007).

I'm working with two high school students now in the burn unit. At a party, their boyfriends decided to pour grain alcohol into a dish to see if it would continue to burn on its own once they lit it. They lit the bottle from which it was poured, and suddenly, the bottle exploded, engulfing the girls in flames. One girl's parents are at the hospital every day, supporting and loving her. The other girl's parents yelled at her, "How could you do this?" She's lying there so badly burned, and her own parents are blaming the victim!

—*From the journal of Melanie Haber, nursing student*

Because individual perceptions vary greatly, no discussion of grieving behavior can really be exhaustive. However, themes emerge across the spectrum of problems. For example, clients and families may experience different reactions on learning of the possibility of a diagnosis of cancer and throughout the course of the disease, with possible impairments and disabilities, such as those listed in Table 7–1.

These feelings and losses are not unique to cancer. They are universal and apply to other life-threatening illnesses or disabilities. Clients with muscular dystrophy, and their families, for example, deal with progressive muscular weakness and with ensuing losses of strength and functional ability. When facing a loss, an individual's sense of personal control and well-being may be replaced by feelings of fear, helplessness, and anger. The latter is often directed at God, health care providers, family, and friends. A person may also encounter anxiety and depression (Maguire, Walsh, Jeacock, & Kingston, 1999). Other people *appear* to be in denial, but they are

| Table 7–1    Reactions to a Diagnosis of Cancer | |
| --- | --- |
| **Upon Learning of the Possibility of a Diagnosis of Cancer** | **After the Diagnosis is Made and Throughout the Course of the Illness** |
| • Fear of death<br>• Fear of disfigurement<br>• Fear of disability<br>• Fear of abandonment<br>• Fear of disruption in relationships and role functioning<br>• Fear of loss of finances<br>• Loss of independence<br>• Denial<br>• Anxiety<br>• Anger | • Loss of control<br>• Anger<br>• Guilt<br>• Fear of abandonment<br>• Fear of pain<br><br>• Psychiatric disorders<br>• Other psychosocial factors |
| (Sussman, 1995) | (Blanchard & Ruckdeschel, 1986) |

actually repressing these thoughts and fears, submerging them in their unconscious mind for the present time. Let us take a closer look at grieving behavior within the context of conceptual models of grieving.

## CONCEPTUAL MODELS OF GRIEVING

Several models of grieving have emerged over the years and have stood the test of time. As you read about the stages of grieving and dying, integrative theory of bereavement, and tasks of mourning models, refer to Table 7–2 for a comparison of the theoretical concepts of grieving.

### Stages of Grieving and Dying

In the second half of the 1960s, Swiss psychiatrist Elisabeth Kübler-Ross began to work with clients who were dying and, before the end of the decade, produced what was to become the

| Table 7–2    Comparative Models of Grieving | | |
| --- | --- | --- |
| **Stages of Grieving and Dying (Kübler-Ross, 1969)** | **Integrative Theory of Bereavement (Sanders, 1989)** | **Tasks of Mourning (Worden, 2002)** |
| 1  Denial | Shock | Accept the reality of loss |
| 2  Anger | Awareness of loss | Experience the pain associated with grief |
| 3  Bargaining | Conservation and withdrawal | Adjust to circumstances created by loss |
| 4  Depression | Healing | Emotionally relocate the person who has died and progress with life |
| 5  Acceptance | Renewal | |

formative work on the subject. *On Death and Dying* (1969) details the emotional process of dying, described in five stages: *denial, anger, bargaining, depression,* and *acceptance.* This widely, though not universally, accepted framework has also become a model for facing a loss in which no death is involved, such as those of functional limitations and disabilities. For example, the diagnosis of lifelong conditions in children, such as type 1 diabetes, may represent multiple losses for parents. On learning of the newly diagnosed diabetes, parents' grief reactions are similar to those of bereavement due to death (Lowes & Lyne, 2000).

## Integrative Theory of Bereavement

In addition to Kübler-Ross' five stages of grieving and dying, another way to understand bereavement is to examine an integrative theory of bereavement (Sanders, 1989). This model also has five phases, which are correlated with emotional, biological, and social factors. In the beginning, the person experiences *shock.* He or she responds to the loss with disbelief: "It can't be happening" or "It's not true." The person numbly moves through this initial phase, often unable to complete the simplest tasks or make any decisions.

During the second phase, the person develops an *awareness of the loss.* Reality is beginning to "set in," and the person is starting to understand the meaning of the loss and the extent of the void caused by it.

In the third phase of *conservation and withdrawal,* the individual may feel fatigued, even listless: "I feel like a rag doll" or "I can barely get through the day. I don't have energy to spare." This is a period of conserving personal resources and avoiding tasks perceived as "extra" or unnecessary. The person may even isolate himself or herself from others and the everyday routine.

As time passes, the fourth phase of *healing* begins. It is a time of adjusting to a new reality. Activities are resumed, and the individual may be surprised to hear his or her own laughter. Sometimes, however, this realization of self-enjoyment can trigger feelings of guilt, and the person may retreat.

Finally, there can be *renewal.* During this fifth phase, the person is reaching resolution of his or her grief and emerging at the other end, engaged in life, often enthusiastically.

The integrative theory of bereavement model recognizes that variables from both the individual and the environment influence the grieving process. Both sets of mediating variables operate from the outset of grief. External mediators include social support, sudden versus chronic illness, socioeconomic status, religion, concurrent crises, culture, and stigmatic death, such as AIDS. In addition, internal mediators are also at work, such as age, gender, personality, health, ambivalence toward the deceased person, and dependency behavior. Outcomes of bereavement in this model are similar to those already discussed above. There may be personal growth (positive), a downward shift in general health or life's activities (negative), or no change in behavior or thinking (neutral).

## Tasks of Mourning

In addition to Kübler-Ross' five stages of grieving and dying and Sanders' five phases in the integrative theory of bereavement, another model to consider is Worden's (2002) tasks of mourning model. Worden believes that grief is a process that involves learning to master four tasks of mourning. First, the person needs to *accept the reality of the loss.* The disbelief that accompanies a loss or a death is compounded if the incident is sudden, such as the unexpected death of a teenager on a basketball court. To accomplish this task, the person comes out of denial (Kübler-Ross' first stage of grieving) and shock (Sanders' first phase).

Once the person accepts the loss as real, the grieving person needs to *experience the pain associated with grief,* the second task of mourning. If the individual is part of a society that does not encourage people to express their feelings and emotions around the loss, there may be a temptation to lightly touch on or even skip this mourning task. Although initial brief denial can comfort and shield a person from the loss, it limits the individual from moving on and completing the process. Avoiding the pain can also lead to depression or other psychiatric problems, as discussed in Chapter 13.

Worden's (2002) third task of mourning is *adjusting to circumstances created by the loss.* This could mean adjusting to life without a right arm or assuming different roles in life that were once fulfilled by the person who has died. A young widow may need to learn to manage a household budget and be "both a mother and a father" to her children. A new sense of self, including one's perceived worth and esteem, may be a healthy by-product. Both physical and emotional tasks need to be mastered.

Finally, the fourth task of mourning in this model is *emotionally relocating the deceased and progressing with life.* Relocating does not connote erasing the person and the corresponding memories from one's life. Rather, it means giving those memories a different emotional role so that the individual may resume life's activities, that is, to "go on" despite the loss. It also means assigning meaning to the loss and integrating it into his or her belief system.

## Common Themes Across the Models

Common themes emerge across the conceptual models of grieving. The initial period involves shock, disbelief, or denial. To progress through the grieving process, a person needs to become aware of the situation and accept the reality of the loss. The grieving individual needs to experience the pain of the reality, which may involve profound distress, including sadness or depression. There is little energy, and personal resources are used sparingly, even to the point of social isolation.

To emerge at the other end of the grieving tunnel with psychological and physical health intact, the person needs to find ways to adjust to circumstances, in light of the loss, to find other means of accomplishing things and discover alternate ways "to be." The goal is to heal, accept, and progress with life, in a word, to be renewed. Across the models, people who are grieving experience many feelings, behaviors, and characteristics, such as denial, anger, bargaining, sadness and depression, acceptance, guilt, anxiety, and diminished problem solving.

**DENIAL**    Denial of the situation, fears, and thoughts can be present even when the circumstances are visible and difficult for *others* to deny. Consider Richard, a 35-year-old man who was unsuccessfully treated for a glioblastoma. His brain tumor resulted in seizures, weakness, and functional limitations. Despite being told that he would not live much longer, he persisted in making long-range plans for when he "got better."

On receiving "bad" news—a diagnosis, prognosis, statement of complications—it is not unusual for a client or someone in the personal support system to react with surprise and *denial.* "It can't be true!" "I just had a mammogram (or electrocardiogram or some other test), and it was fine. You must have someone else's test results." "I will walk again. Can't you see that my toe just moved?"

Denying that there is a change or loss is not a conscious decision; rather, it is a form of self-preservation. Denial is not necessarily counterproductive to accepting one's reality. Like so much else in life, it is a matter of degree of intensity and duration. Initially, denial is a protective reaction, cushioning someone against shocking or discouraging news. It affords time to compose oneself, and in time, employ other defense mechanisms on the road forward. It permits time to adjust to the reality of the loss. When denial goes beyond the initial phase, though, it can be detrimental. Seeking a second medical opinion is wise. "Shopping around for doctors," looking for "good" news, is part of an active denial system, which may ultimately hamper adjustment and acceptance.

Initially, I thought Julia accepted the fact that her child had been born deaf and blind when she said that she would grow up like Helen Keller. I now believe she was in denial. Just because she can't hear or see doesn't mean that she can or will achieve the unusual accomplishments of Ms. Keller, who also couldn't speak. That's a huge leap of faith!
—*From the journal of Matthew Mulcahey, medical student*

Denial is not necessarily a one-time response. It can reappear whenever there are new challenges to face. The unpredictable relapses of a form of multiple sclerosis trigger a new surge of grief, anxiety, anger, and guilt; symptom reduction from a different round of medications adds more denial for the individual and family, as they grapple with what the disease means in their lives (Kalb, 2007).

Although all team members may share the responsibility of dealing with denial, it is generally the purview of the mental health professional (i.e., psychotherapist, psychologist, psychiatric nurse, social worker) to decide how best to manage denial to meet the client's needs. For instance, the mental health professional may decide to confront the denial to mitigate its effect or maintain it as a productive defense mechanism that can be beneficial in adapting to the changed life (Langer, 1994). Both schools of thought have their supporters and detractors, a discussion that is beyond the scope of this book.

It is the job of health care providers to deal with denial within the boundaries of their practice. They can support the person and provide hope. When clients sense that the environment and conditions are safe, denial sometimes begins to dissipate.

**ANGER**   When dealing with loss and grief, anxiety and depression often pale in comparison to anger. Clients may feel anger toward their own bodies for betraying them. They may feel angry at being cheated out of a "normal" life, one without illness, injury, or premature death. At times, anger may also be based on fear. Clients often say, "It can't be me!" or "Why me?" Once the news is absorbed and is beginning to be processed, the client may feel resentment: "What did I do to deserve this? Why couldn't it have been him (or her)?" "Life isn't fair!" Typically, the person feels anger and sometimes even rage. Internalized anger is often allied with feelings of self-blame and guilt. This is particularly true if the client feels responsible for the disability (Gill, 1999), such as John, who blames himself for the car accident that resulted in the death of his girlfriend and the amputation of his left lower extremity.

Martha Beck (1999) shares her personal story of being pregnant with a child who has Down syndrome. In a bookstore, she selected a book on the subject with a cover that horrified her: "two children, lumpish and awkward-looking, stared dully at the camera through small, misshapen eyes. I cannot tell you how much it hurt me to look at that picture . . . . It was like getting my heart caught in a mill saw" (p. 196). After she purchased the book, she hurried into a small elevator where her feelings exploded:

> I . . . hit the stop button with a closed fist. . . . Then, I leaned back against the wall and covered my face with my hands, trying to control myself. I felt as though some evil ogre had killed my "real" baby—the baby I'd been expecting—and replaced him with an ugly, broken replica. My grief at losing that "real" baby was as intense as if he had been 2 years old, or 5, or 10. The whole thing seemed wildly unfair to me: My baby was dead, and I was still pregnant. I was suddenly seized by a rage so strong I wanted to bash in the elevator walls. (p. 196)

Anger can appear when a person no longer fits society's picture of "normal." It may fester when a client can no longer do the same activities in the previous way. The rage and resentment may be displaced onto health care providers, friends, and family, such as the client who blames his wife for his stroke because it happened while they were having sex.

Clients may lash out at health professionals or be excessively demanding. Care providers find it difficult to accept a client's rejection. Ruth Purtilo (1984), a medical ethicist and physical therapist, espouses five plausible reasons for this rejection. First, the client "rejects" the health care provider because of the displaced anger that the client, friends, or family put on the professional. Second, the client may consider that there is no longer a need for the care provider, thinking that he or she has come to terms with the anticipated death or other loss. Third, the client may have little energy and selectively chooses to use it on family and friends. Fourth, the client may have difficulty separating from or showing affection to the health care professional. Finally, the client may be separating from anything or anybody related to the health care setting.

Any one or a combination of these possibilities may explain the apparent rejection. It is natural for the health care provider to feel hurt, rejected, and confused and to suspect that he or she has somehow failed the client. However, it is important for the care provider to understand the behavior rather than judge it or take it personally.

As uncomfortable as it may be for health professionals to witness and deal with anger, deal with it we must. Anger that is not recognized and confronted tends to impede the grieving process. If ignored, it can be camouflaged and appear in other ways, such as in disabling illness, maladaptive behavior, and chronic unhappiness (Cerney & Buskirk, 1991). In Chapter 8, we discuss therapeutic responses to loss and grief. We can help clients acknowledge their anger and make referrals to appropriate team members, if the situation is outside the scope of our practice.

**BARGAINING**    We learn to negotiate early in life. "If I get ready for bed now, can I have a story?" "If I clean my room, can I sleep over at Robin's house?" In clients with illness or injury, bargaining sounds like "If I can just live long enough to walk my daughter down the aisle on her wedding day." This is often a short-term strategy (it is one thing if the wedding is imminent; it is another if the daughter is currently only 7 years old). Bargaining with God, health care providers, family members, or themselves is done to postpone an anticipated loss. Impairments and disabilities often steal some of a person's control over their lives and environment. Bargaining is one way to reassert some control. However, when clients do everything they are "supposed to do," following the prescribed regimen, and continue to have pain, impairment, or a poor prognosis, they often feel that they have lost that control.

**SADNESS AND DEPRESSION**    Grieving behavior also includes sadness and sometimes depression. (See Chapter 13 for a detailed discussion of depression.) Perhaps much of what Kübler-Ross describes as depression may really be profound sadness rather than clinical depression. Everyone feels sadness to a certain degree, but not everyone experiences depression as part of grieving behavior in response to loss. Sometimes there is also a sense of "why bother?"

Depression may coexist with other reactions to loss and hinder adjustment to illness. Clients with end-stage renal disease and their families are overwhelmed by the intrusion, lifestyle adjustments, and significance that kidney dialysis has on their lives (White & Grenyer, 1999). In addition to depression, these clients often experience anger and hopelessness. Although dialysis technology can be life sustaining, it can have a negative impact on lifestyle. Framing the experience differently can help clients cope in positive ways, as described in Chapter 8. It is also interesting to note that depression can be mitigated by physiological changes. Reflect on a woman with end-stage renal disease who is no longer depressed since her electrolytes have been stabilized.

Depression can be an offshoot of loss. It may be clinical depression or depressed bereavement patterns, the ways in which people grieve for their losses (Langer, 1994). Either way, it justifies diagnostic and therapeutic intervention. Between 25 and 79 percent of people who have strokes are depressed (Gordon & Hibbard, 1997). If health professionals fail to identify the depression and provide appropriate intervention, the depression may impede functional and emotional recovery (Hermann, Black, Lawrence, Szekely, & Szalai, 1998). Our role as health care providers is to be able to recognize the signs and make referrals to appropriate team members, such as a psychotherapist, psychologist, psychiatric nurse, or social worker, as indicated.

**ACCEPTANCE**   A client who no longer denies the reality, has come to terms with anger, is not trying to bargain with good behavior to "buy" more time or easier circumstances, and is not depressed is considered by Kübler-Ross (1969) to be in the fifth stage—acceptance. Acceptance, however, is more than the absence of the other stages. It represents an advanced degree on the continuum of personal healing. For people with disabilities, it may be learning how to cope with and adjust to situations. If impending death is the issue, acceptance is not synonymous with joy or satisfaction. It is sometimes a sense of resignation, devoid of feelings. Sometimes, it is a sense of peace.

It is critical to realize that not every person moves through all five stages and that the progression is not linear. The stages actually occur as more of a process. There is also no time sequence that accompanies the passages. These stages, however, are typical, in varying degrees. There is a great deal of back-and-forth movement. People often find themselves in one stage, only to slip back into a previous stage. Not everyone reaches acceptance. Some people remain depressed. Others never stop denying the reality of their situation. Anger becomes a constant and counterproductive companion for other people, while some never cease to bargain and negotiate. In addition to denial, anger, bargaining, depression, and acceptance, it is important to note that other types of grieving behavior may coexist, such as guilt, anxiety, and diminished problem solving.

**GUILT**   Anger and guilt are natural parts of the grieving process. Irrational anger may even be directed toward the deceased. "He left me with all these bills to pay and no insurance policy." "She said she'd take me to buy my prom dress. How could she just leave me like that?" Unresolved feelings of guilt may follow the anger.

Guilt also comes into play on someone's death, if those who are grieving feel as though they have wronged, disappointed, neglected, or been angry with the deceased person. "I should have taken her to chemotherapy." "I could have brought meals over to the house." "I never did give him the money I owed him." "I never told my son that I loved him." If the bereaved person perceives the loss as punishment, guilt may also be a factor. "I should have insisted that she go to the hospital." "If I had used a condom, I wouldn't have AIDS, and I wouldn't be blind."

Guilt and shame often are intertwined. Following acute myocardial infarctions, women may feel guilty and ashamed about being tired and weak (Svedlund & Axelsson, 2000). They often feel "distressed," "vulnerable," and useless, as they grapple with the fear of what their cardiac condition means to them. While adjusting to their heart attacks, they may develop insights about how to adapt and live "normally." It is interesting to note that these women do not always share their thoughts and feelings with their partners, suggesting a lack of communication, perhaps another loss.

**ANXIETY**    Psychological distress complicates one's ability to cope with the physiological changes associated with illness or injury. Although depression is not widely experienced, anxiety may be. Remember that depression and sadness are not synonymous. However, both anxiety and depression can be intermittent or constant, such as that seen over the course of breast cancer and its treatment (Longman, Braden, & Mishel, 1999). They may also persist through the final phase of a terminal illness. Anxiety, as well as depression, may be long lasting. For instance, anxiety and depressive symptoms were still evident 5 years after people underwent coronary artery bypass graft surgery (Lee, 2009).

**DIMINISHED PROBLEM SOLVING**    Any type of loss can result in a period of distress. A person can feel confused and defeated. The feelings of grief that accompany the loss tend to be affiliated with diminished cognitive effectiveness and problem-solving abilities, which vary in intensity and length of time (Caplan, 1990). As such, people who are grieving often have difficulty acquiring, storing, and processing information. Inattention, slower information-processing speed, and diminished verbal fluency are associated with bereavement in older adults (Ward, Mathias, & Hitchings, 2007). Disability and depression can also affect cognitive functioning. Two years after a diagnosis of multiple sclerosis, clients performed slowly on timed tasks, indicating cognitive changes, and cognitive impairment was related to depression (Siepman et al., 2008).

These changes can add to distress. Consider the 36-year-old mother of two young children whose husband recently died. Although she needed to return to work to support her family, she worried that she would not be able to adequately perform her job because she felt "dull."

During the grieving process, people tend to lose some level of ability to clearly define their sense of purpose and meaning in life, as well as the ability to continue in the face of adversity—"I just can't go on," "I can't live without," "I can't handle this." These thoughts and feelings can be associated with diminished energy. Such attitudes and perceptions weaken a person's sense of capability and resolve to "fight the good fight."

The grieving behaviors we have discussed are the more typical responses to loss. However, some clients have maladaptive reactions that diminish their ability to function and can lead to other problems (Bateman et al., 1992). Other types of grief behaviors include medical symptomatology and illness, stemming from a decreased immune system response and resistance to infection; psychophysiological reactions, such as essential hypertension, ulcerative colitis, and neurodermatitis; maladaptive behavior, such as sexual promiscuity and drug use; and neurotic and psychotic manifestations, such as schizophrenic and phobic reactions, which may begin or be exacerbated by severe loss. Therapeutic interventions that acknowledge the importance of psychosocial factors and incorporates them into the plan of care can help minimize a sense of helplessness for the clients and their families. We discuss these issues in Chapter 8.

## GRIEF OUTCOMES

The perception of how severe a functional loss is will be influenced by both psychodynamic and pragmatic issues. The nature and severity of physical obstacles and the dependency caused by the loss affect one's perception. Isolation, loneliness, and loss of social support may result. Consider the college student with paraplegia, secondary to a motor vehicle accident. His primary goal was to ambulate. The reality was that, although he could ambulate very short distances using crutches, the enormous energy expenditure compromised his health status. He was not able to walk functionally. Rather than being able to accept using the wheelchair as a means of mobility, he viewed it as a failure of his rehabilitation team. He also could not accept that there were fewer, and different, available options in life.

The negative reactions of other people also have an impact on a functional loss and how a person copes with it. These factors, acting singly or in combination, can become a social disability, impeding the quality of one's social life. Other contributing aspects may also color how a person responds to a loss, including the person's premorbid personality and coping styles. Prior life history and cultural issues both play a role in a person's perception of loss, as well as strategies to adjust to it. The roles that people have, such as head of the household, athlete, or beauty queen, and the attributes assigned to or assumed by them are part of a person's core identity. Being able to integrate the loss into their current lives is challenging. Sometimes a person will say, "I don't even recognize myself any more. Who is this person I've become?"

Sufficient resources, such as social and economic support, are also key elements that can influence the degree and type of other life stressors (Langer, 1994). Consider the family that cannot afford to make their home wheelchair accessible or purchase a van and is under strain. Socially introverted before the illness that was to change their lives, they lack a network of friends to emotionally or practically help them. Everything is a struggle for them, which adds to their isolation and stress.

Following a loss, three interdependent elements influence outcome: (1) the pain of the loss of attachment and anguish of dealing with the situation, (2) the "handicapping" deprivation of not having what you once had before the loss, and (3) the deterioration of cognitive capabilities, including problem solving, and the will to struggle or live (Caplan, 1990). These three elements, working alone or together in varying degrees, may affect grieving outcomes, which can be positive or negative.

Some individuals may develop an acute adjustment disorder or chronic psychopathology, that is, psychiatric illnesses where they manifest maladaptive behavior to avoid reality or isolate themselves. Another poor outcome of grieving would be the development of a physical illness. Grief is considered pathological when it becomes excessive, protracted, or blocked. This is more likely to occur when social support is lacking. In contrast, these three elements may also produce a healthy grieving outcome, wherein the person enlists effective coping strategies and develops personal fortitude and self-mastery of the situation.

People may develop and affirm negative (perpetually mourning) or positive attitudes (engaging in life to the best of their ability) (Frankl, 1984). However, attitudes are dynamic and, therefore, changeable. People may vacillate between poles or have elements of both positive and negative attitudes concurrently. Lucy Grealy (1994) was diagnosed with Ewing's sarcoma at the age of 9. As a result of this primary malignant bone tumor, she underwent surgery to remove a significant section of her jaw, endured years of radiation and chemotherapy, and had 30 corrective operations that were not cosmetically successful. Self-discovery was difficult:

> I . . . came up with a hand mirror and, with a bit of angling, looked for the first time at my right profile. I knew to expect a scar, but how had my face sunk in like that? . . . Was it possible I'd looked this way for a while and was only just noticing it, or was this change very recent? More than the ugliness I felt, I was suddenly appalled at the notion that I'd been walking around unaware of something that was apparent to everyone else. A profound sense of shame consumed me. (pp. 111–112)

Although Lucy ultimately accepted this as part of the person she was, during active cancer treatment, she established a protective barrier by wearing a large hat. "It hid me, it hid my secret, though badly, and when people made fun . . . or stared . . . I assumed it was only because they could guess what was beneath my hat" (p. 107).

Frears and Scheider (1981) believe that "transcending the loss" is the final stage, wherein the person has done the painful grief work, searched for meaning in the loss and grief, grown and matured, and reintegrated into life. Facing a loss and working through grief can be phenomenally challenging. How it is done can make a difference between moving on with one's life or "staying stuck" in one's grief. It is important to remember that grief is not a finite point on the continuum between loss and adjustment; it is a process. Grieving older women whose husbands have hospice care and die describe a process of "being aware," "experiencing distress," "supporting," "coping," and finally, "facing new realities" (Jacob, 1996). This is congruent with Worden's (2002) tasks of mourning.

Health professionals use a bereavement model to describe the process of loss and readjustment. In a study of people who had strokes and their caregivers and health professionals, the people with strokes acknowledged the losses and disabilities that disrupted their lives (Alaszewski, Alaszewski, & Potter, 2004). To help return their lives to "normal," they established goals to progress toward recovery. Health providers may disagree with the goals set by their clients, believe them to be unrealistic, and perceive that the clients have become "stuck." A valuable message here is that health providers need to clearly and understandably communicate and develop plans of care that work in tandem with the goals and strategies of the clients.

Someone who goes through the loss and bereavement process may discover a new sense of purpose. Actor and director Christopher Reeve, forever known as *Superman* in the movies, came crashing to the ground when the horse he was riding unsuccessfully attempted a jump over an obstacle on a course. Fracturing his cervical vertebrae, Reeve suddenly became a person with high-level quadriplegia. With his catastrophic injury and celebrity status, Reeve developed a new mission, a new purpose in life. He became a major spokesman and fund-raiser for spinal cord injury and created the Christopher and Dana Reeve Foundation, dedicated to curing spinal cord injury. Although he died in 2004 at age 52, this work became his legacy.

Although there are "typical" reactions to loss, people's responses do vary. There are no set, predictable sequences of mourning and no specific time frames. Grief usually lasts 6 months to a year or longer, but the acute pain of it diminishes slowly over time, commonly within the first few months. However, in our society of instant relief, instant satisfaction, and quick studies, people are often impatient with the "schedule" of the grieving. It is not unusual to hear comments like, "When will they get over it?" "When will *I* get over it?" "What's the problem? It's been a year already." "Put the past behind you." For some people, grief can become chronic and even perpetual.

## CHRONIC SORROW

Sadness is a response to loss and is a natural part of the grieving process. There is sadness around acute loss, which can be short lived or prolonged. There is sadness around chronic conditions. There is also sadness that is lifelong, episodic in nature, or progressive. It may be a response to a chronic or terminal illness. It can affect both the individual with a chronic illness or disability, as well as the family members (Rosenberg, 1998). It can be experienced by the parents of a child who faces permanent problems, which is also the loss of the fantasy of the "perfect" child. It can also be part of a spousal relationship. The "it" is chronic sorrow—the grief experienced from continual loss of milestones of life that are not reached, unrelenting loss of future plans, and lifestyle adaptations based on restrictions (Hainsworth, 1995). It is also characterized by antecedent events that cause the sorrow to recur.

Living with certain conditions carries a high risk for living with chronic sorrow, such as multiple sclerosis (80 percent; Hainsworth, 1994) and cancer (90 percent; Eakes, 1993). Over a long period of time, feelings of chronic sorrow occur episodically, triggered by an event that reminds people of the chronicity of their situation. Consider the case study of a woman with multiple sclerosis and her husband that describes chronic sorrow throughout her illness and disability (Hainsworth, Burke, Lindgren, & Eakes, 1993). She endures the progressive loss of bodily functions, the stigma associated with chronic illness, a restricted social life, and loss of future plans. Each functional loss provokes a new episode of sorrow. Chronic sorrow also affects families, including those of clients with multiple sclerosis. Eighty percent of next of kin were identified as having chronic sorrow, enduring losses of "security," "sense of community in family life," and "joy and recreation" (Liedström, Isaksson, & Ahlström, 2008). Recommendations for health care providers are to consider the welfare of caregivers and help them cope with this phenomenon, including support programs as one possible strategy.

Chronic sorrow is experienced by parents in a lifetime of ongoing losses. Parents of children with epilepsy with other existing conditions had higher degrees of anger than parents of children with epilepsy without comorbid problems (Hobdell et al., 2007). Chronic sorrow and coping were similar across groups. The recommendation is for early recognition of the sorrow so that health professionals can help the parents with coping and improve their outlook.

For parents of a child with a disability, each failure to achieve a typical milestone triggers a new episode of grief. This "sadness without end" continues to be an enduring focus in the lives of parents, even when they may no longer be the caretakers of their child (Krafft & Krafft, 1998). However, behavior may differ between parents. For example, mothers of children with developmental disabilities tend to lapse into chronic sorrow, whereas the fathers' behavior leans toward resignation (Mallow & Bechtel, 1999). Activated by health care crises, responses also differ among parents. Affective aspects tend to dominate in mothers, as they feel sadness and grief. In contrast, fathers emphasize cognitive aspects, as they compare social norms in their children with others. It is also interesting to note that children who lose a parent also experience chronic sorrow, when the parent is absent at significant life events.

This chronic sorrow, which is the periodic recurrence of permanent, pervasive sadness and other feelings associated with grief related to a loss, can emanate from mental, as well as physical, illness. An excerpt from a mother's journal (personal communication, February 2, 2001), whose daughter has been living with mental health problems, epitomizes chronic sorrow:

> After a while, it becomes obvious that this disability is forever. She is 18 now and is making her own decisions. She is living away from us and has a very unhealthy lifestyle, and she is not safe. Her doctor told me that I had done a wonderful job taking care of her. It doesn't matter. She is not safe, and I can't help her. I can't fix her.

> I know that the child I had is gone and that I have to grieve this terrible loss. I miss the smart, funny, warm, caring person she used to be. I don't know who she is now.
>
> I have accepted the permanence of this loss, and I have given up the future. She is lost to us as the child who we knew and the relationship that we had. Her doctor and her therapist tell me that things will get better, but I can't go there. I have to accept that she is gone and is not coming back as the child we had. That means that anything that we get from this point on is a gift and not another disappointment.

Chronic sorrow is characterized by lifelong, periodically recurring sadness. One man, whose 10-year-old son died, describes sorrow as a wave in the ocean. He said, "You can be swimming along just fine, when suddenly it hits you. You never see it coming and never know when it will hit." Although people differ in their reactions, in one study, 83 percent of people and their spouse caregivers experienced chronic sorrow (Hainsworth, Eakes, & Burke, 1994). Depression is an expected by-product of chronic sorrow. Although not all clients experience severe depression, most display at least transient evidence of it (Frank, Elliott, Corcoran, & Wonderlich, 1987; Rybarcyzk, Nyenhuis, Nicholas, Cash, & Kaiser, 1995; Wortman & Silver, 1989).

A middle-range theory of chronic sorrow recognizes the phenomenon as a normal response to ongoing "living" loss across the life span that may be progressive, recurring, permanent, or cyclical (Eakes, Burke, & Hainsworth, 1998; Gordon, 2009). This normal response to grief may become pathological and coexist with depression if one's support system is lacking or if there is insufficient assistance for problems with coping, as evidenced in parents experiencing chronic sorrow (Gordon, 2009). Recommendations for health care practitioners are to evaluate chronic sorrow and collaborate with and support people to foster improved coping skills.

Antecedent trigger events play a strong role in chronic sorrow. Comparing the reality of one's situation to the "normal" milestones of life can also precipitate the sorrow. Grief is renewed as each loss is realized, that is, the ability to walk, the ability to procreate, loss of dreams, loss of income (Gill, 1999). Chronic sorrow is not only the province of parents regarding children. Children also experience this if their parent, sibling, or friend dies young and cannot attend a graduation, wedding, or the birth of a child. Consider the earlier example of the father who still grieves for his son who died at 10 years old. The father is not alone in his grief; the boy's brother would have had him be his best man at his recent wedding.

A mother's journal continues:

> It was excruciatingly painful for me to walk into her school. It was so painful; I used to get physically ill. I could not participate in the PTA or be a room mother because I could not bear to hear the other mothers talking about all their children's activities and successes, when our daughter wasn't doing any of those things. All my closest friends have family members with serious illness or disabilities.
>
> A couple of months ago, my mother came to visit. She wanted to buy my daughter a birthday present, so we went to [the department store]. She ended up trying on prom dresses, even though she is not going to the prom, and she is not going to graduate on time. She has never been to a single high school dance or football game or any of those things. I had to leave the store and sit in my car and cry. I wasn't crying about the prom. It was the prom that opened the door for everything.

We cannot expect chronic sorrow to resolve with final acceptance, which typically occurs in other forms of grief, because the chronicity of the disability serves as a constant reminder of the loss (Burke, Hainsworth, Eakes, & Lindgren, 1992). However, a distinction is made between chronic sorrow and pathological grief. Pathological grief is characterized by unrelenting feelings of sadness, guilt, or anger, whereas the presence of chronic sorrow still allows for an adaptation, characterized by a highly functional lifestyle.

## Summary

This chapter introduced the continuum of loss, grief, and coping as a process rather than finite stages. Everyone experiences loss in their lives, and clients are challenged by additional losses from injury, disease, disability, and death. Primary and secondary types of losses were discussed, both of which can cause psychological distress. These losses pose issues for the client, as well as for the personal and professional caregivers.

In response to loss, there is the universal human phenomenon of grief, a psychological and physiological process that occurs in response to loss in every age group and culture. It is a painful process during which people, we hope, can understand the meaning of the loss and accept its place in their lives. Reactions to loss are as varied as the people who experience them, but there are common themes.

Following a loss, many variables affect the outcome, including the anguish of the loss, the deprivation experienced by the loss, and the diminution of cognitive capabilities. We explored the types of grief, including anticipatory, acute, chronic, delayed, and suppressed grief. We also described grieving behaviors, emphasizing that the outward behavior of a grieving person can be deceiving.

Three models of bereavement were presented: the widely known stage theory of Kübler-Ross, the integrative theory of bereavement, and the tasks of mourning. Because grief is also a natural response to a loss of meaning in one's life, adjustment necessitates finding a new meaning and purpose or reframing them. It may require creating a harmony between one's losses here and now and the possibilities for future opportunities.

We also explored the lifelong, episodic, and progressive sadness characteristic of the phenomenon of chronic sorrow. In the next chapter, we will study therapeutic responses to loss and grief and how the health care provider can assist in the process of coping.

## Reflective Questions

1. a. What activities, functions, or people are most important to you?
   b. Which are you most afraid of losing? Why?
   c. What would this loss mean to you?
   d. How do you think you might react to this loss?
2. Consider the multiple combined problems facing people as they age.
   a. What do you think it would be like to wonder what you might "lose" next?
   b. What could you do to maintain meaning in your life?
   c. What would motivate you to get out of bed in the morning?
3. Of the three models of grieving presented in this chapter, which one feels most valid to you? Explain why.

4. Out of fear of doing or saying the "wrong" thing, people often avoid those who are grieving.
   a. What are some verbal and nonverbal responses or actions that might be supportive or helpful to a person who is grieving?
   b. What responses might be detrimental?
5. What behaviors might you observe in a person who is experiencing grief that are indicative of
   a. denial?
   b. anger?
   c. guilt?
   d. bargaining?
   e. sadness or depression?
   f. anxiety?
   g. diminished problem-solving?

## Case Study

Cynthia Osbourne is a survivor. In a fiery blaze at a nightclub that killed 100 people and injured hundreds more, she lost her fiancé and was burned over more than 30 percent of her body. First rushed to a nearby hospital, then moved to an out-of-state burn center and then another hospital, she was kept unconscious so that she would not have to endure the unbearable pain from the burned areas. During this time, surgeons performed 10 skin grafts on her body, including her hands.

Three months after the fire, she was transferred to a rehabilitation hospital, still in a neighboring state. Her 10-year-old and 7-year-old sons have been in the care of their grandparents. Now that she is out of the induced coma, Cynthia has flashbacks to the flames, the screaming in the inferno, and seeing piles of bodies being trampled as people tried to exit the building.

Lying in bed for 3 months resulted in heterotrophic ossification in both knees and an elbow, caused by a buildup of calcium that accumulated due to inactivity. Unable to bend her knees, she had generalized limited function, mobility, range of motion, and strength. She doubted that she would ever walk again. In addition, scar tissue on her hands limited her ability to feed herself and perform other self-care activities. Therapy included very painful stretching, attempts at standing, and eventually walking a few steps. Because she could not flex her knees, she had to descend stairs backwards and had difficulty getting into and out of a car from/to a wheelchair.

Throughout this difficult period in Cynthia's life, the physical therapist, physical therapist assistant, and occupational therapist were able to make Cynthia laugh. She credits their supportive, nurturing care in helping her to reach this point in time and "not be crazy." Although Cynthia was the youngest person at the rehabilitation center, she was close in age to the therapy team, who would "break up the day" by dropping in to visit her.

Because everything in her life is now different, she has had moments of weeping and sadness. However, she has maintained a positive attitude throughout the hospitalization part of the ordeal. Cynthia and her fiancé were planning a wedding and shopping for a home. She has had to grieve her situation, as well as the loss of her partner.

1. a. Describe Cynthia's losses.
   b. Identify which losses are internal losses and which are external losses. Provide a rationale for your decisions.
   c. Identify which losses are primary and which are secondary types of losses. Provide a rationale for your decisions.
2. Discuss the impact of Cynthia's losses and limitations on her self-esteem, independence, and social roles, including those of parenting and vocation.
3. a. What phase of grieving might Cynthia now be experiencing in each of the three models described in the text: stages of grieving and dying, integrative theory of bereavement, and tasks of mourning.
   b. Provide a rationale for each of your decisions.
4. In what ways are the therapeutic team members influencing possible outcomes of Cynthia's grief?

## References

Alaszewski, A., Alaszewski, H., & Potter, J. (2004). The bereavement model, stroke and rehabilitation: A critical analysis of the use of a psychological model in professional practice. *Disability Rehabilitation, 26* (18), 1067–1078.

Axelsson, B., & Sjoden, P. O. (1998). Quality of life of cancer patients and their spouses in palliative home care. *Palliative Medicine, 12*(1), 29–39.

Bateman, A., Broderick, D., Gleason, L., Kardon, R., Flaherty, C., & Anderson, S. (1992). Dysfunctional grieving. *Journal of Psychosocial Nursing and Mental Health Services, 30*(12), 5–9.

Beach, S. R., Schulz, R., Yee, J. L., & Jackson, S. (2000). Negative and positive health effects of caring for a disabled spouse: Longitudinal findings from the Caregiver Health Effects Study. *Psychology and Aging, 15*(2), 259–271.

Beck, M. N. (1999). *Expecting Adam.* New York, NY: Berkley.

Berger, S. A. (2009). *The five ways we grieve: Finding your personal path to healing after the loss of a loved one.* Boston, MA: Shambala Publications.

Billings, D. W., Folkman, S., Acree, M., & Moskowitz, J. T. (2000). Coping and physical health during caregiving:

The roles of positive and negative affect. *Journal of Personality and Social Psychology, 79*(1), 131–142.

Blanchard, C. G., & Ruckdeschel, J. C. (1986). Psychosocial aspects of cancer in adults: Implications for teaching medical students. *Journal of Cancer Education, 1*(4), 237–248.

Boelen, P. A., & Prigerson, H. G. (2007). The influence of symptoms of prolonged grief disorder, depression, and anxiety on quality of life among bereaved adults: A prospective study. *European Archives of Psychiatry and Clinical Neuroscience, 257*(8), 444–452.

Boss, P. (1999). *Ambiguous loss.* Cambridge, MA: Harvard University Press.

Boss, P., & Couden, B. A. (2002). Ambiguous loss from chronic physical illness: Clinical interventions with individuals, couples, and families. *Journal of Clinical Psychology, 58*(11), 1351–1360.

Bowlby, J. (1980). *Attachment and loss: Vol. 3. Loss: Sadness and depression.* New York, NY: Basic Books.

Breitbart, W. (1990). Cancer pain and suicide. In K. Foley, J. J. Bonica, & V. Ventafridda (Eds.), *Advances in pain research and therapy* (Vol. 16, pp. 399–472). New York, NY: Raven Press.

Breitbart, W., Chochinov, H., & Passik, S. (1998). Psychiatric aspects of palliative care. In D. Doyle, G. Hanks, & N. MacDonald (Eds.), *Oxford textbook of palliative medicine* (pp. 933–954). New York, NY: Oxford University Press.

Breitbart, W., & Rosenfeld, B. (1999). Physician-assisted suicide: The influence of psychosocial issues. *Cancer Control, 6*(2), 146–161.

Bruce, C A. (2007). Helping patients, families, caregivers, and physicians in the grieving process. *Journal of the American Osteopathic Association, 107*(12), ES33–ES40.

Burke, M., & Flaherty, M. J. (1993). Coping strategies and health status of elderly arthritic women. *Journal of Advanced Nursing, 18*(1), 7–13.

Burke, M. L., Hainsworth, M. A., Eakes, G. G., & Lindgren, C. L. (1992). Current knowledge and research on chronic sorrow: A foundation for inquiry. *Death Studies, 16*, 231–245.

Cable, D. G. (1998). Grief in the American culture. In K. Doka & J. Davidson (Eds.), *Living with grief: Who we are, how we grieve* (pp. 61–71). Philadelphia, PA: Hospice Foundation of America.

Caplan, G. (1990). Loss, stress, and mental health. *Community Mental Health Journal, 26*(1), 27–48.

Cerney, M. S., & Buskirk, J. R. (1991). Anger: The hidden part of grief. *Bulletin of the Menninger Clinic, 55*(2), 228–237.

Cheng, J. O., Lo, R. S., Chan, F. M., Kwan, B. H., & Woo, J. (2010). An exploration of anticipatory grief in advanced cancer patients. *Psychooncology, 19*(7), 693–700.

Cheville, A. L. (2000). Cancer rehabilitation and palliative care. *Rehabilitation Oncology, 18*(1), 19–20.

Clark, A., Stedmon, J., & Margison, S. (2008). An exploration of the experience of mothers whose children sustain traumatic brain injury and their families. *Clinical Child Psychology and Psychiatry, 13*(4), 565–583.

Clukey, L. (2008). Anticipatory mourning: Processes of expected loss in palliative care. *International Journal of Palliative Nursing, 14*(7), 316, 318–325.

Coser, R. L. (1963). Alienation and the social structure. In E. Friedson (Ed.), *The hospital in modern society* (pp. 231–265). Glencoe, IL: Free Press.

Coughlin, R. (1993). *Grieving: A love story.* New York, NY: Random House.

Drench, M. E. (1992). A phenomenological study of the lived experience of health care professionals working with people with acquired immune deficiency syndrome. *Dissertation Abstracts International, 53*(5), 25.82B. (University Microfilms No. 9226096)

Drench, M. E. (1995). Coping with loss—Adjusting to change. *International Society for Behavioral Science in Physical Therapy, 7*(2), 1–4.

Drench, M. E. (1998). *Red ribbons are not enough: Health caregivers' stories about AIDS.* Wilsonville, OR: BookPartners.

Eakes, G. G. (1993). Chronic sorrow: A response to living with cancer. *Oncology Nursing Forum, 20*(9), 1327–1334.

Eakes, G. G., Burke, M. L., & Hainsworth, M. A. (1998). Middle-range theory of chronic sorrow. *Image Journal of Nursing Scholarship, 30*(2), 179–184.

Eriksson-Mangold, M., & Carlsson, S. G. (1991). Psychological and somatic distress in relation to perceived hearing disability, hearing handicap, and hearing measurements. *Journal of Psychosomatic Research, 35*(6), 729–740.

Erlandsson, S. I., Hallberg, L. R., & Axelsson, A. (1992). Psychological and audiological correlates of perceived tinnitus severity. *Audiology, 31*(3), 168–179.

Evans, R. L., Bishop, D. S., & Ousley, R. T. (1992). Providing care to persons with physical disability. Effect on family caregiving. *American Journal of Physical Medicine and Rehabilitation, 71*(3), 140–144.

Fairclough, D. L. (1998). Quality of life, cancer investigation, and clinical practice. *Cancer Investigation, 76*, 478–484.

Feldstein, M. A., & Gemma, P. B. (1995). Oncology nurses and chronic compounded grief. *Cancer Nursing, 18*(3), 228–236.

Figley, C. R. (Ed.). (1995). *Compassion fatigue: Coping with secondary traumatic stress disorder in those who treat the traumatized.* New York, NY: Brunner/Mazel.

Folkman, S., & Moskowitz, J. T. (2000). Positive affect and the other side of coping. *American Psychologist, 55*(6), 647–654.

Frank, R. G., Elliott, T. R. Corcoran, J. R., & Wonderlich, S. A. (1987). Depression after spinal cord injury: Is it necessary? *Clinical Psychology Review, 7*, 611–622.

Frankl, V. E. (1984). *Man's search for meaning: An introduction to logotherapy* (3rd ed.). New York, NY: Simon & Schuster.

Frears, L. H., & Schneider, J. M. (1981). Exploring grief and loss in a wholistic framework. *Personnel and Guidance Journal, 59*(6), 341–345.

Fulton, G., Madden, C., & Minichiello, V. (1996). The social construction of anticipatory grief. *Social Science and Medicine, 43*(9), 1349–1358.

Garner, J. (1997). Dementia: An intimate death. *British Journal of Medical Psychology, 70*(Pt. 2), 177–184.

Gill, M. (1999). Psychosocial implications of spinal cord injury. *Critical Care Nursing Quarterly, 22*(2), 1–7.

Gilliland, G., & Fleming, S. (1998). A comparison of spousal anticipatory grief and conventional grief. *Death Studies, 22*(6), 541–569.

Gordon, J. (2009). An evidence-based approach for supporting parents experiencing chronic sorrow. *Pediatric Nursing, 35*(2), 115–119.

Gordon, W. A., & Hibbard, M. R. (1997). Post-stroke depression: An examination of the literature. *Archives of Physical Medicine and Rehabilitation, 78*, 658–663.

Grealy, L. (1994). *Autobiography of a face.* Boston, MA: Houghton Mifflin.

Hainsworth, D. S. (1998). Reflections on loss without death: The lived experience of acute care nurses caring for neurologically devastated patients. *Holistic Nursing Practice, 13*(1), 41–50.

Hainsworth, M. A. (1994). Living with multiple sclerosis: The experience of chronic sorrow. *Journal of Neuroscience Nursing, 26*(4), 237–240.

Hainsworth, M. A. (1995). Helping spouses with chronic sorrow related to multiple sclerosis. *Journal of Gerontological Nursing, 21*(7), 29–33.

Hainsworth, M. A., Burke, M. L., Lindgren, C. L., & Eakes, G. G. (1993). Chronic sorrow in multiple sclerosis: A case study. *Home Healthcare Nurse, 11*(2), 9–13.

Hainsworth, M. A., Eakes, G. G., & Burke, M. L. (1994). Coping with chronic sorrow. *Issues in Mental Health Nursing, 15*(1), 59–66.

Hall, J. (1997). Nursing stress: Applying the wisdom of the wounded healer. *Lamp, 54*(8), 24–25.

Hermann, N., Black, S. E., Lawrence, J., Szekely, C., & Szalai, J. P. (1998). The Sunnybrook stroke study: A prospective study of depressive symptoms and functional outcomes. *Stroke, 29*, 618–624.

Herth, K. (1998). Integrating hearing loss into one's life. *Quality Health, 8*(2), 207–223.

Hobdell, E. F., Grant, M. L., Valencia, I., Mare, J., Kothare, S. V., Legido, A., & Khurana, D. S. (2007). Chronic sorrow and coping in families of children with epilepsy. *Journal of Neuroscience Nursing, 39*(2), 76–82.

Holley, C. K., & Mast, B. T. (2009). The impact of anticipatory grief on caregiver burden in dementia caregivers. *Gerontologist, 49*(3), 388–396.

Horowitz, M. J., Siegel, B., Holen, A., Bonanno, G. A., Milbrath, C., & Stinson, C. H. (2003). *Diagnostic criteria for complicated grief disorder, Focus 1* (pp. 290–298). Washington, DC: American Psychological Association.

Hunfeld, J. A., Wladimiroff, J. W., & Passchier, J. (1997). Prediction and course of grief four years after perinatal loss due to congenital anomalies: A follow-up study. *British Journal of Medical Psychology, 70*(Pt. 1), 85–91.

Jackson, V. A., Mack, J., Matsuyama, R., Lakoma, M. D., Sullivan, A. M., Arnold, R. M., & Block, S. D. (2008).JaJ A qualitative study of oncologists' approaches to end-of-life care. *Journal of Palliative Medicine, 11*(6), 893–906.

Jacob, S. R. (1996). The grief experience of older women whose husbands had hospice care. *Journal of Advanced Nursing, 24*(2), 280–286.

Kalb, R. (2007). The emotional and psychological impact of multiple sclerosis relapses. *Journal of the Neurological Sciences, 256*(Suppl. 1), S29–S33.

Kash, K. M., Holland, J. C., Breitbart, W., Berenson, S., Dougherty, J., Ouellette-Kobasa, S., & Lesko, L. (2000). Stress and burnout in oncology. *Oncology (Williston Park, NY), 14*(11), 1621–1633; discussion 1633–1634, 1636–1637.

Krafft, S. K., & Krafft, L. J. (1998). Chronic sorrow: Parents' lived experience. *Holistic Nursing Practice, 13*(1), 59–67.

Kübler-Ross, E. (1969). *On death and dying.* New York, NY: Macmillan.

Langer, K. G. (1994). Depression and denial in psychotherapy of persons with disabilities. *American Journal of Psychotherapy, 48*(2), 181–194.

Lee, G. A. (2009). Determinants of quality of life five years after coronary artery bypass graft surgery. *Heart and Lung, 38*(2), 91–99.

Lev, E. L., & McCorkle, R. (1998). Loss, grief, and bereavement in family members of cancer patients. *Seminars in Oncology Nursing, 14*(2), 145–151.

Liedström, E., Isaksson, A. K., & Ahlström, G. (2008). Chronic sorrow in next of kin of patients with multiple sclerosis. *Journal of Neuroscience Nursing, 40*(5), 304–311.

Longman, A. J., Braden, C. J., & Mishel, M. H. (1999). Side effects burden, psychological adjustment, and life quality in women with breast cancer: Pattern of association over time. *Oncology Nursing Forum, 26*(5), 909–915.

Loos, C., & Bowd, A. (1997). Caregivers of persons with Alzheimer's disease: Some neglected implications of the experience of personal loss and grief. *Death Studies, 21*(5), 501–514.

Lowes, L., & Lyne, P. (2000). Chronic sorrow in parents of children with newly diagnosed diabetes: A review of the literature and discussion of the implications for nursing practice. *Journal of Advanced Nursing, 32*(1), 41–48.

Maguire, P., Walsh, S., Jeacock, J., & Kingston, R. (1999). Physical and psychological needs of patients dying from colorectal cancer. *Palliative Medicine, 13*(1), 45–50.

Mallow, G. E., & Bechtel, G. A. (1999). Chronic sorrow: The experience of parents with children who are developmentally disabled. *Journal of Psychosocial Nursing and Mental Health Services, 37*(7), 31–35.

Maslach, C., Schaufeli, W. B., & Leiter, M. P. (2001). Job burnout. *Annual Review of Psychology, 52*, 397–422.

Maxeiner, A. M., Saga, E., Downer, C., & Arthur, L. (2009). Comparing the psychosocial issues experienced by individuals with primary vs. secondary lymphedema. *Rehabilitation Oncology, 27*(2), 9–15.

Ormel, J., Kempen, G. I., Penninx, B. W., Brilman, E. I., Beekman, A. T., & van Sonderen, E. (1997). Chronic medical conditions and mental health in older people: Disability and psychosocial resources mediate specific mental health effects. *Psychological Medicine, 27*(5), 1065–1077.

Peteet, J. R. (2000). Cancer and the meaning of work. *General Hospital Psychiatry, 22*(3), 200–205.

Pilkington, F. B. (1999). A qualitative study of life after stroke. *Journal of Neuroscience Nursing, 31*(6), 336–347.

Pound, P., Gompertz, P., & Ebrahim, S. (1998). A patient-centered study of the consequences of stroke. *Clinical Rehabilitation, 12*(4), 338–347.

Prigerson, H. G., & Jacobs, S. C. (2001). Traumatic grief as a distinct disorder: A rationale, consensus criteria, and a preliminary empirical test. In M. S. Stroebe, R. O. Hansson, W. Stroebe, & H. Schut (Eds.), *Handbook of bereavement research: Consequences, coping, and care* (pp. 613–647). Washington, DC: American Psychological Association.

Prigerson, H. G., Shear, M. K., Jacobs, S. C., Reynolds, C. F., Maciejewski, P. K., Davidson, J. R. T., . . . Zisook, S. (1999). Consensus criteria for traumatic grief. *British Journal of Psychiatry, 174*, 67–73.

Purtilo, R. (1984). *Health professional/patient interaction* (3rd ed.). Philadelphia, PA: W. B. Saunders.

Rosenberg, C. J. (1998). Faculty–student mentoring. A father's chronic sorrow: A daughter's perspective. *Journal of Holistic Nursing, 16*(3), 399–404.

Rybarcyzk, B., Nyenhuis, D. L., Nicholas, J. J., Cash, S. M., & Kaiser, J. (1995). Body image, perceived social stigma, and the prediction of psychosocial adjustment to leg amputation. *Rehabilitation Psychology, 40*(2), 95–105.

Sanders, C. M. (1989). *Grief: The mourning after*. New York, NY: Wiley.

Shear, K., Monk, T., Houck, P., Melhem, N., Frank, E., Reynolds, C., & Sillowash, R. (2007). An attachment-based model of complicated grief including the role of avoidance. *European Archives of Psychiatry and Clinical Neuroscience, 257*(8), 453–461.

Siegal, B. S. (1986). *Love, medicine and miracles: Lessons learned about self-healing from a surgeon's experience with exceptional patients*. New York, NY: Harper & Row.

Siepman, T. A., Janssens, A. C., de Koning, I., Polman, C. H., Boringa, J. B., & Hintzen, R. Q. (2008). The role of disability and depression in cognitive functioning within 2 years after multiple sclerosis diagnosis. *Journal of Neurology, 255*(6), 910–916.

Sirki, K., Saarinen-Pihkala, U. M., & Hovi, L. (2000). Coping of parents and siblings with the death of a child with cancer: Death after terminal care compared with death during active anticancer therapy. *Acta Paediatrics, 89*(6), 717–721.

Smith, L. N., Norrie, J., Kerr, S. M., Lawrence, I. M., Langhorne, P., & Lees, K. R. (2004). Impact and influences on caregiver outcomes at one year post-stroke. *Cerebrovascular Disease, 18*(2), 145–153.

Sullivan, M. D. (2003). Hope and hopelessness at the end of life. *American Journal of Geriatric Psychiatry, 11*(4), 393–405.

Sussman, N. (1995). Reactions of patients to the diagnosis and treatment of cancer. *Anticancer Drugs, 6*(Suppl. 1), 4–8.

Svedlund, M., & Axelsson, I. (2000). Acute myocardial infarction in middle-aged women: Narrations from the patients and their partners during rehabilitation. *Intensive Critical Care Nursing, 16*(4), 256–265.

Vilhjalmsson, R. (1998). Direct and indirect effects of chronic physical conditions on depression: A preliminary investigation. *Social Science and Medicine, 47*(5), 603–611.

Viorst, J. (1986). *Necessary losses: The loves, illusions, dependencies and impossible expectations that all of us have to give up in order to grow.* New York, NY: Fawcett Gold Medal.

Ward, L., Mathias, J. L., & Hitchings, S. E. (2007). Relationship between bereavement and cognitive functioning in older adults. *Gerontology, 53*(6), 362–372.

Weiss, L., Frischer, L., & Richman, J. (1989). Parental adjustment to intrapartum and delivery room loss: The role of a hospital-based support program. *Clinical Perinatology, 16*(4), 1009–1019.

Wess, M. (2007). Bringing hope and healing to grieving patients with cancer. *Journal of the American Osteopathic Association, 107*(12), ES41–ES47.

White, Y., & Grenyer, B. F. (1999). The biopsychosocial impact of end-stage renal disease: The experience of dialysis patients and their partners. *Journal of Advanced Nursing, 30*(6), 1312–1320.

Worden, J. W. (2002). *Grief counseling and grief therapy* (3rd ed.). New York, NY: Springer.

Wortman, C. B., & Silver, R. C. (1989). The myth of coping with loss. *Journal of Consulting Clinical Psychology, 57,* 349–355.

Yardley, L. (1994). Contribution of symptoms and beliefs to handicap in people with vertigo: A longitudinal study. *British Journal of Clinical Psychology, 33*(Pt. 1), 101–113.

# Coping

When I first looked at Diane sitting in her wheelchair by the edge of the pool, I only saw a woman "crippled" by her condition. (Honestly, that's the word that came to mind; so much for people-first language.) Scleroderma had stretched her skin so taut that I thought it would tear. It pulled with such force that her facial features were distorted into a perpetual smile, and her hands and feet were deformed. She was a 20-year-old woman, though she looked at least 40, and was frozen in place. There was nothing she could functionally do for herself. On Saturday mornings, though, she was transformed as she "swam" in the community pool. As her volunteer pool buddy this week, I carefully lifted her tight body off the chair and lowered her into the water. Almost inaudibly, she said, "This is what heaven feels like. It's the one time all week that I feel like a human being."

It seemed like being in the pool gave her a small sense of control and an important way for her to cope with her life.

—*From the journal of Paul Rodriguez, physical therapist student*

Albert Camus, Nobel laureate for literature, said, "In the depth of winter, I finally learned that within me there lay an invincible summer." On the continuum of loss and grief and adjustment, there is coping—an adaptation to new circumstances, awareness, knowledge, and growth. Individuals may need to adapt to changes in relationships with family and friends or deal with employment, financial, and insurance issues. This chapter discusses coping behavior, psychosocial adaptation strategies, and implications for health care professionals.

## COPING BEHAVIOR

As we discussed in the previous chapter, there are many types of personal losses and grief responses. Sometimes we experience a collective grief. The public united in collective horror at the sudden attack on the United States one September morning in 2001. Terrorists hijacked commercial airplanes and used them to crash into and destroy the World Trade Center in New York and part of the Pentagon in Washington, D.C. A third terrorist mission was aborted by passengers and crew who diverted their airplane and crashed it into a field in Pennsylvania instead. The terrorists killed thousands of people that morning. The world community faced incomprehensible shock and grief in January 2010, when a devastating earthquake suddenly and swiftly killed hundreds of thousands of people in Haiti.

The passage of time may dull the intensity of emotions, but memories can become embedded in our common psyche. Most of us are untrained in how to cope with loss and grief. In contemporary society, people create artificial timetables and expect themselves and others to conform to them. We believe that grieving should only last so long. We should resume life's activities and return to the workplace within a prescribed period of time. Try to have another baby. Start dating. While a structured routine fills the often endless hours with activities and thoughts other than grieving, it does not put closure on bereavement. Because the loss and grief experience is distinct for every individual, people have their own unique timetables for responding.

Value judgments are often made about the way people grieve, as if there is a "right" way. People assess losses and determine the validity of a loss and subsequent grief. For instance, the loss of a 3-month-old child is considered a valid reason to grieve. On the other hand, not everyone understands the full significance of a miscarriage, stillbirth, or neonatal death. They may not even consider it a "real" loss and, therefore, not support the grieving person.

Other losses that may be trivialized or not validated through social recognition include the death of a pet or of someone in a relationship that is not socially sanctioned, such as a partner in a gay or extramarital relationship. The manner of death also has an impact on the social support offered to grieving people. Death resulting from suicide or substance abuse may be perceived as a choice, or the individuals may be blamed for their weaknesses. Yet, the loss is real to those left behind, and they still need supportive care. Often they feel isolated and alone because the social stigma attached to their loss prevents "normal" levels of social support. They may also experience negative and hurtful messages about the manner of death.

Illness, impairment, and disability do not have the same finality as death, and people may use different coping behavior. Many factors contribute to how a person emotionally responds, including one's premorbid personality, experience with previous illness and grief experiences, and the impact of the illness, such as how far reaching the changes will be and how long the disruption lasts. Other influences that contribute to how a person responds and copes include expectations, life responsibilities and aspirations, age, and support available to help one deal with the stressful situation. For example, the late Senator Ted Kennedy taught his eldest son that nothing is impossible. At his father's funeral, Ted Kennedy, Jr., who had his leg amputated secondary to bone cancer when he was 12 years old, told the story that months after his surgery, his father suggested that they sled down their driveway to enjoy the snowfall. Ted Jr. recalls:

> I was trying to get used to my new artificial leg. . . . As I struggled to walk, I slipped, and I fell on the ice. And I started to cry, and I said, "I can't do this. I'll never be able to climb up that hill." And he lifted me up in his strong, gentle arms and said something I will never forget. He said, "I know you can do it. There is nothing that you

can't do. We're going to climb that hill together, even if it takes us all day." . . . At age 12, losing your leg pretty much seems like the end of the world. But as I climbed on his back, and we flew down the hill that day, I knew he was right. I knew I was going to be OK. You see, my father taught me that even our most profound losses are survivable . . . it is what we do with that loss, our ability to transform it into a positive event (Kennedy, 2009).

To cope optimally with change, the person first needs to accept the loss, grieve the loss, and then learn to adapt to the changes. Coping involves cognitive and behavioral changes to lessen, control, or accept situational demands, in other words, to manage them. It is a mechanism and a process that is used to shield oneself from psychological harm and difficult situations. It is a way to control the impact of stressors. There are many means of coping, and everybody adds their own "spin" to it, creating their unique style.

Coping strategies can differ with regard to success. Some may be inadequate, such as "giving up," especially if the person has a pattern of learned helplessness. Other maladaptive forms of coping include blaming others, self-indulging, blaming oneself, and using defense mechanisms (Weiten, Lloyd, Dunn, & Hammer, 2009). In contrast, adaptive coping is healthier and more successful and includes dealing with problems, being realistic in the assessment of stress and coping, identifying and confronting unhealthy emotional responses to stress, and controlling, to the degree possible, detrimental behavior.

In their foundational work, Lazarus and Folkman (1984a) said that two elements need to exist for stress to affect a person: A person identifies a circumstance as threatening or challenging *and* deems that he or she does not have resources to deal with the circumstance. Pearlin and Schooler (1978) delineate three functions of coping in their classic work: Eradicate or reduce stressful circumstances, manage the meaning of the stressors and situation, and reign in emotional effects. Coping is a way to deal with life challenges. For example, clients with diabetes cannot eradicate the stressor of this chronic disease, but they can learn to manage it.

Lazarus and Folkman (1984a) designed a paradigm of the three steps in a coping process. The initial step or primary appraisal is when a person evaluates the stress (i.e., "Am I in trouble?"); the next step or secondary appraisal is when a person contemplates ways of coping (i.e., "What, if anything, can I do about it?"); and the third step, tertiary appraisal, is when coping options are put into action. These actions do not necessarily lead to immediate success; more commonly, they have to be tried, evaluated, and modified. They called these coping strategies *problem focused* if they focused on action, and *emotion focused* if they focused on feelings and reduced emotional distress.

## Coping Skills

People who experience loss and subsequent grief use different means to cope in order to "get through the day." The word *skill* is often paired with *coping*, which connotes an active process that can be learned. Coping is "defined as the thoughts and behaviors used to manage the internal and external demands of situations that are appraised as stressful" (Folkman & Moskowitz, 2004, p. 745). As such, it is a step in adapting to changed circumstances and not a situation of one-size-fits-all. Rather, "effective" coping is situation and person specific. To make matters more complex, the word *effective* is a value judgment. Three classic models for constructive coping with stresses have been developed and modified (Lazarus & Folkman, 1984a, 1984b; Moos & Billings, 1982;

Moos & Schaefer, 1986). Their contention is that people employ strategies that are appraisal focused, problem focused, emotion focused, or a combination of these approaches.

**APPRAISAL-FOCUSED COPING**    Appraisal-focused coping helps an individual seek out the *meaning* in a situation that might be threatening or negative and look for the positive. It is a logical cognitive process that entails assessment and mental practice, definition and reframing, and avoidance or denial. Individuals divide an overpowering situation into smaller manageable parts, rather than absorbing the entire situation at once, which can be incredibly overwhelming (Drench, 2003a, 2003b). They evaluate what is happening in the present and integrate how well they may have handled challenging situations in the past.

Appraisal-focused coping entails examining or reframing situations to assess the meaning associated with a crisis. It helps a person understand the current circumstances. Receiving unfortunate medical news, the client can think, "It could be worse." When someone close dies, people often say, "Well, he lived a long life." Some of the strategies used in appraisal-focused coping include examining one's values, considering the meaning of life, and reassessing spiritual or religious beliefs (Folkman, 2008). Negative or maladaptive appraisal-focused coping can amplify the extent and significance of a problem and involve catastrophic thinking. It may take the form of a person framing his or her experience with illness as "payment for his or her sins." In contrast, positive, or adaptive, appraisal-focused coping is more rational and hopeful and promotes productive coping.

When a person is grieving, it often helps to find some meaning in what is happening. For some, this meaning comes in the context of spirituality or a belief in divine intervention or purpose. For others, it involves becoming an instrument of hope or a resource in coping for others. For clients with cancer, for example, religious and spiritual coping strategies can help with long-term adjustment, by sustaining self-esteem and helping them to find a purpose or meaning in their illness (Baldacchino & Draper, 2001). For others, spirituality may be a source of hope and provide a sense of well-being (Thuné-Boyle, Stygall, Keshtgar, & Newman, 2006).

Appraisal-focused coping that involves reframing or redefining circumstances is a rational process that incorporates identifying negative understandings and reinterpreting them into positive meanings. For example, a man diagnosed with cutaneous lymphoma considered himself in a better position than another client with non-Hodgkin's lymphoma. By comparing himself to another, he realized that his situation "wasn't so bad."

In addition, some people reframe the grief experience and perceive it as a gift, enabling them to grow in positive ways. Candy Lightner, founder of Mothers Against Drunk Driving, believes that although death takes something precious away, it can also give something back. She became a crusader for driving while sober after her child was killed by a drunk driver. This tragedy became the motivating factor for her to create an organization that has significantly raised the public's awareness about drunk driving.

After grief work, some people develop greater compassion and awareness that enables them to help themselves and others. Illness can also be a catalyst for changing priorities and values. Some people develop dissatisfaction or a sense of urgency in their lives, whereas others become empowered to do things that they might otherwise not have contemplated. They may seek different jobs, homes, or relationships.

Appraisal-focused coping can also involve denial or avoidance. People may minimize or deny the severity or existence of a situation, in order to protect themselves from fully recognizing the stress. They may even distance themselves from the circumstances. This allows them to unconsciously "stall," providing time for additional coping skills to be developed or called on. After a young National Hockey League hopeful sustained a substantial eye injury during a game, he initially said he planned to pursue his dream and would play at that level again. A year later, despite the fact that he maintained his overall physical fitness and underwent multiple eye treatments, it became obvious to him that his optimistic outlook would not be realized. He would need to pursue other career goals.

**PROBLEM-FOCUSED COPING**    Problem-focused coping emphasizes the practical aspects of a situation, and, as the name implies, is directed at solving the problem at hand and altering situations that clients view as controllable or amenable to change. To be effective, the problem(s) must first be identified; alternative options for *action* need to be recognized and evaluated; and an action needs to be selected and implemented. In other words, the individual describes the problem to be solved, comes up with possible solutions, and evaluates the pros and cons of each.

To begin, the person garners information and support, learning the facts about the situation and courses of action, and then explores the possible consequences. As adaptive as this is when it is balanced, excessive intellectualization can be maladaptive. After collecting information and support, a person who is engaged in problem-focused coping will move into action, which can include scheduling rehabilitation appointments, arranging transportation to a clinic or Meals-on-Wheels, structuring the day around care and rest periods (Drench, 2003b), or managing nutrition and medication for a person with diabetes (Grey, 2000). It can also involve getting help from others, managing time wisely, practicing self-control, and using only productive, assertive behavior. Consider Sheila, who was recently hospitalized for an opportunistic infection related to AIDS. She asked each of seven friends to be available to care for her children one day a week, so that she would not have to worry about that detail if she required emergency care at any time.

Developing alternative measures of satisfaction or success is another aspect of problem-focused coping skills. When the challenges of Parkinson's disease reportedly became too significant for actor Michael J. Fox to continue with the demands of a popular television show, he stopped working and redirected his energy toward raising awareness and funds for the disease. He also balanced his schedule so he could spend more time with his family. By making these changes in his life, he created other avenues of satisfaction and measures of success.

**EMOTION-FOCUSED COPING**    In addition to appraisal- and problem-focused coping skills, people also use emotion-focused coping strategies, which involve managing the *emotions* associated with a critical situation. These strategies are used to reduce emotional distress and make life less overwhelming and "easier to bear." As such, they may be helpful in dealing with the pain or discomfort associated with a particular form of treatment. These strategies regulate the emotional components of stressful situations and are best suited for those over which the client has little control.

Lazarus and Folkman (1984a) believe that emotion-focused coping strategies can be productive, particularly when an individual perceives that there is nothing that can be done to alter the stressor or that the stressor will be fleeting. These skills can ease frustration and stress. An example of this is the healthy use of humor (see Chapter 5). In addition, "actively processing and expressing emotion" improved adjustment and health status for women with breast cancer, as evidenced by fewer physician visits for cancer-related problems, better health and energy, and less distress than women who did not use these coping strategies (Stanton et al., 2000). Further, emotion-focused coping helps lessen the negative feelings about stressors in people with spinal cord injury (i.e., bowel and bladder accidents; secondary disability, illness, and injury; public embarrassment, degradation, and discrimination) and makes them "feel better," even though it does not resolve the stress itself (DeGraff & Schaffer, 2008).

Everyone does not agree, however, that emotion-focused coping is productive; in fact, it can be maladaptive. People can keep emotions pent-up, abuse drugs or alcohol, and, at its worst, attempt or complete suicide. Detractors of emotion-focused coping think that although the person feels better, the problems still exist, and the stress associated with them is still present or can reoccur. For example, the use of emotion-focused strategies by clients coping with the stress of traumatic maxillofacial injury, necessitating emergency intervention, correlates with more problems of acute stress disorder (Auerbach et al., 2008). Similarly, in a study of patients with breast cancer and their spouses, use of emotion-focused strategies (i.e., ventilation and avoidance) by either or both of them was associated with increased distress and lower levels of psychosocial adjustment (Ben-Zur, Gilbar, & Lev, 2001). When people are emotionally overwhelmed, they may not have the resources to adequately address and find solutions to problems (Ben-Zur et al., 2001). Individuals may rely more on emotion-focused behaviors to alter how they perceive the situation, which is not always productive. For instance, in clients with multiple sclerosis, depression correlates with emotion-focused responses (Aikens, Fischer, Namey, & Rudick, 1997; Jean, Paul, & Beatty, 1999).

Various studies of people with diabetes have shown that coping can have either positive or negative metabolic effects on glycosylated hemoglobin levels, functional status, symptom intensity, body mass index, and body weight. Psychosocial outcomes, including adjustment, depression, and quality of life, are also affected (Grey, 2000). Teenagers may not test their blood glucose or take insulin injections as often as required. This reluctance to deal with their disease may relieve the stress of being different from their friends. However, it can be as ineffective as some other emotion-focused strategies that Lazarus and Folkman (1984a) discuss, such as minimizing the extent of the circumstances, distancing oneself from the situation, and using selective attention. Emotion-focused coping has been found to have negative outcomes in some people with spinal cord injuries. They may withdraw, abuse substances, such as drugs or alcohol, throw tantrums, sleep late or nap excessively, or view pornography (DeGraff & Schaffer, 2008).

Affective regulation, part of emotion-focused coping, helps people control and modulate their emotions in the face of a crisis. Consider the expectant parents who have wallpapered and equipped a nursery, in preparation for bringing their newborn home. When the infant dies in the hospital shortly after birth, it takes a period of time until they are emotionally ready to dismantle the room and donate the gifts from the baby shower. In effect, they are regulating their affect and emotions by controlling their environment and exposure to stressful activities.

Emotional discharge, the release of suppressed feelings and emotions, is another facet of this form of coping. It may be adaptive and take the form of crying, yelling, or joking, or be maladaptive, such as overeating or drinking. Consider 12-year-old Gregory, who suddenly became unruly in school and then started skipping it altogether. He had remained silent for years about the neglect he felt while his parents devoted all their time and attention to his sister with cystic fibrosis.

In resigned acceptance, another element of emotion-focused coping behavior, a person accepts the reality as it is perceived, believing that there is nothing that can change it. This can be a form of surrender, with varying outcomes. In adults with diabetes, this strategy has been associated with negative outcomes, measured by loss of weight and poor metabolic control

(Grey, 2000). In contrast, consider parents who decided they needed to remove their 19-year-old son from their home. His refusal to take medication to treat his schizophrenia resulted in behavior that endangered the safety and well-being of the family. In this situation, the family had no ability to manage the young man's illness or behavior and chose to accept the situation. By doing so, they could protect the remaining family members, especially the other children.

Resigned acceptance is not the same as "letting go." In this situation, individuals accept the reality of their condition and choose to live at peace with the consequences. Their lives are not the same as before, but they no longer struggle to change what is unchangeable. They find ways to live with their new reality and reorder their priorities.

These coping skills may be used individually or in various combinations. Although certain circumstances may preclude constructive use of one or more strategies (i.e., an atheist may be poorly equipped to utilize appraisal-focused coping), using these measures in adaptive ways leads to the best outcomes. People can release emotion in healthy ways, ask for help to solve problems, and place the problem into a framework that can be managed. For example, a woman who is diagnosed with breast cancer may use emotion-focused coping to release pent-up emotions, expressing sadness or anger. She may also use appraisal-focused coping to analyze the situation and psychologically prepare herself for possible outcomes. Using problem-focused coping, she must consider the risks and benefits of a lumpectomy versus a mastectomy and the value and consequences of chemotherapy, radiation, or a combination of treatment options. These coping modes are not mutually exclusive. In this instance, she may have first employed emotion-focused coping, then appraisal-focused coping, and then became problem focused to collect information and find support from friends, family, health care providers, support groups, or counseling. She is now ready to face making difficult decisions.

Our role as health care professionals is to facilitate the use of adaptive coping strategies, helping to line up necessary resources and make referrals as needed. Table 8–1 gives examples of adaptive and maladaptive behaviors associated with these coping strategies.

**Table 8–1**    Examples of Adaptive and Maladaptive Behaviors Associated with Coping Strategies

| Appraisal-Focused Coping Strategies | | Problem-Focused Coping Strategies | | Emotion-Focused Coping Strategies | |
|---|---|---|---|---|---|
| **Adaptive** | **Maladaptive** | **Adaptive** | **Maladaptive** | **Adaptive** | **Maladaptive** |
| Reframing | Blaming God/ others | Information gathering | Intellectualization | Early denial | Continuous denial |
| Spirituality | Harmful beliefs | Questioning | Avoidance | Emoting | Drinking |
| Meditating | Fanaticism | Problem solving | Excessive behavior | Social support | Drugs |
| Painting | Excessive behavior | Adherence | Nonadherence | Counseling | Self-injury |
| Dancing | | Writing | | Companionship | Suicide |
| Long walks | | Helping others | | | Promiscuity |
| | | Doing | | | Isolation |

## Defense Mechanisms

Sigmund Freud, an Austrian neurologist, physiologist, and psychologist, developed the theory and practice of psychoanalysis. Although his well-known theories of the unconscious mind, anxiety, and ego-defense mechanisms were published in the late 19th century (Freud, 1894), they are still utilized today. Since Freud's time, other defense mechanisms have been described. The common elements of all are that they (1) protect the individual from tension, hurt, anxiety, pain, and psychic disorganization and (2) tend to be unconscious. It is not uncommon to use some defensive mechanisms, individually or in combination with others, to deal with daily life, but they can become maladaptive if they are the primary way to deal with stress and are used in excess. Sometimes, the person can use rational strategies to defend himself or herself, such as crying, "venting" to others, finding support, and laughing. These are types of emotion-focused strategies, as described earlier in this chapter. Although these can be influenced by learned behavior, they often become automatic parts of the ways we cope. At other times, the person makes use of irrational protective approaches that lessen anxiety, but they can be self-deceptive and distort reality. These strategies are known as defense mechanisms, and they are used subconsciously to protect the self from external threats, such as having to deal with the sudden loss of a loved one. Defense mechanisms protect a person from conscious thoughts and feelings by transforming reality. Because defense mechanisms are generally used subconsciously, the individual may feel anxious, fearful, or uncomfortable, without understanding the reason behind the feelings. The full range of defense mechanisms is too numerous to detail, but some are highlighted here.

- *Denial of (or minimizing) reality*    This is a refusal or inability to acknowledge that which has happened or will happen. It protects the person from having to face unpleasant topics, situations, and thoughts. Perhaps the most primitive of the defense mechanisms, denial can sound like "I don't have an eating problem; I'm just stressed out studying for exams." When faced with a serious diagnosis, for example, the thought that "this isn't happening to me" can protect oneself from the full measure of the situation until such time that the person can better deal with it.
- *Fantasy*    We all fantasize to some degree, working out problems, dreaming of what "could be," picturing ourselves in various situations with different people. Fantasy becomes a maladaptive form of coping when it becomes a continual replacement for reality. In its extreme, it is a total escape from reality, where an imaginary world that is less menacing is an alternate to the real one.
- *Repression/suppression*    Freud (1894) considered repression to be the primary defense mechanism because it is the foundation of others that are more complex. Negative experiences, thoughts, feelings, and actions are rejected from one's awareness, disregarded and forgotten, with no conscious memory of what has been repressed. A person who is raped can have selective amnesia of the events. However, even though the information is "below the radar" of conscious awareness, the memory still exists. In contrast to repression, suppression is consciously obstructing a thought, word, or deed or choosing to avoid it, such as the desire to copy another student's answers on a test.
- *Rationalization*    With this mechanism, acceptable, though inaccurate, reasons replace real ones. Faulty logic can be used to justify behavior or temper disappointment. The phrase "sour grapes," from the Aesop's fable "The Fox and the Grapes," is often used to illustrate rationalization. When the fox couldn't reach the grapes he wanted, he said that they were probably sour anyway. There are those who think that ice cream sodas made

with diet beverages are not "so bad" because they are cutting calories. Sometimes, individuals try to convince themselves that they have sound reasoning when, in fact, they do not.

- *Projection*   In projection, individuals see positive or negative traits of themselves and put them outside of the self, onto other people. Generally, a lack of insight and self-responsibility are factors. Freud (1894) thought that projection was a key defense mechanism in people who were paranoid or who had antisocial personalities. With negative projections, responsibility can be shifted to others: "I lost all those points on the essay question because the teacher didn't cover that material well." Someone who is not a team player may accuse others on the team of not being team players and wanting to make all the decisions unilaterally.

- *Reaction formation*   If a reaction is too painful, negative, or threatening, a person can reform the reaction, accepting attitudes, feelings, impulses, and thoughts that are the opposite of his or her true feelings. A client may be very angry with a clinician but act excessively nice rather than show irritation. By doing this, there is no conscious threat or awareness of the negative feelings. Some people who campaign against gambling, alcohol, smoking, homosexuality, or other issues may have a history of personal struggles with these same behaviors.

- *Displacement*   In displacement, the person shifts a symbolic meaning, emotion, thought, or impulse from someone or something for which it was directed to another person or thing. A teenager being demeaned at home kicks the dog or bullies someone at school, which may be safer than directing that anger and hostility at the parents. Sometimes, the feelings are turned inward, and people can blame or deflate themselves and emotionally "beat themselves up." As with other defense mechanisms, the anxiety, fear, and issues remain, though not consciously, and are displaced onto other people and circumstances, which can create other issues.

- *Sublimation*   A cousin of displacement, sublimation involves redirection of inappropriate emotions, thoughts, or impulses into acceptable ones. When feeling anxious, for example, a person goes for a walk rather than smoking a cigarette. Christopher Reeve, the late actor, who sustained a high-level spinal cord injury, redirected feelings over his disability into creating a research foundation, channeling his emotions and energy in positive directions.

- *Emotional insulation*   To protect oneself from hurt, pain, frustration, and disappointment, the person can become emotionally isolated, passively accepting what life offers and diminishing involvement with others. The man who has been looking for a job for a year may resign himself to this seemingly hopeless situation, becoming increasingly apathetic. In the extreme, the person can become alienated and uninvolved in life's activities, which would be recognized as depression. On one hand, this defense mechanism protects, on the other, it is unhealthy to withdraw from life.

- *Withdrawal*   This is a form of isolation when the individual withdraws from people and events that can trigger reminders of anxious or painful feelings and thoughts. In so doing, the person absents himself or herself from activities, such as talking with friends, listening to music, or watching television. He or she may become quiet and detached or resort to addictive behaviors, such as abusing alcohol and drugs. In its extreme, withdrawal can result in greater estrangement, which may also be a red warning flag of depression.

- *Intellectualization*   This strategy helps the individual evade a painful situation or feeling by using a rational explanation that removes the emotion and hurtful meaning. A person can become quite detached from his or her feelings. Richard Galli wrestled with his decision to remove his son Jeffrey from a ventilator, following a high-level spinal cord injury, using the same reasoning processes developed over years as an attorney.

- *Undoing (atonement)* This is used to nullify wrongdoings or inappropriate impulses, behaviors, or thoughts. Asking for forgiveness, apologizing, or being punished are ways of undoing. One celebrity actor/comedian used to bring his wife expensive jewelry or crystal to atone for his infidelity.

- *Acting out* This occurs when an individual reacts with a radical physical behavior rather than emotionally expressing thoughts and feelings. A student punched her fist into a concrete wall rather than express her emotions at failing another test. Her short-term release of pent-up tension and anxiety resulted in broken hand bones. Temper tantrums in children are a form of acting out.

- *Regression* The concept of moving backwards and using a response that the person has outgrown may provide short-term protection but is limited in maturity. A 4-year-old child may resume bed-wetting when a new sibling enters the family. A college freshman may move home when problems with roommates arise. To defend the self, a person reverts to a "place" that may be more gratifying (i.e., parental attention) or safe, with fewer expectations. As with other defense mechanisms, this can be helpful , but it can also be taken to extreme.

- *Compensation* To counteract real or imagined weaknesses, failures, or inadequacies, a person can emphasize other strengths. In the movie *Forrest Gump*, the young Forrest cannot keep up with the other children and is taunted because of this and for wearing long leg braces. He works hard to overcome this and later no longer needs the braces and becomes a runner. In real life, Wilma Rudolph overcame the childhood impairments of poliomyelitis and became the first American woman to win three gold medals in the Rome Olympics. Not all compensatory reactions are so grand. An unathletic, science "geek" in school can strengthen his academics and go on to develop computers or space programs. However, not all reactions are positive. For example, some people may act out to bolster their insecurity. Some may demean others to appear stronger or better. In the extreme, a person may become eccentric to gain attention or participate in antisocial activities.

- *Identification* Feelings of self-worth and self-esteem may be boosted by identifying with a person or place in a good position. People can identify with the prestige, strengths, power, and abilities associated with marrying into the "right" family, working at a well-known institution, or attending an illustrious university, because they take these characteristics as their own. For individuals with a lower sense of self, this support can be very attractive. However, when there is a blemish of some kind, tainting the source of identification, such as corporate wrongdoings that become public, economic failure, divorce, or a losing team, an individual may experience a loss of self-value.

- *Introjection* A close cousin of identification, introjection integrates another's standards and values, even when they were not those that the person previously had. A classic illustration of this is "If you can't beat them, join them." For example, in the event of a new political regime, a change of corporate leadership, or an altered family structure, it may help to adopt others' attitudes, beliefs, and values.

- *Dissociation* In dissociation, a person can disengage from time, person, and place to enter another world or dimension. When dissociated, the individual does not have the emotions, thoughts, and memories that he or she finds so unacceptable or painful. This can happen as a result of child abuse or trauma associated with a violent event. In the extreme, this can result in an individual thinking there is more than one self in their body (i.e., dissociative identity disorder).

- *Compartmentalization* A distant cousin to dissociation, compartmentalization is when certain parts of a person are disconnected from other behaviors and values of which the person is aware. A classic example of this is the person who is otherwise honest, but defrauds the government on tax returns, consciously unaware of the incongruency. It can also be used to compartmentalize certain troublesome aspects of one's life from other areas. For example, while at work, a person may not focus on the problems at home; at home, one may not think about the problems at work.

In summary, defense mechanisms are generally learned behaviors that people employ to protect themselves from problems and pain. As such, they can conceal a wide range of feelings, thoughts, and impulses. Used too long, these reactions can become instinctive, so that a person no longer may know what he or she really feels or thinks. Some, as described, not only cause stagnation but can create other issues. In the short run, they may be helpful coping measures, but ultimately, it is healthier to be able to rely less on them and face one's issues. This may be difficult to identify or to change, and referral to a skilled psychotherapist may be useful.

## PSYCHOSOCIAL ADAPTATION STRATEGIES

Although coping behavior helps reduce or eliminate psychological distress, it is only one part of adapting to changed circumstances. To achieve successful adjustment, various psychosocial adaptation strategies can be employed. Some common strategies include stress management, acquiring skills, developing peer support, making occupational accommodations, and using cognitive reframing (Drench, 2003b). Ideally, stressors (allostatic load) are balanced by the effective use of available resources, as illustrated in Figure 8–1.

Adequate information and resources are necessary to manage a condition or illness and are vital to adjustment. For example, it may be necessary to obtain essential equipment, counseling services, and practical supports, such as help from homemakers, nurses' aides, and personal care attendants. Caregivers also need emotional and practical support from friends and health professionals. This kind of support provides respite to family caregivers, who need both time for other aspects of their lives and opportunities for venting their feelings and concerns. Adjustment also has an active component, something one needs to "do." Susan Nessim survived cancer as a teenager and founded Cancervive, a national support group that addresses challenges of survivorship. She discovered that being cured of cancer did not mean that she was released from its stigma. "There was more to overcoming this disease than surviving the hardships of treatment. Instead, the end of treatment marked the beginning of a new and unexpected challenge: adapting to life after cancer" (Nessim & Ellis, 1991, p. xix). These strategies are all examples of problem-focused coping, described earlier in this chapter.

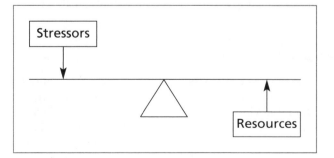

**FIGURE 8–1** Stressors and Resources in Balance

Many people equate disability, loss, and dependence with a life that is not worth living. Yet, even clients with a significantly disabling condition, such as amyotrophic lateral sclerosis (ALS), commonly referred to as Lou Gehrig's disease, can find beneficial adaptation strategies. Health providers need to understand that catastrophic physical limitations do not necessarily rob clients of their purpose in living and the potential for a high quality of life. Consider Morrie Schwartz, the professor and mentor who guides his former student, Mitch, through one last private discourse on "The Meaning of Life." Every Tuesday, until his death marks graduation day, Morrie holds a private seminar in his home. He calls these sessions "his last class," where he informs Mitch not just about how to die but also how to live:

> ALS is like a lit candle: It melts your nerves and leaves your body a pile of wax. Often, it begins with the legs and works its way up. You lose control of your thigh muscles, so that you cannot support yourself standing. You lose control of your trunk muscles, so that you cannot sit up straight. By the end, if you are still alive, you are breathing through a tube in a hole in your throat, while your soul, perfectly awake, is imprisoned inside a limp husk, perhaps able to blink, or cluck a tongue, like something from a science fiction movie, the man frozen inside his own flesh. *Do I wither up and disappear, or do I make the best of my time left?* he had asked himself. He would not wither. He would not be ashamed of dying. Instead, he would make death his final project, the center point of his days. He could be research. A human textbook. *Study me in my slow and patient demise. Watch what happens to me. Learn with me.* (Albom, 1997, pp. 9–10)

Foley and associates (2007) found that the meaning of the quality of life for people with ALS is defined by cognitive and behavioral strategies and is individual and multidimensional. In appraising their life circumstances, people consider what aspects of their lives they can control and which they cannot. Central themes that came to light were taking pleasure in life, the value and role of faith, and the significance of family, support, and unselfishness. Other key themes were the meaning of dignity, the need to preserve their dignity and control, a sense of loss, and struggling with the disease. Instead of being overwhelmed by all the aspects and potential sequelae of their progressive disease, they try to focus on each day's concerns. They believe that professional services are a factor in their well-being.

Stress can be managed in many ways. Some people use relaxation techniques, such as meditation, visualization, guided imagery, or prayer. Others may engage in activities that "nourish their souls," such as playing an instrument, dancing, knitting, or gardening. Changing parts of a lifestyle to regain control over parts of life is another form of action. This can occur through activities, such as eating a healthier diet, exercising, making changes at work, or seeking professional help.

## Cognitive Reframing

Reframing, or altering the way one perceives fears and concerns, can not only be beneficial but also be transforming. It is important to remember that grieving is a requisite step on the loss-to-adjustment continuum. Individuals first need to mourn the loss. Then, they need to put it into perspective and integrate it into their lives. Reframing helps put meaning to the loss and makes it not only bearable but perhaps even positive. To be able to integrate a loss, Kushner (1981) suggests that people need to change the questions they are asking. "In the final analysis, the question of why bad things happen to good people translates itself into some very different questions, no longer asking why something happened, but asking how we will respond, what we intend to do now that it has happened" (p. 147).

Along the loss–grief–adjustment continuum, people frequently redefine the meaning of their illness, disability, and life. "Being better" means different things to different people. It could indicate an improvement or resolution of the disorder, an adjustment to working around the condition, or an adaptation to living with the problem. It could also mean finding meaning in the loss that changes one's beliefs and perspectives. In their research of the meaning of recovery in people with work-related musculoskeletal disorders of the upper extremity, Beaton and colleagues (2001) called this "resolution, readjustment, and redefinition." They found that the concept of "getting better" was influenced by people's perceptions of how justifiable the disorder was, their definition of health and illness, and their coping styles. In short, while individuals' physical conditions may not improve, they may consider themselves "better" (Drench, 2003b).

Furthermore, clients may seek meaning in death (Yedidia & MacGregor, 2001) or redefine the meaning of life amidst a new set of circumstances. In a study of 10 women newly diagnosed with breast cancer, awareness of the meaning of existential issues was a central phenomenon. These existential issues included varying levels of life expectations, including battling against death and life related to future outlook. Religious beliefs and doubts and an enhanced understanding of values in life also had important effects. A core finding was the significance of the will to live. The investigators suggest that if health professionals increase their awareness of existential issues linked to the will to live, they can better help women and their families cope (Landmark, Strandmark, & Wahl, 2001).

The personal crisis and interruption of work that results from having a life-threatening illness may also endanger an individual's identity regarding wellness and ability. In a small pilot study of three women diagnosed with breast cancer, the main message was that "doing equals living," demonstrating a powerful connection between meaningful occupation and a perception of oneself as healthy and capable (Vrkljan & Miller-Polgar, 2001). This theme was also evident in the story of Lance Armstrong. Lance was a 23-year-old professional bicycle racer when he was diagnosed with stage IV testicular cancer. After undergoing grueling surgery and chemotherapy, he continued to keep moving. His philosophy was "if you can move, you are still alive" (Armstrong & Jenkins, 2000). Remaining active or resuming activities may be the catalyst for people to reconstruct the meaning of life, a process of reclaiming control and a sense of normalcy (Vrkljan & Miller-Polgar, 2001).

## Emotional and Practical Support

Impairments, limitations, and disabilities affect both the individual and their significant others and families. They challenge all types of relationships. Some individuals become stronger in the face of adversity; some relationships do not endure. Support from families and friends has been shown to contribute to survival in aging adults (Giles, Glonek, Luszcz, & Andrews, 2005) and has an important impact on adaptation (Drench, 2003b). In a study of parents of children who survived a brain tumor, the effects of uncertainty and loss resulted in alterations in parenting and the meaning and purpose of life, as well as sorrow, isolation, and grief (Forinder & Lindahl Norberg, 2010). A social network that supports the parents helps them cope with a new reality, one in which they will continue to live with uncertainty and the sequelae of the disease and its treatment.

The most frequently described coping resource for people living with spinal cord injuries is relationships with family, friends, and personal assistants (DeGraff & Schaffer, 2008). African American couples combine their strengths to actively cope with and survive the diagnosis of breast cancer, doing things jointly, such as "walking," "praying," "seeking," "trusting," "adjusting," and "being together." Culturally sensitive clinicians can assist clients and families in coping by integrating these aspects into therapeutic encounters (Morgan et al., 2005). Similarly, African American adolescents who are coping with breast cancer of a parent say that "we are survivors, too," as they deal with an uncertain future. Researchers recommend that care be family centered and age appropriate. A support group comprised of peers facing the same issues can foster family strengths and combat feelings of aloneness and apprehension (Davey, Tubbs, Kissil, & Niño, 2010).

Health providers can be very effective in supporting coping. They can assist clients to encourage and accept external support from friends, provide an ear for them to give voice to their emotions and worries, and prioritize their decision making. Focusing on functional adaptation to a changed physical situation is another part of adjustment. This is what rehabilitation professionals are most comfortable doing. Further, in a study of people living with spinal cord injuries, the third most frequently described coping resource is exercise (DeGraff & Schaffer, 2008). Outcomes of exercise may include improved physical independence, as well as enhanced self-esteem (Drench, 2003b).

Clients and families often feel the loss of professional support once they leave a clinical setting or the health care system. Family members may have been partners in care for a loved one, only to feel adrift once the individual is discharged from care or dies. Perhaps they have completed their own course of treatment or rehabilitation and feel "over their heads" without the daily care and support of professionals. Some agencies and institutions provide follow-up telephone calls and letters for the immediate period following the loss of this professional support. Unfortunately, this is not a universal practice. A significant benefit of this bridge of communication is that it maintains continuity of care. Sensitive discussion can elicit questions and evaluate adjustment responses (Kaunonen, Aalto, Tarkka, & Paunonen, 2000).

## Counseling

I can't seem to get through to Bill, he's just so angry. He's the star quarterback for his high school team, a big man on campus. At least he was until the thresher accident. He was working on his family's farm, and his right arm got pulled into the grain machine. It tore his arm off above the elbow. I guess if I were him, I'd be angry, too. Even as I sit here and type this, I'm using two hands.

*—From the journal of Walter Johnson, occupational therapy student*

Clients and their significant others grieve many kinds of losses and experience varied reactions to them. Health professionals can encourage counseling for people to express their feelings about concerns, such as progressive loss, dependence on others, and, perhaps, anticipated death (Drench, 2003b). Providing the opportunity to talk about the changes and losses is sometimes sufficient to help people feel less isolated and adjust more successfully. Other times, formal counseling is indicated, which can also deal with maladaptive coping and its destructive behavior. Counseling can help highlight the negative consequences of choices and reinforce productive pursuits (DeGraff & Schaffer, 2008). It can also facilitate addressing anxieties and fears and guide in the development of constructive coping strategies. Counseling skills include listening and attending to clients, as well as verbal counseling approaches (Drench, 2003b). Whereas the latter are the purview of mental health disciplines, such as counselors, social workers, psychologists, and psychiatrists, all health providers play a role in listening and attending to clients. Recognizing what the client needs and wants is part of being effective.

The purpose of counseling is to enable people to recognize and use their own coping resources. Clients and significant others need the time, opportunity, and permission to grieve (Budin et al., 2008). It is often helpful to let them tell what happened and how they feel about it. Health providers can encourage clients to talk about their memories, concerns, and fears. This also places the situation in a very real context. Acknowledging the fears can be a precursor to dealing with them (Goudsmit, Ho-Yen, & Dancey, 2009). Putting feelings into words can be healing.

Health care providers facilitate a person's autonomy by supporting his or her goals and helping the person reach them. Providing comprehensive and compassionate care requires integrating psychosocial issues into every aspect of assessment and treatment. A study of clients with breast cancer and their partners demonstrated that those receiving education and counseling for emotional adjustment had better social and vocational outcomes and well-being (Budin et al., 2008). Comprehensive presurgical counseling, with the spouse present, for people who were going to have laryngectomies was more effective than the preoperative information previously given by surgeons (Keith, Linebaugh, & Cox, 2009).

Wise health professionals adapt their interventions to the clients' stress level so that the education is more helpful. People who are highly flustered or frightened will not be able to receive information and learn. For example, perioperative nurses do the most comprehensive teaching for clients who they evaluate to have mild stress levels; they give less information but fuller consideration to specific areas for those clients who they assess to have moderate stress levels. For clients with severe stress levels, the nurses give the most basic information and provide a fuller opportunity for the clients to talk about their fears and concerns (Garbee & Gentry, 2001). Other health care providers may consider using this strategy when educating clients.

Grief counseling can help people work through their issues, prevent or mitigate unresolved grief and destructive feelings of anger and guilt, and facilitate personal growth (Worden, 2002). Professional counseling can address issues that need to be recognized and worked through if adjustment is to occur. Denial can either be confronted or sustained, depending on the need of the client and assessment of the health care provider (Wess, 2007). Anger can forestall the grieving process and may result in maladaptive behavior, illness, and lack of joy in life (Worden, 2002). It can also release long-repressed feelings and allow the grieving person to move forward in life. Different counseling approaches may be indicated for different situations. Although these may not be within your scope of practice, it is recommended that health care providers become knowledgeable about the types of resources available in their community and be ready to make referrals as needed.

## Support Groups

Sharing practical information and "success" stories with others are additional rehabilitation and psychosocial strategies (Oliffe et al., 2008). Learning *how* others cope can open a door to reality and pragmatic information and strategies. Knowing *that* others cope can open a world of possibilities. The pain and difficulty of surviving a loss or an illness can be overwhelming. It can be tremendously healing to be in the presence of others who have experienced the same losses. Knowing that you are not alone can be very powerful in minimizing or removing isolation, loneliness, and the sting of stigma. It is also comforting to be in a place where you feel like you "belong." Belonging is the key theme in a study of clients' experiences of social relationships during pulmonary rehabilitation for chronic obstructive pulmonary disease (Halding, Wahl, & Heggdal, 2010). It is also helpful to know there are others more experienced than yourself who you can call on for advice, information, or even a shoulder on which to cry. Seeing the success of others as they gain, or regain, skills can provide hope.

Some groups have been developed by communities, agencies, and health facilities that recognize the benefit of peer support and are organized by diagnosis, age group, role (i.e., parents, families, children), and other common denominators. Various types of psychoeducational group intervention programs provide support and information. Although the methodologies vary, they all generally work to foster coping and optimize adaptive strategies. Leadership, led by either peers or professionals, is important for successful recruitment and retention of participants and effective outcomes (Oliffe et al., 2008). Support groups for clients and family caregivers can meet simultaneously, when everyone is available. Seasonal camps and year-round programs are opportunities for children to get together, play, and talk with others with physical disabilities, which aids in coping and adjustment (McMillan & Coulter-O'Berry, 2008).

Peer support for clients with chronic kidney disease, for example, motivates their self-management and results in better health outcomes. Clients can gain invaluable practical information from others who are living the same experience. They can then apply this information to their own decision making about treatment (Hughes, Wood, & Smith, 2009). In addition, they share empathy and collective understanding, which creates a bond and a sense of belonging; the clear message is that they are not alone in their experience. Further, peer supporters are positive role models, helping others adjust to living with chronic illness, for example, giving a sense of empowerment and hope, as they follow through with taxing treatments. Important caveats to remember regarding peer support are to make careful, prudent choices when matching peers with others and to provide effective training (Hughes et al., 2009).

## Hope

"Hope is the ability to invest our energy and vision in a reality beyond our sight in the present moment, the capacity to yearn for and expect a meaning deeper and an outcome better than the circumstances seem to allow" (Phillips, 1989, p. 31). Hope plays a central role in healing. Establishing and maintaining hope can be critically important in the adjustment process and is a key role of the health provider (Wess, 2007). However, it is important to provide realistic hope rather than offer false promises. For example, when a mother asks if her 3-year-old son, who has lead poisoning, will develop "normally," the clinician has to tread carefully. Rather than promising that things will be perfect, or that stating the outlook is grim, he or she can say, "We have a lot of work to do together." Fostering hope begins with the development of an open, trusting, forthright relationship with the client and family. The second step in promoting hope is analyzing the client's and family's ability to accomplish the tasks of hoping.

In a seminal study on the process and tasks of hoping (Wright & Shontz, 1968), four cognitive-affective tasks were identified: reality surveillance, encouragement, worry, and mourning. Reality surveillance is a cognitive function that integrates hope with reality, as it is perceived by the individual. Adults need to base their hopes in reality. Conversely, because children rely on adults to be responsible for their welfare, they can verbalize hopes without considering the reality and possibility of future outcomes. Whereas reality surveillance, the first task of hoping, is a cognitive function, the other three tasks—encouragement, worry, and mourning—are affective (Wright & Shontz, 1968). Reality surveillance checks and tests reality to see if the hopes are possible.

**BOX 8–1    How Health Providers Help Clients with Fact-Based Reality**

- *Validate or shed accurate light on the patient's/client's beliefs:* "I thought that if I could get into that special eye and ear clinic, my macular degeneration could be cured, and I'd see again."
- *Guide the patients/clients in assessing their physical, emotional, and interpersonal strengths and weaknesses:* "I can no longer use my hands to paint, but I could try mouth-painting."
- *Help them make accurate comparisons to complete the evaluation of their assets:* "I thought I was the worst one off here, until I met Joe."
- *Help the patient/client perceive the positive growth opportunities from the situation:* "It's funny to think of this accident as a good thing in my life, but I've slowed down, learned to listen more, and feel good hugging my kids."
- *Seek verification of statements with the patient/client:* "Your shoulder motion is still very limited. Have you been working with the home exercise program as much as you need to? I want to stress to you why it is so important."
- *Equip patients/clients with accurate information and reassure them while they face their challenges and take responsibility for themselves:* "I can't bury my head in the sand any longer. I'm ready for the biopsy."
- *Practice empathetic communication while helping people face what may lie ahead:* "We'll certainly keep working to maintain the strength of Mark's muscles, but with your son's type of muscular dystrophy, we also need to consider other ways to help him be mobile."
- *Help the patient/client be optimistic and yet realistic:* "Your wound is looking better. With your diabetes, though, we need to continue our close monitoring and dressing changes."
- *Provide current information and indicate that newer treatments may be developed:* "Clinical trials are being conducted that use a combination of newer antiviral medications."
- *Help sustain hope by professing its value:* "There are no guarantees of what tomorrow will bring. Nothing is written in stone."

*Source:* Kim (1989).

Encouragement is the feeling side of reality surveillance. It helps people know that they do have a basis for hope and, therefore, it is both motivating and comforting. In contrast, worry works in tandem with the cognitive process when it is uncertain. The client takes another look at the perceived reality. The fourth task of hoping, mourning, is accomplished when a hope has to be abandoned. It is a necessary step if the person is going to be able to reevaluate the situation and develop other hopes to replace the one that had to be surrendered.

Health care practitioners can provide information that is honest and accurate, while allowing the client opportunity to hope. Consider Mr. Fox, who asked his physician if he would live the 6 months needed to see his son graduate from high school. By hearing that it was possible, even though not likely, Mr. Fox could still hope that this would happen. Health providers can assist clients in evaluating their fact-based reality (Kim, 1989) (see Box 8–1).

## IMPLICATIONS FOR HEALTH CARE PROVIDERS

Many people have difficulty dealing with the concepts of illness, disability, or death, making it difficult for them to offer solace to a person who is experiencing a health-related crisis. They may say nothing or offer meaningless, though well-intended, remarks, such as "I know what you're going through." Because each experience of loss and grief is unique, and the meaning of the loss distinct, no one can really know what another person is feeling. Health care providers are no exception. We process all of our similar personal and professional experiences and offer consolation, but we really cannot understand what another person is feeling at the deepest level. We can, however, be authentic about our own experiences and allow the client to see that we, too, know how painful losses can be. We do not always have to verbalize or explain this; our tone of voice and nonverbal messages say so much.

We may want to avoid people who are grieving because we are at a loss about what to say or are embarrassed or uncomfortable by their open display of emotions. We may feel overwhelmed by their sadness and feel we may get lost in the sadness, as well. Perhaps we find ourselves changing the subject or "selling" the idea that keeping busy is the answer to moving through grief and adjustment. A better approach would be to acknowledge the person's loss or pain and show concern. We might open a dialogue by saying, "This must be a difficult time for you. Do you want to talk?" or "How are you doing today?"

We often see clients and families when they are at their worst, when their coping behavior and dynamics are sorely challenged. Yet, we may label them as "nonadherent" or as "problems." We may expect them to follow our advice, work hard, and make progress—in short, to "get with it." It is critical that we examine our own motivation, patience, and understanding of the situation. If our tunnel vision only focuses on a specific piece of the puzzle, overlooking the cognitive and affective dimensions of care, we are not providing the most compassionate care possible.

For the ultimate loss (life), people, including health professionals, often fall short of knowing what to say and how to act. For example, in Leo Tolstoy's classic story of Ivan Ilych (1886/1971), the "client" is alone in dealing with his dying, in the face of his family's code of silence. Instead of discussing death or providing him the opportunity to express himself and confront his mortality, they pretend that Ivan is not dying. Health care providers may also abandon the client to face death or loss alone. Their code of silence may even be disguised by meaningless chatter and averted eyes. In addition, people tend to use euphemisms for death and try to "cheer up" the grieving individual. They steer the conversation away from death and loss or use platitudes, such as "God wanted her by His side," "He lived a full life," and "It's better this way. He's out of pain." This creates a barrier between the professional and the person who is grieving.

When health care providers understand the stages of grief, as described in the previous chapter, they are in a good position to be able to help their clients work through many of the feelings associated with grief. For example, they can encourage outward expressions of grief, such as crying or yelling, as a healthy, warranted response to loss. It is important to be aware that confronting the pain associated with grief can take many forms. Consider the siblings whose idea it was to "play funeral" with their 6-year-old brother, who was dying of leukemia. The children gave the role of funeral director to their social worker. She was able to honestly answer their questions and let them express their feelings in a safe environment. By dealing with their grief in the "here and now," they will be less likely to have adjustment problems later. Compare this example to a home where little if anything is said about dying, and the children use their imagination in place of real information. This can be far more scary.

Health care providers can encourage adjustment at a pace that is comfortable for the individual. Their role also includes nurturing the people, fortifying their strength, and reinforcing positive growth. A new sense of self, including one's perceived worth and esteem, may be a healthy by-product of this task. Health professionals can assist significant others by their empathetic "presence" and coaching, by encouraging people to express their feelings and perceptions and collaborate in problem solving. This, in turn, helps them identify and manage personal, client, and other family issues.

Individualized interventions may sometimes be unorthodox, but they can have a significant impact on the well-being of the client. One debilitated client could not eat very much, except for grilled-cheese sandwiches. The nurses began to cancel some of his food trays and instead prepared several grilled-cheese sandwiches for him during each shift as part of their care plan (Drench, 1998). At times, although the therapeutic opportunity may be missed, the lesson can still be learned, as in the case of a nurse who was caring for a dying woman:

> She had a little girl whom she hadn't been able to spend much time with. I went in one day and she said, "My little girl, I wanted to make her a Cinderella." I knew right away that she wanted to buy her a party dress and dress her all up. She was feeling really bad that she hadn't. It was too late, and it didn't happen. The next time there was a woman here and a child involved, I made sure that things like that happened. (Drench, 1998, p. 136)

As a footnote, before being able to help others cope, health professionals need to cope well and maintain their personal health. Emotional roller-coasters do not elude health care providers, especially those working with people who have frequent losses. Although there may be a temptation to share problems with clients, this adds to their burdens and is not client-centered care. Similar to the value of support groups for clients and their families (McMillan & Coulter-O'Berry, 2008), health care providers can also benefit from support groups to weather the emotional toll of professional losses and prevent burnout (Drench, 1996). A designated liaison can be helpful to the staff, such as a psychiatric nurse (Drench, 1998) or psychiatrist. This consultant can meet weekly with staff groups to discuss and clarify psychological issues that are inherent in working with certain client populations.

## Summary

This chapter addressed the third part of the loss–grief–adjustment continuum, highlighting coping behavior, psychosocial adaptation strategies, and the implications for health care providers. To cope with the stresses of an illness, people use strategies that are appraisal focused, problem focused, emotion focused, or a combination of these approaches. These strategies are key elements in how people adjust to the changes in their lives and are influenced by many factors.

The need for positive psychosocial adaptation strategies cannot be underestimated. These strategies incorporate counseling, health care personnel, and emotional and practical support for the caregivers, as well as the affected individuals. Some of the other adaptation strategies discussed include sharing practical information, returning to work or other life activities, stress management,

support groups, and hope. Listening actively and compassionately, inviting feelings to be expressed, and facilitating an understanding of the situation are parts of the helping relationship. Encouraging individual expressions of grief and honoring culturally-appropriate rituals are also vitally important. In addition, health care providers assist the person in accepting a new reality, finding relevant coping strategies, connecting with a support system, and following-through with the identified ways to cope.

Health care providers can offer information and education to clients and caregivers and help them articulate their emotions and worries. This includes discussing grief, remaining supportive, arranging resources, and being alert to changes in the clients. In addition to providing practical assistance, it helps to establish empathetic presence and comfort. We explored strategies for health care providers to facilitate adaptation, emphasizing that their interventions can positively influence the physical, mental, and emotional health and adjustment of others. By helping people express their feelings, by educating and supporting clients, and by adapting the client's environment, health care providers facilitate a person's autonomy and clarify positive indicators of the healing process.

## Reflective Questions

1. As a response to illness or injury, what adaptations and adjustments would be most difficult for you to make?
2. Everyone needs support to cope with losses.
   a. What kind of supportive responses might *you* find most helpful?
   b. What kind of supportive responses might *you* find least helpful?
3. a. How can you determine what types of support to offer to clients who are grieving?
   b. What kind of feedback could you use to determine if your support has been effective?
4. In this chapter, we discussed an empathetic presence. Describe a situation when this might be beneficial.
5. When working with a client who is terminally ill, how can you communicate realistic expectations while maintaining the client's hope?

## Case Study

*Note:* Because loss, grief, and coping are presented on a continuum as a process rather than finite stages in time, this case study is a continuation of the Chapter 7 case. Before proceeding, therefore, you should reread the case study about Cynthia Osbourne in Chapter 7.

Six weeks after entering the rehabilitation hospital, Cynthia returned to her own state, to the home of her parents. She is struggling to reclaim her life. She is unable to bicycle or play pickup basketball with the children, but her vision is sufficiently improving, enabling her to resume reading, an area of enjoyment for her.

She is hopeful that recent surgery on her hands will enable her to return to work as a ward secretary at a hospital. The therapists are assisting Cynthia in identifying strategies and resources that will help her overcome her difficulties. As much as she would like to return to her "old self," her physicians have told her "to forget that person," a thought that she rejects. She rejoices at small improvements in walking, although she is beginning to accept that things will never be "perfect." She is also hopeful that she may be able to do more in the future. In the meantime, her low endurance and limited flexibility remain factors, and she continues to descend stairs in a backwards position. Every time she plays with her children, doing what she is able, she rejoices in her small pleasures.

1. What factors might be contributing to how Cynthia is coping with her situation?
2. Discuss in what ways Cynthia is using or has used appraisal-focused, problem-focused, and emotion-focused coping behaviors.
3. a. Discuss psychosocial adaptation strategies that Cynthia employed and their effect on her.
   b. Identify other possible psychosocial adaptation strategies that you believe would have been or still might be useful to Cynthia. Provide a rationale for your beliefs.
4. a. What role is hope playing in Cynthia's life?
   b. How might the therapeutic team members help Cynthia be realistic yet hopeful?

## References

Aikens, J. E., Fischer, J. S., Namey, M., & Rudick, R. A. (1997). A replicated prospective investigation of life stress, coping, and depressive symptoms in multiple sclerosis. *Journal of Behavioral Medicine, 20*(5), 433–445.

Albom, M. (1997). *Tuesdays with Morrie.* New York, NY: Doubleday.

Armstrong, L., & Jenkins, S. (2000). *It's not about the bike.* New York, NY: Berkley Books.

Auerbach, S. M., Laskin, D. M., Kiesler, D. J., Wilson, M., Rajab, B., & Campbell, T. A. (2008). Psychological factors associated with response to maxillofacial injury and its treatment. *Journal of Oral and Maxillofacial Surgery, 66*(4), 755–761.

Baldacchino, D., & Draper, P. (2001). Spiritual coping strategies: A review of the nursing research literature. *Journal of Advanced Nursing, 34*(6), 833–841.

Beaton, D. E., Tarasuk, V., Katz, J. N., Wright, J. G., & Bombardier, C. (2001). "Are you better?" A qualitative study of the meaning of recovery. *Arthritis and Rheumatology, 45*(3), 270–279.

Ben-Zur, H., Gilbar, O., & Lev, S. (2001). Coping with breast cancer: Patient, spouse, and dyad models. *Psychosomatic Medicine, 63*, 32–39.

Budin, W. C., Hoskins, C. N., Haber, J., Sherman, D. W., Maislin, G., Cater, J. R., . . . Shukla, S. (2008). Breast cancer: Education, counseling, and adjustment among patients and partners: A randomized clinical trial. *Nursing Research, 57*(3), 199–213.

Davey, M. P., Tubbs, C. Y., Kissil, K., & Niño, A. (2010, March 3). "We are survivors too": African American youths' experiences of coping with parental breast cancer. *Psychooncology*. Advance online publication. doi: 10.1002/pon.1712

DeGraff, A. H., & Schaffer, J. (2008). Emotion-focused coping: A primary defense against stress for people living with spinal cord injury. *Journal of Rehabilitation*. Retrieved from http://findarticles.com/p/articles/mi_m0825/is_1_74/ai_n25378304/?tag=content;col1

Drench, M. E. (1996). Too many rides on the AIDS rollercoaster: Understanding and preventing job burnout. In M. L. Galantino (Ed.), *Issues in HIV rehabilitation* (pp. 301–316). Alexandria, VA: American Physical Therapy Association, Oncology Section.

Drench, M. E. (1998). *Red ribbons are not enough: Health caregivers' stories about AIDS*. Wilsonville, OR: BookPartners.

Drench, M. E. (2003a). Loss, grief, and adjustment: A primer for physical therapy, Part I. *PT Magazine, 11* (6), 50–52, 54–61.

Drench, M. E. (2003b). Loss, grief, and adjustment: A primer for physical therapy, Part II. *PT Magazine, 11* (7), 58–70.

Foley, G., O'Mahony, P., & Hardiman, O. (2007). Perceptions of quality of life in people with ALS: Effects of coping and health care. *Amyotrophic Lateral Sclerosis, 8*(3), 164–169.

Folkman, S. (2008). The case for positive emotions in the stress process. *Anxiety, Stress, and Coping, 21*(1), 3–14.

Folkman, S., & Moskowitz, J. T. (2004). Coping: Pitfalls and promise. *Annual Review of Psychology, 55*, 745–774.

Forinder, U., & Lindahl Norberg, A. (2010). "Now we have to cope with the rest of our lives." Existential issues related to parenting a child surviving a brain tumour. *Supportive Care in Cancer, 18*(5), 543–551.

Freud, S. (1894). *The neuro-psychoses of defence. The standard edition of the complete psychological works of Sigmund Freud, Volume III (1893–1899): Early psycho-analytic publications* (pp. 41–61).

Garbee, D. D., & Gentry, J. A. (2001). Coping with the stress of surgery—Patient strategies. *Association of PeriOperative Registered Nurses Journal*. Retrieved from http://findarticles.com/p/articles/mi_m0FSL/is_5_73/ai_74571582

Giles, L. C., Glonek, G. F., Luszcz, M. A., & Andrews, G. R. (2005). Effect of social networks on 10 year survival in very old Australians: The Australian longitudinal study of aging. *Journal of Epidemiology and Community Health, 59*(7), 574–579.

Goudsmit, E. M., Ho-Yen, D. O., & Dancey, C. P. (2009). Learning to cope with chronic illness: Efficacy of a multi-component treatment for people with chronic fatigue syndrome. *Patient Education and Counseling, 77*(2), 231–236.

Grey, M. (2000). Coping and diabetes. *Diabetes Spectrum, 13*(3), 167–170.

Halding, A.-G., Wahl, A., & Heggdal, K. (2010). Belonging: Patients' experiences of social relationships during pulmonary rehabilitation. *Disability and Rehabilitation, 32*(15), 1272–1280.

Hughes, J., Wood, E. & Smith, G. (2009). Exploring kidney patients' experiences of receiving individual peer support. *Health Expectations, 12*(4), 396–406.

Jean, V. M., Paul, R. H., & Beatty, W. W. (1999). Psychological and neuropsychological predictors of coping patterns by patients with multiple sclerosis. *Journal of Clinical Psychology, 55*(1), 21–26.

Kaunonen, M., Aalto, P., Tarkka, M. T., & Paunonen, M. (2000). Oncology ward nurses' perspectives of family grief and a supportive telephone call after the death of a significant other. *Cancer Nursing, 23*(4), 314–324.

Keith, R. L., Linebaugh, C. W., & Cox, B. G. (2009). Pre-surgical counseling needs of laryngectomees: A survey of 78 patients. *The Laryngoscope, 88*(10), 1660–1665.

Kennedy, T., Jr. (2009). *Full speech: Ted Kennedy, Jr. pays tribute to his father and recalls his encouragement after amputation*. Retrieved from http://abcnews.go.com/print?id=8443171

Kim, T. S. (1989). Hope as a mode of coping in amyotrophic lateral sclerosis. *Journal of Neuroscience Nursing, 21*(6), 342–347.

Kushner, H. S. (1981). *When bad things happen to good people.* New York, NY: Avon Books.

Landmark, B. T., Strandmark, M., & Wahl, A. K. (2001). Living with newly diagnosed breast cancer: The meaning of existential issues. A qualitative study of 10 women with newly diagnosed breast cancer, based on grounded theory. *Cancer Nursing, 24*(3), 220–226.

Lazarus, R., & Folkman, S. (1984a). Stress, appraisal, and coping. New York, NY: Springer.

Lazarus, R. S., & Folkman, S. (1984b). Coping and adaptation. In W. D. Gentry (Ed.), *The handbook of behavioral medicine* (pp. 282–325). New York, NY: Guilford.

McMillan, A., & Coulter-O'Berry, C. (2008). Literature review: Comparison of surgical options, function, and psychosocial issues in treatment of children with solid tumors of the lower extremity. *Rehabilitation Oncology, 26*(2), 15–19.

Moos, R., & Billings, A. (1982). Conceptualizing and measuring coping resources and process. In L. Goldberger & S. Breznitz (Eds.), *Handbook of stress: Theoretical and clinical aspects* (pp. 212–230). New York, NY: Macmillan.

Moos, R. H., & Schaefer, J. A. (1986). Life transitions and crises: A conceptual overview. In R. H. Moos (Ed.), *Coping with life crises: An integrated approach* (pp. 3–28). New York, NY: Plenum Press.

Morgan, P. D., Fogel, J., Rose, L., Barnett, K., Mock, V., Davis, B. L., . . . Brown-Davis, C. (2005). African American couples merging strengths to successfully cope with breast cancer. *Oncology Nursing Forum, 32*(5), 979–987.

Nessim, S., & Ellis, J. (1991). *Cancervive: The challenge of life after cancer.* Boston, MA: Houghton Mifflin.

Oliffe, J. L., Halpin, M., Bottorff, J. L., Hislop, T. G., McKenzie, M., & Mroz, L. (2008). How prostate cancer support groups do and do not survive: British Columbian perspectives. *American Journal of Men's Health, 2*(2), 143–155.

Pearlin, L. I., & Schooler, C. (1978). The structure of coping. *Journal of Health and Social Behavior, 19*, 2–21.

Phillips, J. (1989). Sustaining our hope. In J. B. Meisenhelder & C. L. LaCharite (Eds.), *Comfort in caring: Nursing the person with HIV infection* (pp. 31–40). Boston, MA: Scott, Foresman.

Stanton, A. L., Danoff-Burg, S., Cameron, C. L., Bishop, M., Collins, C. A., Kirk, S. B., . . . Tillman, R. (2000). Emotionally expressive coping predicts psychological and physical adjustment to breast cancer. *Journal of Consulting and Clinical Psychology, 68*(5), 875–882.

Thuné-Boyle, I. C., Stygall, J. A., Keshtgar, M. R., & Newman, S. P. (2006). Do religious/spiritual coping strategies affect illness adjustment in patients with cancer? A systematic review of the literature. *Social Science and Medicine, 63*(1), 151–164.

Tolstoy, L. (1971). *The death of Ivan Ilych and other short stories* (L. Maude & A. Maude, Trans.). London, UK: Oxford University Press. (Original work published 1886)

Vrkljan, B. H., & Miller-Polgar, J. (2001). Meaning of occupational engagement in life-threatening illness: A qualitative pilot project. *Canadian Journal of Occupational Therapy, 68*(4), 237–246.

Weiten, W., Lloyd, M. A., Dunn, D. S., & Hammer, E. Y. (2009). *Psychology applied to modern life: Adjustment in the 21st century* (9th ed.). Belmont, CA: Wadsworth Cengage Learning.

Wess, M. (2007). Bringing hope and healing to grieving patients with cancer. *Journal of the American Osteopathic Association, 107*(12), ES41–ES47.

Worden, J. W. (2002). *Grief counseling and grief therapy* (3rd ed.). New York, NY: Springer.

Wright, B. A., & Shontz, F. C. (1968). Process and tasks in hoping. *Rehabilitation Literature, 29*, 322–331.

Yedidia, M. J., & MacGregor, B. (2001). Confronting the prospect of dying: Reports of terminally ill patients. *Journal of Pain Symptom Management, 22*(4), 807–819.

# Understanding Family Needs, Roles, and Responsibilities

Mrs. Casey paced back and forth in the waiting room. Her husband was seated in a wheelchair, breathing heavily and in apparent pain. I watched as she approached the clerk at the emergency room desk for the third time. She said, "We've been waiting over an hour. My husband's blood pressure is very high. I'm afraid he might be having a heart attack. When will somebody see him?" The clerk, obviously annoyed, responded, "We'll see him as soon as we can. Please be seated and stay out of the corridor." As her husband lowered his head and closed his eyes, Mrs. Casey looked even more distressed. She saw a nurse hurrying by and shouted, "Please help my husband! I'm afraid he's having a heart attack!" I could see the nurse wasn't happy about this and grudgingly decided to take the client into the examination room. When Mrs. Casey started to come with him, the nurse held up her hand, stopping her. She actually told his wife to sit down until she was called. Mrs. Casey began to shake. She tried to explain that she had his nitroglycerin with her if he needed it. The nurse curtly told her that they had their own and repeated that she should sit down. Exasperated, Mrs. Casey found a seat in the waiting room, where she waited alone for the next two hours until the nurse called her in to the examination room.

Observing this whole interaction made me feel very uncomfortable. I didn't know what to do. I understood that Mrs. Casey was upset, and that her husband was not as ill as she thought he was. The doctors and nurses were appropriately triaging clients and establishing priorities. It was just that Mrs. Casey reminded me of my grandmother. I understood her worry and concern. She was trying to help and protect her husband and was afraid of losing him. I wished there were something I could have done to comfort her.

—*From the journal of Rebecca Soren, social work student*

Family caregivers play a significant role in the health care system in emotional, practical, and economic terms. Illness or injury of one member affects the entire family system. This chapter discusses the resulting changes in family members' roles and responsibilities, client and caregiver needs, and caregiver burden. Strategies to develop caregiver skills and minimize burnout are explored.

## FAMILY SYSTEMS

The "nuclear family" of the 1950s and 1960s consisted of a mother and father and one or more children. Grandparents often lived nearby and were available to assist with child care and other family responsibilities. In today's society, families have become more mobile and varied. Children grow up and move away from old neighborhoods. Grandparents may no longer live nearby. Blended families from remarriages and nontraditional family groupings have become more common. The family into which one is born or adopted has been known as the *family of origin;* the *family of creation* is the social group that an individual develops outside the fold of the family of origin. Families of creation include friends, significant others, roommates, coworkers, and other individuals with whom one develops a relationship. These families of creation may be as, or even more, important as those of origin in assuming caregiver responsibilities (Randall & Boonyawiroj, 1999).

The family system is comprised of a group of individuals who work together to adapt to outside influences. Individuals relate to each other in predefined ways. Power and decision-making responsibilities are understood among group members. Illness, injury, or disability of one family member affects the entire family, changes family dynamics, and may cause increased stress among all members. This may necessitate reassigning roles and changing established communication patterns. In an attempt to maintain a sense of equilibrium, some group members may resist change, increasing tension within the group (Qualls, 2000). Family issues will vary depending on an individual's life stages and the nature of earlier relationships among the group. Sibling rivalries may resurface. Families who failed to communicate prior to the illness or injury may have difficulty expressing emotions and acknowledging new losses or grief (Keeling, Dolbin-Macnab, Hudgins, & Ford, 2008).

In the traditional biomedical approach to health care, health care providers were viewed as the experts. Diagnoses and treatment plans were based on medical symptoms, and clients' psychological, social, and cultural experiences were disregarded (Garden, 2008). Clients who asked questions or who did not comply with suggested treatment regimens were considered "difficult." They were expected to do what the "professional" told them to do. During the past decade, public and quasi-public institutions, such as the Institute of Medicine and the Joint Commission, formerly the Joint Commission on Accreditation of Healthcare Organizations, have pushed the health care system to become more client centered rather than disease centered. Public grant funding was made available to help achieve the goal of cultivating more welcoming and shared environments of care that include collaboration with clients and families and respect for their beliefs and health care preferences. Studies show that when clients and families are kept informed and involved in decision making, client care is better coordinated, clients are more adherent with treatment protocols, and clients and family members feel more comfortable and supported. In addition, client, family, and staff stress decreases, and medical outcomes improve (Davidson et al., 2007; Davis, 2009; McCullagh, Brigstocke, Donaldson, & Kalra, 2005).

Children with special health care needs require more health-related services than those without such needs. Parents face additional medical costs and child care challenges, as well as excessive time and work demands. They are often forced to choose between staying home with a child or going to work. Although staying home has been shown to positively benefit both the child and parent, parents state it negatively compromises job performance and finances (Schuster et al., 2009). Increased demands may lead to stress, depression, and anxiety among caregivers, negatively affecting their ability to cope with their children's illnesses (Brehaut et al., 2009).

The personal costs of caregiving continue, even as children reach adulthood. According to Ghosh and Greenberg (2009), fathers of adult children diagnosed with schizophrenia were found to have lower self-esteem and marital satisfaction, higher levels of depression, and twice as many chronic conditions and limitations as parents of healthy children. Providing the parents of adult children who have physical and/or psychological disabilities with education and support services may assist them in better meeting their own health care needs, as well as those of their adult children.

Today, many children may be living with and being cared for by grandparents. Many of these children have previously been living in adverse conditions, which put them at risk. They may have lived in poverty or had parents who abused alcohol and/or drugs, had psychological problems, or abused or neglected them. Health care providers can assist by identifying and referring children to appropriate resources, where they can get help dealing with their feelings, and by providing adequate support services to grandparents (Sands, Goldberg-Glen, & Shin, 2009).

Military service can affect family systems, and going off to fight a war, especially for a lengthy period, has a major impact on service men and women and their families. Stress may occur before, during, or after a deployment and extend well beyond an individual's military service. Deployment of one spouse leads to changes in family roles and responsibilities, uncertainty about safety, and fear of the future. Once family members have accepted their newly assigned roles, reintegration of the returning veteran may further exacerbate family stress (Rentz et al., 2007). In previous military conflicts, individuals who experienced serious physical or psychological trauma often did not survive. Today, advances in military equipment, medical technology, and rapid delivery of emergency services post-injury have drastically increased survival rates (Franklin, 2009). As a result, more returning veterans will need health care services to assist them in dealing with post-traumatic stress disorder and traumatic brain injuries, as well as physical and psychological conditions, including depression, anxiety, substance abuse, and spousal and child abuse (Feczer & Bjorklund, 2009; Martin et al., 2007; Radomski, Davidson, Voydetich, & Erickson, 2009). Health care providers may assist veterans and their family members by developing an understanding of military culture and the challenges these individuals face and by providing them with appropriate education and resources to meet their needs (Savitsky, Illingworth, & DuLaney, 2009).

As the U.S. population ages and health care costs continue to rise, family-centered care continues to evolve. The infrastructure to provide the assistance needed for people to remain in their own homes, in spite of declining health, has been strengthened, and the growth in family caregiving has been associated with longer life expectancies and reluctance of family members to seek outside assistance (Adams, 2006). Types of care provided by family or friends include transporting members to and from appointments, managing medications and dressing changes, monitoring vital signs, supervising home programs, and assisting with activities of daily living (Bookman & Harrington, 2007; Schumacher, Beck, & Marren, 2006). Health care providers need to recognize that family roles have expanded, leading to a higher demand for collaboration between them, clients, and family members (Bookman & Harrington, 2007; Dokken & Ahmann, 2006). It is important to view family members as partners in the health care delivery system who are interested in learning how they can best assist their loved ones. The value of family caregiving in the overall plan of care should not be underestimated. Our ability to care effectively for children, as well as the aging baby boomer population, depends on successful achievement of a strong community-based health infrastructure, with care coordinated primarily by families (Brehaut et al, 2009; Davidson et al., 2007).

The fastest growing age group in the United States is people over the age of 85, estimated to be 13 million by the year 2037. Many of these individuals will be dependent on others to assist them with their daily lives. With the increasing life expectancy and a declining birth rate in the United States, fewer family members will be available to care for elderly people at home. Employers will need to offer employees leaves of absence, flexible work schedules, job sharing, and on-site family day care in order to attract and retain future workers who have caregiving responsibilities (Bookman & Harrington, 2007; Pavalko & Henderson, 2006; Schuster et al., 2009; Spillman & Pezzin, 2000).

Family caregiving is what sustains the majority of frail elders and adults with disabilities. Approximately 44 million Americans ages 18 or older provide some type of unpaid assistance and support to older people and individuals with disabilities. Caregivers face physical, emotional, and financial hardships while caring for family members. Reducing caregiver stress levels has been shown to significantly avoid or defer client nursing home admissions, resulting in lower costs for care (Spillman & Long, 2009). If caregivers do not receive adequate support, they may require medical and psychological assistance to treat conditions resulting from caregiver burden, placing increasing economic demands on the health care system (National Alliance for Caregiving & AARP, 2004).

## Working Together, Working Apart

Busy health care professionals may view family members as being overly concerned and "in the way." Conversely, family members may view health care providers as being aloof and uncaring. Although both health professionals and family members want what is best for the client, they may have different views, which can place them in adversarial roles. Professionals value medical and technical expertise and may fail to recognize that family members can also be experts about their loved one's problems. Family members may be the first to note changes in a client's condition, based on knowledge developed over years of caring; yet, they may be perceived as challenging health care professionals' authority or a health care facility's policies and procedures, especially if they assert themselves and disrupt the routine of care.

Consider Mrs. Brown, who has been assisting her 95-year-old father with his activities of daily living for more than 20 years because he has had multiple cerebrovascular accidents (strokes). Whenever she takes him to visit a new care provider, she encounters the same scenario. Because he cannot hear, she offers to accompany him into the examination room and assist with communication. Over the years, many well-meaning health providers have informed her that they need to talk directly to her father and ask her to remain in the waiting room. Repeatedly frustrated, she no longer argues and waits until they discover that they are unable to communicate with him. When they then ask for her assistance, she enters the treatment room, and the examination is able to begin.

When a client is ill or dying, health care providers are often uncomfortable surrounded by the emotions that families express. They may prefer to distance themselves from emotional involvement and avoid contact with dying clients and their families. In addition, in today's health care environment, some providers fear litigation from family members and, as a result, avoid communication at all costs (Levine & Zuckerman, 2000). However, health care professionals may need to rely on family members. For example, as the acuity level of hospitalized clients increases, nurses are required to spend most of their time attending to the needs of those who are critically ill. When clients are transferred from specialized units, such as intensive care or coronary care, family members become more important in providing comfort measures and monitoring the needs of their loved ones. Discharges from one setting to another, even within the same facility, often trigger the need for family caregivers to become client advocates to ensure that appropriate care is provided (Bookman & Harrington, 2007).

Consider Mr. Gainey, who was visiting his wife in the intensive care unit when he was informed that she was being transferred to another floor. He accompanied his wife and the nurse to the medical/surgical unit. The nurse informed him that she would update the head nurse as to Mrs. Gainey's condition and that the nurse would be in to meet her and monitor her vital signs. Mrs. Gainey was left in a wheelchair inside the room. Shortly thereafter, a dietary aide dropped off a lunch for her, leaving it on a table out of her reach. Mr. Gainey retrieved the meal and fed his wife her lunch. Then, after waiting 2 hours, he approached the nurses' station, where he learned that the staff had forgotten about her. Only after he had expressed concern was Mrs. Gainey monitored and assisted into bed. Mr. Gainey reluctantly left for home that evening, worrying that his wife would be alone and unable to call for help if needed.

The length of stay in hospitals has become very brief, and clients are often unstable on discharge. Health care professionals rely on family members to carry out procedures at home that used to be performed only by licensed personnel, such as providing wound care, monitoring respirators, administering medications, giving injections, and completing chemotherapy infusions (Bookman & Harrington, 2007; Levine & Zuckerman, 2000). Family members who suddenly find themselves in the role of "home care provider" may be terrified that their lack of expertise and education will adversely affect their loved one's health. In addition, although some home care agencies provide case managers, it is frequently the responsibility of a family member to coordinate home-based health care services. This may include evaluating and purchasing medical equipment; ordering, monitoring, and reordering prescriptions; locating and hiring home health aides; and transporting clients to follow-up appointments.

As the human body ages, comorbid conditions become more common. Because most physicians today are specialists, family caregiver responsibilities increase even further, with the need to coordinate visits to multiple providers, such as a primary care physician, orthopedist, oncologist, ophthalmologist, physical therapist, and psychiatrist. This can be a very time-consuming and frustrating task (Bookman & Harrington, 2007). These new responsibilities increase the burden of family members, who may already be overextended with household chores, child care, and careers. The worry and concern they experience can further drain available emotional resources.

## Family Caregivers: Who Are They? From Where Do They Come?

Anyone can become a family caregiver. Some people are prepared to assume this responsibility and plan ahead, whereas others assume this role quite unexpectedly. A sudden car accident, stroke, diagnosis of peripheral vascular disease, or the birth of a child with a disability can lead to the need for someone to assume the caregiver role. Research has shown that both gender and ethnicity influence who will be expected to take on the caregiver role. In some cultures, caregiving is seen as "women's work," and women are responsible, unless there are no female relatives available. Members of some minority cultural groups have been shown to feel stronger obligations to care for parents than those of the majority White culture in the United States; because children from higher socioeconomic groups can better afford to hire formal caregivers, they may experience less stress than those who cannot afford this accommodation (Szinovacz & Davey, 2007).

When asked how they became a caregiver, people often respond, "I had to. There was no one else available." Caregiving has been described as a "career," though often unintended, unplanned, and unselected. There are little or no wages, and family caregivers cannot resign, even if they might choose to do so.

According to the National Alliance for Caregiving (NAC) and the American Association for Retired People (AARP, 2004), approximately 25 percent of American households participate in some type of caregiving for adults over the age of 50. That constitutes 44.4 million informal caregivers, about 83 percent of whom are providing services for a relative, usually a spouse or parent. Although this care is generally unpaid, it has been estimated that it is valued at $257 billion annually. Caregivers' time commitments range from a few hours per week to 40 or more hours per week, essentially providing constant care. Statistics regarding who the caregivers are vary among sources. According to Schumacher and associates (2006), the majority of caregivers are women, approximately age 46, with some college education. Wolff and Kasper (2006) indicate that although the majority of family caregivers are adult children, spouses also constitute a significant proportion of caregivers, wives more often than husbands. Research shows that when husbands and sons are called on to provide care, they report less caregiver burden than wives or daughters (NAC & AARP, 2004). This may be because men tend to be less emotional about caregiving and use a problem-solving approach. It is also likely that many sons are married and that their wives assume a share of the caregiver duties (Faison, Faria, & Frank, 1999; Hoffmann & Mitchell, 1998; Laditka & Laditka, 2000). Yet, when called on to be caregivers, men may lack the peer support, work flexibility, or skills necessary to take on caregiver tasks (Keeling et al., 2008). Interestingly, the life expectancy for men is escalating at a faster rate than it is for women, which raises the likelihood that husbands may increasingly take on the caregiver role, relieving their daughters of this responsibility (Hirst, 2001). Because the prevalence of dementia among elderly women is also increasing, many of these men will be caring for wives who have cognitive deficits (Ducharme et al., 2006).

Relationships among family members change when caregiver roles are assumed (Honea et al., 2008). Whereas caring for a spouse may bring partners closer together, it may change traditional marital roles and responsibilities and decrease a caregiver's satisfaction with life. Caring for a parent may result in an adult child spending less time with his or her own children or spouse or spending financial resources on the parent, negatively affecting his or her personal relationships. Furthermore, the responsibilities of the adult child may interfere with his or her relationships with siblings. Family members may not recognize the magnitude of the caregiver's responsibilities. They may avoid contact with both the caregiver and the receiver and fail to understand how ongoing deterioration of the care receiver places additional burdens on the family caregiver. This may lead to increased feelings of anxiety, frustration, and burden (Keeling et al., 2008). Ongoing resentment of an aging parent may be exacerbated when an adult child who was the victim of child abuse is asked to care for his or her former abuser (Van Volkon, 2006).

When working with families, health care providers need to identify the primary caregiver, so they can communicate and work with that person to develop appropriate care plans. Sometimes, working with the "wrong" person may increase family conflict and negatively affect client outcomes (Keeling et al., 2008). However, in today's mobile society, families may experience frequent changes in the caregiving network. Szinovacz and Davey (2007) found that one-fourth of primary adult children caring for parents were replaced by a sibling, as one caregiver dropped out and another assumed the responsibility. Exchange of one caregiver for another has been found to be higher among people who are African American and Hispanic than White. Providers should recognize that information may need to be disseminated to multiple family members as caregiving roles fluctuate. Strategies to accomplish this goal may include conference calls, video-conferences, e-mails, telephone calls, and use of online resources (Keeling et al., 2008).

## CAREGIVER NEEDS

Family caregivers are often unseen, untrained, and lack support systems. They make up what has been called a "shadow workforce." They serve as client "case managers, medical records keepers, paramedics and patient advocates to fill dangerous gaps in a system that is uncoordinated, fragmented, bureaucratic and often depersonalized" (Bookman & Harrington, 2007, p. 1005). A review of the literature indicates that family caregivers seek information, education, trust, and understanding from their health care providers. They further need support systems, the ability to speak on behalf of their family members, and assistance navigating the health care system (Brehaut et al., 2009; Bookman & Harrington, 2007; Schuster et al., 2009; Smith & Smith, 2000; Szinovacz & Davey, 2007). Health care professionals need to recognize these issues and provide clients and family caregivers with mechanisms to obtain what they need to improve outcomes.

### Information and Education

Family caregivers want honest information about their loved ones' diagnoses and prognoses. They need to understand the tests, diagnosis, treatment options, and prognosis for recovery. They require appropriate training so they can respond to disease-related issues as illnesses progress (Bookman & Harrington, 2007; Honea et al., 2008). Caregivers want to understand care plans and recognize what the future might hold. It is wise to individualize this information, based on client and family culture, needs, and questions (Pasacreta, Barg, Nuamah, & McCorkle, 2000).

Many caregivers indicate that the way information is delivered is important. For example, if they are provided with information when their loved one is in the hospital, they do not remember much when they return home because of the stress of the moment, and this can create a sense of fear and feelings of frustration (Smith & Smith, 2000; Zwygart-Stauffacher, Lindquist, & Savik, 2000).

Timing is important. Providing too much information to clients or family members when they are under stress will probably be ineffective. They simply will be overloaded and will not remember what they heard. Cultural issues (see Chapter 3) may also affect communication and education. Another consideration is literacy level. Surprisingly, some individuals who read poorly believe they read and comprehend information well. They will be unlikely to ask questions about information they do not understand, often because they are embarrassed to do so.

A study of clients in home settings indicated that 85 percent of written client educational materials was inappropriate. Presented in full-text format, materials did not identify or emphasize "need-to-know" information. Instructions were not summarized, were handwritten, and were difficult to read. When interviewing clients and caregivers, health professionals need to assess their ability to read and understand written instructions. Materials should be in larger print, and writing should be at a fifth- or sixth-grade reading level to ensure consumer comprehension (Wilson, 2000).

Zwygart-Stauffacher and colleagues (2000) note that health providers, clients, and their caregivers may disagree about the type of knowledge needed. Whereas health providers want to disseminate factual information, clients and family caregivers may also want information related to alternative therapies. Conducting an individualized needs assessment for clients and family members can help providers determine what type of information is desired.

Family members also report that health professionals do not understand or address families' fears of the future and the unknown. Caregivers express their frustration that many providers do not speak with one another and are only familiar with one aspect of a client's medical history. They stress the need for continuity of care so they can develop relationships with their family member's health providers. Furthermore, because clients and family members often think of questions once they are home, newer methods of communication, such as e-mail, telephone hot lines, listservs, and websites, are needed to augment information disseminated in the acute care and rehabilitation settings (Bookman & Harrington, 2007; Zwygart-Stauffacher et al., 2000).

Some interventions may be more helpful than others to family caregivers. In a study related to caregiver burden on family members caring for clients with cancer, researchers found that caregivers benefited from educational programs that provided self-help strategies. Effective programs encouraged caregivers to challenge their own negative thoughts and replace them with positive thoughts, participate in pleasant and positive activities, and develop better problem-solving abilities focusing on time management (Honea et al., 2008). Religious organizations, pastoral counseling, adult day care, counseling, and respite care can also be helpful. Findings indicate that positive spiritual well-being plays an important role in caregivers' mental health (Yeh & Bull, 2009).

Health care providers should be aware of services in their area and provide clients with information on accessing such services. However, providers must also recognize that many services may be inaccessible or underutilized because of limited availability, cost, stigma, cultural insensitivity, lack of transportation, caregiver reluctance to delegate the responsibility of caring for their loved one to strangers, and limitations in the energy needed to take advantage of such programming (Keeling et al., 2008).

Educational workshops and peer support groups have also been shown to be effective. They provide individuals with information as problems arise and improve communication and cooperation among family members. In addition, they help caregivers develop confidence in their skills and abilities. Providing a day care center for clients to attend, concurrent with the workshop sessions for their caregivers, reduces stress and allows caregivers the opportunity to participate without needing to find someone to care for their family member (Ostwald, Hepburn, Caron, Burns, & Mantell, 1999). Studies show that the switch from a client-centered approach to a client-*and caregiver*-centered approach empowers caregivers and results in better long-term outcomes (McCullagh et al., 2005).

### Trust

Family caregivers want to be able to trust health providers, but fears related to errors of omission or commission cause them to avoid leaving loved ones alone in hospital settings. Many errors of judgment and practice have been observed and publicized. In addition, overlooking basic elements of a nurturing environment, failure of professionals to respond to clients' needs in a timely manner, and not giving meaningful responses can all create distrust. This is especially true when clients have been diagnosed with disabling conditions that may leave them unable to protect themselves (Smith & Smith, 2000).

One caregiver discussed how she felt the need to personalize her father in the eyes of the hospital staff. She taped pictures of him in his younger days to the hospital walls. She wanted the staff to see him as a person, not simply as a "sick old man." She felt it was important, especially since he was nonverbal, that the staff recognize and understand his identity as a person (Keeling et al., 2008).

Consider Mr. O'Donnell, an 84-year-old man who had been married to his wife for 57 years. Following abdominal surgery, Mrs. O'Donnell told her husband that she was in pain. He contacted the nurse and asked for medication. When the nurse asked the client how she felt, she responded, "Fine." The nurse indicated that, based on the client's response, no pain medication was needed. Mr. O'Donnell became agitated. "You don't understand. I know my wife. She needs medication! She just doesn't want to complain." Frustrated and busy, the nurse then asked the woman to rate her pain on a one-to-ten scale. When Mrs. O'Donnell replied, "Ten," the nurse agreed to the medication. Because Mr. O'Donnell believed he could not trust the hospital staff to adequately care for his wife, he believed it was necessary for him to become her advocate. This is neither a welcome nor a desired role, and many caregivers need advice and guidance on how to best advocate for their family members.

## Advocacy

Elements of effective advocacy include knowledge of federal, state, and local regulations regarding health care services, insurance, and special education delivery; assertive communication skills; negotiation skills; and conflict resolution abilities. Because it is challenging to advocate for clients' welfare when dealing with bureaucracies, caregivers benefit from validation and encouragement, as well as emotional and social support.

Clients with cognitive or emotional deficits may have unrealistic goals or behavior problems, which require caregiver involvement (Smith & Smith, 2000). Caregivers' decisions may conflict with the goals and desires of other family members or even with those of the client. If the client is over the age of 18, a legal process may be required to allow a family member to assume decision-making responsibilities. Some caregivers may need to become surrogate decision makers if the people in their care are under the age of 18; are frail, elderly, or diagnosed with dementia; or have physical, cognitive, or emotional deficits that render them unable to make their own decisions.

Consider the case of Denis Rockwell and his 16-year-old son Jeff. Because he continually "acted out" in school, Jeff had been suspended several times before finally being expelled. He had been arrested for shoplifting on numerous occasions and attacked his mother, causing her to leave the family home. When Jeff began talking about suicide, Mr. Rockwell tried to discuss his concerns with school professionals and the family doctor. They considered Jeff a "problem child" who merely needed more structure in his life. Mr. Rockwell, however, believed that something more serious was being overlooked. He continued to be an advocate and located a physician who admitted the young man to a psychiatric hospital, against his son's wishes. While there, the son was diagnosed with depression, placed on medication, and attended counseling sessions and peer support groups. When he returned home, his father needed to advocate with the school system to provide appropriate educational support so that Jeff could successfully complete high school, which he was able to do. This would not have been possible had Mr. Rockwell not served as his son's spokesperson and advocated for him, obtaining the necessary medical interventions.

## Identification of Resources

Another need expressed by family caregivers is assistance in dealing with the health care system and obtaining necessary resources (Bookman & Harrington, 2007; Smith & Smith, 2000).

Families caring for members who need home care services require professional advice and coordination. For example, they may not realize that, in addition to nursing and rehabilitation services, home health care agencies can provide home health aides to assist clients with activities of daily living. Programs like Meals-on-Wheels serve home care clients one meal daily. A raised toilet seat, grab bars in the hallway, or other accommodations may be installed to assist the client in safely maneuvering in the home.

Many family caregivers discuss the difficulties involved in finding appropriate services. For example, one client spoke about the fact that she could no longer read, one of her favorite activities. She needed to get to an ophthalmologist for a new eyeglass prescription but did not have transportation, and the mechanisms available seemed too complex. Although a transport van was available through elder services, the driver was not allowed to enter the home to help her up and down the stairs. In an effort to avoid duplication of services, home health and community services may be uncoordinated, resulting in the client being unable to leave the home or access required services (Bookman & Harrington, 2007). It is the role of the health care team to identify needs and collaborate with the client, family caregivers, and community service organizations to help clients navigate the health care system and acquire needed resources. When this does not happen, family caregiver burden is increased and, along with it, rising levels of frustration, anger, and loss of trust.

As time progresses, the needs of clients and family caregivers may change. Health providers need to remain in contact to assist them through times of transition. For example, if a client is no longer able to independently remain at home, family members may require counseling in how to adapt to this new situation. Perhaps it will be necessary for the client to move in with a family member and attend a day care center while the family member is at work. Depending on the client and family situations, a long-term care facility may be more appropriate. It is difficult for families to make these decisions, and providing brochures describing available long-term care facilities is insufficient. Family caregivers need guidance and support when assessing agencies and services to help them make informed decisions (Bookman & Harrington, 2007).

## DEVELOPING CAREGIVER SKILLS

Years ago, the role of family caregivers was similar to that of a nurse's aide. Today, they are expected to complete complicated, highly skilled tasks, with limited training and, sometimes, few, if any, resources. To become licensed health care professionals, students complete lengthy educational programs and pass examinations; yet, there are no such requirements for family caregivers. Imagine how family caregivers must feel when they are first put in the situation of caring for a loved one (Bookman & Harrington, 2007; Pasacreta et al., 2000).

Alone with their family member or friend in the home setting, caregivers may not know what to do. Perhaps they wonder, "Is nausea and vomiting to be expected?" or "How soon should I expect my son to be able to dress independently?" The client may lack an appetite and not want to eat or drink. Respecting his or her wishes, a family caregiver may unknowingly allow the client to become dehydrated.

Some family caregivers may telephone health care professionals daily, asking questions and clarifying concerns, whereas others are reluctant to call, afraid that they are being bothersome. How do we respond to these individuals? Do we lose patience with constant callers or do we educate them to alleviate their concerns? Do we become angry at the person who failed to call, unwittingly putting a family member at risk? Caregivers state they have difficulty watching their family members become sicker and not knowing how to help. Many worry about how to handle future problems, which adds to caregiver burden.

Developing caregiver skills requires education, time, patience, and practice. Caregiving demands that family members monitor clients and observe subtle changes, interpret verbal and nonverbal cues, analyze information, make decisions about actions, keep track of what to do and when to do it, provide direct care, make adjustments as needed, manage treatment schedules, administer medications, seek outside help as needed, and negotiate the health care system (Keeling et al., 2008; Schumacher, Stewart, Archbold, Dodd, & Dibble, 2000).

Competent caregiving involves understanding health care plans. Most family caregivers want to provide excellent care. It is the role of health care professionals to determine what skills caregivers need and work with them to help them develop these skills so they can provide care efficiently and effectively (Schumacher et al., 2000). Developing shared decision-making models, consistently communicating with families, honoring culturally appropriate requests for truth-telling and informed refusal, and providing spiritual support to families are all strategies that will assist family members in developing their caregiver skills (Davidson et al., 2007).

## ROLES AND RESPONSIBILITIES WITHIN THE FAMILY SYSTEM

Within each family system, everyone has roles and responsibilities, knows what is expected, and reacts to other family members according to his or her defined role. However, when a member of the family becomes ill or disabled, responsibilities and roles change. It is important to note the difference between these terms. *Responsibilities* are jobs that family members perform, such as cooking meals, paying bills, doing laundry, and going to school. *Roles* are more complex and difficult to define. Established over many years, they include who you are, how people see you, and what people expect of you. Roles can include that of parent, money manager, head of the household, child, and caregiver. Whereas some may be able to afford to hire people to fulfill household responsibilities, changing the roles within a family system is much more difficult.

### Caring for a Spouse or Partner

When a husband, wife, or partner becomes ill or disabled, the relationship is altered. Responsibilities change, and each may assume a new role. Sometimes, individuals must give up their independence. For example, if someone who becomes ill had been responsible for paying the bills and managing the household, the person who is well may feel overwhelmed when he or she must assume these activities. The partner who is ill or has a disability may not realize his or her deficits or not want to relinquish responsibilities. He or she may feel that the partner is "taking over." It takes everyone in the family, including the person who is ill or has the disability, time to adjust. As they grieve, they try to adjust to the new "self" and the changing roles and responsibilities within the family system.

Some illnesses and disabilities are more difficult than others on spousal/partner relationships. Traumatic brain injury is a good example because the person who sustains the injury may experience personality changes. Family caregivers frequently find these changes extremely difficult, if not impossible, to accept. This particular disability is associated with distress in the entire family. Family therapy may be helpful in assisting members to understand the disruption in family roles, to alleviate strain experienced by caregivers, and to assist family members in developing coping skills and appropriate communication techniques. Referral to support groups, where family members can share experiences with others in similar situations, may also alleviate burden and stress (Gan, Campbell, Gemeinhardt, & McFadden, 2006).

Consider Mrs. Benedetto, a 35-year-old woman, who sustained a traumatic brain injury in a motor vehicle accident. It is not surprising that her husband and two young children are devastated. In addition, Mr. Benedetto is angry with her for driving to an aerobics class during a snowstorm when he specifically asked her not to do so. Her health status and inability to work add considerable financial strain on the family. In addition, Mrs. Benedetto sometimes behaves inappropriately because of the effects of the brain injury, and this causes great embarrassment for the family. The children no longer have their friends visit, and her husband is uncomfortable taking her out in public. They see their friends less often and are becoming socially isolated. Mr. Benedetto misses the companionship and intimacy of his partner. They are both depressed, and the marriage is breaking apart.

Any significant illness or disability will place demands on family members (Gan et al., 2006). Spouses may experience grief, anger, and chronic sorrow (see Chapter 7). Although he or she has "lost" the partner once known, the spouse is still alive, and there is no sense of closure. These problems are universal responses to loss and change within the family system.

According to Banja (1992), health care providers need to integrate the psychosocial dimensions with the clinical phenomenon. "Patients and families who are in the midst of tragedy not only will want superior clinical skills, they will want the company of providers who have opened themselves up to the experience of tragedy and who are willing to share their humanity in the rehabilitation process" (p. 114). When clients and family members appear to be "difficult" or unmotivated, health professionals must try to understand the changes they are experiencing and work with them to help them adjust to their new roles and responsibilities. Accommodation can be a lengthy process.

As illnesses progress and clients reach the end of life, roles and responsibilities shift again. Health providers need to understand that caring for a spouse, partner, or child who is terminally ill often requires round-the-clock coverage and can be intensely demanding and emotional. In addition to helping the health care receiver, the healthy individual is attempting to deal with his or her anticipated loss and the upcoming changes in life. Studies confirm that older spouses may experience more caregiver burden and stress than adult children caring for parents. This may be related to the fact that adult children have alternative roles outside of the parents' home that might help buffer them from caregiver stress, whereas spousal activity may be limited to the caregiving experience within the home. In addition, adult children will not be experiencing normal aging and physical decline to the same degree as their older parents (Pinquart & Sorensen, 2003).

## Caring for a Parent

In today's society, women often postpone childbearing to continue careers. As a result, they, and even younger parents, may find themselves caring for older parents at the same time they are tending to their own young children. They comprise what has become known as the "sandwich generation" (Martine & Stephens, 2003; Spillman & Pezzin, 2000). Conflicting responsibilities may increase stress within the family. Husbands may resent time their wives spend away from home. Women may feel guilty—either they are not spending enough time at home or not spending enough time with parents. Chronic sorrow (see Chapter 7) may be experienced. The same is true for adult sons who assume caregiver roles. They may have difficulty taking over the roles and responsibilities their parents once performed. Although they "grew up" depending on their parents, their parents may now be the dependent ones. The caregivers' own children may sense tension in the home, feel neglected, or "act out" to seek attention. As a result of the stress associated with caregiving, both men and women caregivers are susceptible to developing their own health problems.

When a younger parent becomes ill or disabled, more responsibilities may be placed on children who still live at home. It is difficult to estimate the number of minor children responsible for caring for parents or other family members, because health professionals may be unaware of the services the children provide. Affected children are often referred to as the "unrecognized caregivers" (Baago, 2004; Jacobson & Wood, 2004; Valiakalayil, Paulson, & Tibbo, 2004). Younger children may be upset because parents may no longer be able to play with them as they once did due to pain, fatigue, or other limitations (Poole, Willer, & Mendelson, 2009). Older children may be expected to care for their parent and younger siblings. They may worry about their family's future and their parents' health. At a time when they should be preparing to assert their independence from parents, they find themselves becoming the caregivers (Asal, 2009). They do not seek support and often do not socialize with peers for fear of disclosure of family secrets or intervention of social services. They often feel they have no other options (Williams, Ayres, Specht, Sparbel, & Klimek, 2009). Assigned tasks and responsibilities can range from routine age-appropriate household tasks to complicated responsibilities that would be more fitting for adult caregivers. These responsibilities may be carried out with or without adult supervision (Becker, 2007) and may involve providing both physical and emotional care. Young caregivers may become depressed, socially isolated, and feel financially strained. The high level of responsibility, coupled with a lack of authority and role uncertainty, can be extremely demanding (Williams et al., 2009).

When adults need to rely on children for support, parents may experience depression, and conflict is a common result. As a result, children may internalize their own problems and develop maladaptive coping behaviors, either keeping their feelings to themselves or expressing anger toward others. Health care professionals can assist children who are placed in the caregiver role by helping to facilitate discussion among family members. Parents need to be open with children, providing them with accurate information about their illness or disability. Family counseling and support groups may be recommended. Parents also need to recognize that their depression and conflict affect their children. Therefore, they need to be encouraged to seek help to deal with their own feelings, for the benefit of the entire family.

## Caring for a Child

I was so excited this morning! It was my first day on the maternity ward. I love babies, and I was really looking forward to being a part of the birthing process. This would be a happy rotation, filled with expectant mothers and fathers looking forward to experiencing the birth of an infant. My days would fly by, and I'd be anxious to return to work the next day.

Boy was I wrong! My very first client was in trouble. She had been in labor for a long time and was in severe pain. The doctor finally determined that she would have to perform a Cesarean section. Although the baby was safely delivered, the umbilical cord was wrapped around his throat. Instead of handing the child to the mother to breastfeed, the doctors rushed the baby into the neonatal intensive care unit for further evaluation. Rather than experiencing tears of joy, the parents were sobbing uncontrollably, awaiting some word of their child's status. I quietly stood in the background, not knowing what to say or do.

—*From the journal of Michelle Crowley, nursing student*

Men and women enter parenthood with the expectation that they will love and raise healthy children who will grow up to be independent and live on their own. This is not always the case. When a child is ill or has a disability, parents need to take on the role of advocate for their child, negotiating with the educational, social, and health care systems to obtain services that their child needs. Along the way, they will face many difficult decisions. Blurring of responsibilities among health providers and family caregivers can place tremendous stress on families. Conflict may occur if family members and professionals disagree on what is best for the child (Hartman, DePoy, Francis, & Gilmer, 2000).

Children who are ill or have a disability may require painful, invasive procedures, which cause parents stress before, during, and after the procedures have been completed. Parents want to protect their children from pain, but that is not always possible. Lack of control increases stress levels. Health providers can assist parents by showing them how they can be involved in treatments, such as describing procedures to children, instructing them in deep-breathing and relaxation exercises, or even holding their hand during a procedure.

Parents' needs may be neglected when they care for children who have chronic illnesses or disabilities. They may experience emotional loss and feel responsible for the onset of a child's illness or disability. They will need to mourn the loss of the child they expected, and the experience of chronic sorrow is not uncommon. Sometimes, they may perceive that they are in control. At other times, they may feel depression, anger, guilt, lack of control, powerlessness, and despair. Stress may increase when developmental milestones are not met at anticipated times. Anxiety levels may be further exacerbated as a result of financial loss, due to the expenses of care, equipment, and time away from work. Health professionals can help parents manage their own stress, which will have a positive impact on the child's well-being.

Career mobility may be limited if parents choose to live in a geographical area where a child's health needs can be better met. They may be unable to change jobs, remaining in positions in order to retain their health care coverage or primary care physicians. Financial resources can be even further strained if a parent must quit his or her job to stay home and care for a child who is ill.

Children with disabilities may not achieve independence as quickly as other children. Parents may wonder who will care for their child when they are no longer able. They may feel angry, depressed, and envy families with more "typical" children, and it is not uncommon for parents to feel too guilty to go out and have fun if their child is unable to do so. Support systems that allow independent living away from the family are not always available or desirable (Hartman et al., 2000).

Research has shown that it may be helpful for parents of children with disabilities to envision the child growing up, by making plans for the future. While the details of the plan are not as important as the overall picture, and plans may need to be revised over time, parents indicate that starting the process early helps them to better prepare for the transitions to come. Encouraging children to be independent and do things for themselves is often difficult but of the utmost importance. Families voice frustration over the move from pediatric care to that of adult primary care providers when children turn 18 years old. Most pediatricians no longer care for adult children, and parents miss the bond they have developed with their health care providers over the years. It is not uncommon for primary care physicians who care for adults to be relatively ignorant about the research and treatment for young adults who have childhood-onset illnesses or disabilities (Reiss, Gibson, & Walker, 2005).

Health professionals can help by understanding that families may go through recurring periods of emotional crisis. At times, they might be angry or hostile. Educating families about what to expect may help prevent or alleviate anger. Keeping the lines of communication open is also extremely important. Health care professionals should ask questions to help resolve issues and determine what a family needs or wants and then assist them in obtaining the appropriate social and educational support.

Sometimes, parents are in the difficult position of having to care for children who are faced with life-threatening conditions. Caregiver burden may include time spent providing care, physical and emotional tasks, financial costs, and the potential for their own physical and mental health risks. Health providers may assist family caregivers by maintaining open and honest communication, discussing options for death and dying, supporting home-based hospice if requested, and demonstrating empathy (Rabow, Hauser, & Adams, 2004).

Decisions about whether to initiate or disconnect life-support systems must sometimes be made, and such decisions involve family decision making. Values and spiritual beliefs come into play as do other issues, such as quality of life, the age of the child, cognitive abilities, and pain. Family relationships are additional factors. Family members should be asked open-ended questions about what they understand about the client's condition. Providers should repeat what they have heard to ensure that they fully understand the decisions they are being asked to make. Shared decision making may reduce family stress, and significant support will be needed before, during, and after a death (Davidson et al., 2007). As discussed in Chapter 4, health care chaplains become important members of the team when family members are facing the death of a loved one.

## Sibling Roles and Responsibilities

When a child is ill, the primary focus of parents is necessarily placed on that child. What happens to the siblings living at home? They are undoubtedly experiencing the family stress caused by the complexities associated with caring for a child who is seriously ill or who has a disability. Siblings may experience guilt because they are healthy. Lack of parental support leaves siblings at risk of developing anxiety, depression, and acting out or other behavioral problems (Bellin, Bentley, & Sawn, 2009). Older children may be enlisted to care for younger siblings, while parents attend to the needs of the child who is ill or has the disability. The older child may resent these changes in roles and responsibilities.

The onset, course, expected outcomes, and uncertainty of an illness may also impact siblings. When a child is born healthy and later develops a life-threatening illness, siblings may have more difficulty dealing with the situation. They have already developed a bond with their brother or sister. They may fear that their sibling will die and no longer be available to them. They may be yearning for life as it once was (Batte, Watson, & Amess, 2006). Siblings of children born with congenital conditions may react quite differently. Although an occasional crisis may occur, their early bonding and feelings of warmth and compassion may promote more positive outcomes. They are more likely to feel protective of their brother or sister (Rolland & Williams, 2005). Studies show that many siblings attempt to ease the burden on their parents, avoiding doing anything that may cause further disruptions in family life (Woodgate, 2006).

Just as adult caregivers need adequate information regarding a client's diagnosis and prognosis, siblings also express a desire to understand more about the illness or disability their brother or sister is experiencing. Health providers can teach and support parents to communicate openly with all of the children in the family and invite siblings to be involved in the care plan. A family-centered approach to health care that emphasizes shared decision making and partnerships between the health care provider and the family has been linked to positive outcomes for the child, parents, and other family members. This model supports the fact that a child's psychosocial health is interrelated with that of the surrounding family members (American Academy of Pediatrics, 2003).

Health professionals should encourage parents to cultivate an environment in which all family members, including children, feel free to talk about their feelings, without fear of consequences, and they should answer questions honestly. Whereas all members of the family may be required to take on additional responsibilities, adults need to assure children that they will be treated as children and not as adult caregivers (Fleitas, 2000). Parents should be encouraged to spend as much time with the healthy children as possible to decrease disruption in family life, and health providers can help parents understand that their reaction to the child's illness will affect their other children's responses and behaviors.

## CAREGIVER BURDEN

Following initial diagnoses, accidents, or injuries, there may be an abundance of family and friends to help both client and caregiver. However, as time progresses, people return to their own lives, and caregivers may be left alone to adjust to *their* altered lives. Caring for a family member may offer many rewards (Honea et al., 2008). Some caregivers report developing a strong bond with their "clients" and feel good about themselves as a result of the experience (Rabkin, Wagner, & DelBene, 2000). However, the intensity of providing long-term care can lead to "caregiver burden," resulting in caregiver depression. When caregiver burden is not addressed, it can progress, causing physical and mental health problems (Honea et al., 2008). Caregiver burden has been described in studies of families who care for loved ones with a variety of diagnoses. It encompasses both objective and subjective components. Objective burden refers to the tasks caregivers must perform and the changes that occur in their lives as a result, such as dressing, bathing, feeding, and transporting clients. Subjective burden results from the emotional factors stemming from caregiving responsibilities, such as fatigue, stress, anger, depression, social isolation, fear, and role adjustment. Lack of resources and financial strain can also affect caregiver burden (Honea et al., 2008; McCullagh et al., 2005; Pinquart & Sorensen, 2003).

When friends or family members become caregivers, their lives are disrupted. They must rearrange schedules to meet the needs of the client. Some people make this adjustment easily; others do not. Studies indicate that the quality of the relationship between the caregiver and the client has an impact on the perceived levels of burden and satisfaction with the caregiver role (Snyder, 2000). If the premorbid relationship was characterized by open communication, shared interests, and a family orientation, perceived burden is low, and satisfaction is high. This is true even when objective burden is high. Although health care providers cannot change family histories or relationships, they may assist burdened caregivers by referring them to family counselors or therapists who may be able to help.

Clients may require more assistance over time, especially if the illness or disability is progressive or chronic. When this occurs, caregivers have less time for themselves. Overload and burnout may occur. They may lose sleep if they are frequently interrupted during the night to provide assistance. Contact with former friends may be lost, leaving caregivers feeling socially and emotionally isolated, as they watch their loved ones decline. At the same time, they may also experience anger, resentment, and frustration because their own lives have been disrupted. Some caregivers may resort to maladaptive practices, turning to prescription and nonprescription drugs or alcohol to help them face each day (Gan et al., 2006). Others postpone taking care of their own health needs because they are so busy caring for someone else (Stein et al., 2000). Failure to alleviate stress and burden can ultimately lead to increased doctors' visits, medical expenses, and even more stress (O'Brien, 2000). As discussed in Chapter 15, high caregiver burden, frustration, burnout, and inability to provide adequate care can increase risk for abuse (DeHart, Webb, & Cornman, 2009; Shinan-Altman & Cohen, 2009).

## CARING FOR THE CAREGIVER

The literature suggests that well-informed caregivers, who are confident in their abilities and have developed appropriate coping strategies, exhibit lower stress levels and less caregiver burden. Health care professionals can help by educating family members about common stresses associated with caregiving *before* caregiver burnout begins. Helping them identify available resources for themselves and the client and teaching them to develop healthy approaches for coping will help ensure that clients will receive the best possible support in the home (Bookman & Harrington, 2007; Keeling et al., 2008; McCullagh et al., 2005; Parks & Novielli, 2000; Schumacher et al., 2006).

### Respite Care

The amount of care provided and the duration of an illness influence caregiver burden. It is important for the caregiver to receive some relief from his or her duties. Respite care, as a social service, is designed to support family caregivers by providing temporary daytime or overnight relief. It affords caregivers important time away from their responsibilities (Honea et al., 2008). Originally designed to assist with crisis intervention and avoid institutionalization (Lawton, Brody, & Saperstein, 1989), it is a beneficial system that supports both clients and family caregivers on an ongoing basis and has been shown to reduce caregiver stress and burden (Keeling et al., 2008; Sorenson, Pinquart, & Duberstein, 2002).

Health professionals can assist caregivers by helping them identify appropriate resources. Some local governments have volunteer "sitters" for short periods of time. Formal and informal adult day care programs provide opportunities for caregivers to work, do errands, or just take a break from everyday duties. Bus services may be available to transport individuals to and from day care facilities. Religious organizations may have volunteers available to assist with respite care and transportation. Other family members can be asked to provide care for short periods of time. Although primary caregivers may be uncomfortable giving up "control," health providers can help them understand that it is in everyone's best interest.

### Counseling and Support Groups

Counseling and support groups for both clients and caregivers have been shown to have significant impact on long-term psychosocial interventions and to reduce caregiver burden (Chien & Norman, 2009; Drentia, Clay, Roth, & Mittelman, 2006; Sorenson et al., 2002). As discussed in other chapters, individual counseling and peer support groups can be an effective adjunct for both clients and caregivers. They provide a forum for participants to discuss problems, successes, and feelings regarding their individual roles. This provides the opportunity for everyone to share ideas and strategies for the future.

As technology continues to advance, its role in health care continues to expand. An alternative to support groups is an Internet-based psychotherapeutic support group involving interventions for family caregivers. One study described a model designed to replicate traditional face-to-face support groups. Following implementation of a user-friendly website, a health professional facilitated 10 support group sessions. Later, caregivers were assigned to self-help group discussions, each led by a participating group member. This allowed caregivers to remain at home and still participate in support group discussions. Follow-up interviews revealed that participants reported positive experiences. Respondents indicated they learned to use computers and negotiate websites, knew how to find disease-specific information on the Internet, and were better prepared to use technology to communicate. In addition, they bonded with group members, providing mutual support and guidance to each other. Overall, the online support group assisted participants in better coping with the stresses of caregiving without having to leave their loved ones unattended (Marziali, Damianakis, & Donahue, 2006).

### Humor

As discussed in Chapter 5, humor has been shown to help people maintain balance in their lives. Developing and maintaining a sense of humor can help caregivers feel less overwhelmed and may assist in preventing or overcoming caregiver burden (Keeling et al., 2008). The strategy can be as simple as reading a humorous book or watching funny movies to relieve stress. Some caregivers might feel guilty devoting time to laughter, particularly if their loved one is in pain or uncomfortable, yet those who understand the importance of self-care are less likely to feel guilt. The use of appropriate humor has been shown to ease interpersonal communications and interactions, increase personal satisfaction, and help accomplish goals (Wanzer, Booth-Butterfield, & Booth-Butterfield, 2005).

Although humor can reduce stress, be aware that it can also serve as a barrier to effective communication (Bethea, Travis, & Pecchioni, 2000). Careful judgment is needed. Caregivers may use humor to describe problems or situations to health providers. Anecdotal accounts and jokes may help alleviate uneasiness. Conversely, a caregiver may be using humor because he or she is unable to express a need. In those cases, the caregiver may actually be conveying a serious cry for help. Health providers need to ask probing questions to determine the extent of potential problems and offer appropriate assistance, when indicated.

## RELATIONSHIPS BETWEEN PROFESSIONAL AND FAMILY CAREGIVERS

Families involved in long-term caregiving emphasize the importance of having a good relationship with a competent and caring professional. The effective professional relates well to a family, demonstrates an appreciation for the caregiver's knowledge and skills, and stresses the importance of developing a shared partnership between professional and family caregivers to promote optimal outcomes (Schumacher et al., 2006; Wolff, Rand-Giovannetti, et al., 2009; Wolff, Roter, Given, & Gitlin, 2009). People know when they are in the hands of a person who cares, and the feeling of support is an important source of encouragement and hope.

Caring professionals understand and appreciate the needs of family caregivers and include them in treatment planning. Inexperienced health professionals sometimes make the mistake of maintaining too much control. Being able to relinquish control and decision making to clients and their families encourages them to take responsibility for their own care and can be very empowering.

In the acute care setting, planning for home care needs to begin on admission to the hospital, with communication occurring among clients, family members, and health providers. Although busy health providers have limited time to communicate with family members, it is well worth the effort in terms of clients' health status, staffing needs, and health care dollars.

In a study of clients hospitalized for heart failure, family caregivers who reported a high level of involvement in discharge planning were more satisfied with care than those who did not have the same high level of involvement. In addition, these caregivers felt more prepared to take care of their family member and more accepting of their caregiver role (Bull, Hansen, & Gross, 2000). It is the responsibility of health care providers to ensure that caregivers feel competent in their roles, have realistic expectations, know what to do in case of emergencies, and know who to contact about questions after discharge.

When working with family caregivers in the home, health care professionals must remember that they are in the family's domain. Here it is especially important for interventions to reflect the family values and belief systems. Some families are comfortable with their homes being converted into miniature hospitals; others resist this, minimizing disruption of home and family life. It is important to actively listen to caregivers, view them as experts in the care of family members, and validate their strategies (Toth-Cohen, 2000).

For example, some clients might be comfortable having grab bars and a raised toilet seat installed in the bathroom, whereas others might find it embarrassing when they have visitors. Work with clients and family members to develop an acceptable solution that ensures safety. Consider alternative options. A portable commode could be used in the bathroom on a daily basis and put away when visitors are present. Let clients and caregivers know who they should contact if they experience a decline in function and need additional equipment, support, or resources.

## Summary

This chapter addressed the effects of illness and disability on members of a family system. The role of the family in health care was discussed, and the importance of an interdependent relationship between professional and family caregivers was presented. Family caregivers are at risk for developing depression, caregiver burden, and burnout. Strategies to assist caregivers and optimize client outcomes were explored.

## Reflective Questions

1. a. What comprises a "family" to you?
   b. Who comprises your family of origin?
   c. Who comprises your family of creation?
   d. What roles have been "assigned?"
2. Assume that one of your parents became seriously ill or disabled today.
   a. In your family, who do you think would accept the primary caregiving role?
   b. What burdens would be imposed on this person?
   c. What kind of supports would be available?
   d. What health provider behaviors do you think would be most helpful?
3. a. What conflicts might occur in your family if a decision needed to be made regarding the care of someone who was ill or had a disability?
   b. What conflicts might develop between your family and health care providers?
   c. How might these conflicts be resolved?
4. Imagine that you are 5 years old and your younger brother has just been born with a disability.
   a. What effects might this have on your family?
   b. How might the relationships change?
   c. What additional roles and responsibilities might you need to assume?
   d. How might this have changed your life as a 5-year-old? 10-year-old? 15-year-old?
5. How can you instill trust in clients and family caregivers in the current health care climate?

## Case Study

Yvette is a third-year physical therapist student, who is living on the East Coast with her grandparents while she attends college. Her parents and brother live on the West Coast, and her mother is the only child of the grandparents. Recently, Yvette's grandmother was hospitalized following a cerebrovascular accident (stroke). She is currently receiving home care services. Because Yvette is the only one in the family to attend college, is majoring in a health care profession, and lives at the house with her grandparents, the family expects her to be its advocate.

The grandfather is not happy with the services that are being provided. Although the nurse comes once each week, he believes that she should be there daily. The grandmother is receiving physical therapy services three times each week for strengthening, conditioning, and ambulatory activities, but the grandfather thinks the therapist is "pushing" his wife too hard. A home health aide comes in every day to assist the grandmother with activities of daily living, but the grandfather feels that she is invading his wife's privacy. The occupational therapist has suggested changes in the home environment, including removal of scatter rugs, installation of grab bars in the bathtub, and a commode and hospital bed for the bedroom. Yvette thinks that although the clinicians are providing technically competent care, they are insensitive to the psychosocial needs of her family.

1. How are the family dynamics affected by the circumstances?
2. How are the roles and responsibilities of each family member altered?
3. What can be done to bridge the geographical distance that exists?
4. What steps can be taken to develop a trusting relationship with each family member?

## References

Adams, K. B. (2006). Transition to caregiving: The experience of family members embarking on the dementia caregiving career. *Journal of Gerontological Social Work, 47*(3/4), 3–29.

American Academy of Pediatrics, Committee on Hospital Care & Institute for Family-Centered Care. (2003). Family-centered care and the pediatrician's role. *Pediatrics, 112,* 691–696.

Asal, A. (2009). When a mother has cancer: Myriad issues for children and adolescents. *Clinical Journal of Oncology Nursing, 13*(2), 238–239.

Baago, S. (2004). The unrecognized caregiver: Children of dementia. *Perspectives, 27*(4), 3–4.

Banja, J. D. (1992). Tragedy and traumatic brain injury. *Journal of Head Trauma Rehabilitation, 7*(4), 112–114.

Batte, S., Watson, A. R., & Arness, K. (2006). The effects of chronic renal failure on siblings. *Pediatric Nephrology, 21,* 246–250.

Becker, S. (2007). Global perspectives on children's unpaid caregiving in the family. Research and policy on "young carers" in the UK, Australia, and the USA, and Sub-Saharan Africa. *Global Social Policy, 7,* 23–48.

Bellin, M. H., Bentley, K. J., & Sawn, K. J. (2009). Factors associated with the psychological and behavioral adjustment of siblings of youths with spina bifida. *Families, Systems & Health, 27*(1), 1–15.

Bethea, L. S., Travis, S. S., & Pecchioni, L. (2000). Family caregivers' use of humor in conveying information about caring for dependent older adults. *Health Communication, 12*(4), 361–376.

Bookman, A., & Harrington, J. (2007). Family caregivers: A shadow workforce in the geriatric health care system? *Journal of Health Politics, Policy and Law, 32*(6), 1005–1041.

Brehaut, J. C., Kohen, D. E., Garner, R. E., Miller, A. R., Lach, L. M., Klassen, A. F., & Rosenbaum, P. L. (2009). Health among caregivers of children with health problems: Findings from a Canadian population-based study. *American Journal of Public Health, 99*(7), 1254–1262.

Bull, M. J., Hansen, H. E., & Gross, C. R. (2000). Differences in family caregiver outcomes by their level of involvement in discharge-planning. *Applied Nursing Research, 13*(2), 76–82.

Chien, W. T., & Norman, I. (2009). The effectiveness and active ingredients of mutual support groups for family caregivers of people with psychotic disorders: A literature review. *International Journal of Nursing Studies, 46,* 1604–1623.

Davidson, J. E., Powers, K., Hedayat, K. M., Tieszen, M., Tiesen, M., Kon, A. A., . . . Armstrong, D. (2007). Clinical practice guidelines for support of the family in the patient-centered intensive care unit: American College of Critical Care Medicine Task Force 2004–2005. *Critical Care Medicine, 35*(2), 605–622.

Davis, M. A. (2009). A perspective on cultivating clinical empathy. *Complementary Therapies in Clinical Practice, 15*, 76–79.

DeHart, D., Webb, J., & Cornman, C. (2009). Prevention of elder mistreatment in nursing homes: Competencies for direct-care staff. *Journal of Elder Abuse and Neglect, 21*, 360–378.

Dokken, D., & Ahmann, E. (2006). The many roles of family members in "family centered care." *Pediatric Nursing, 32*(6), 562–565.

Drentia, P., Clay, O. J., Roth, D. L., & Mittelman, M. S. (2006). Predictors of improvement in social support: Five-year effects of a structured intervention for caregivers of spouses with Alzheimer's disease. *Social Science & Medicine, 63*, 957–967.

Ducharme, F., Levesque, L., Lachance, L., Zarit, S., Vezina, J., Gangbe, M., & Caron, C.D. (2006). Older husbands as caregivers of their wives: A descriptive study of the context and relational aspects of care. *International Journal of Nursing Studies, 43*, 567–579.

Faison, K. J., Faria, S. H., & Frank, D. (1999). Caregivers of chronically ill elderly: Perceived burden. *Journal of Community Health Nursing, 1*(4), 243–253.

Feczer, D., & Bjorklund, P. (2009). Forever changed: Posttraumatic stress disorder in female military veterans: A case report. *Perspectives in Psychiatric Care, 45*(4), 278–291.

Fleitas, J. (2000). When Jack fell down, Jill came tumbling after: Siblings in the web of illness and disability. *American Journal of Maternal Child Nursing, 25*(5), 267–273.

Franklin, E. (2009). The emerging needs of veterans: A call to action for the social work profession. *Health and Social Work, 34*(3), 163–167.

Gan, C., Campbell, K. A., Gemeinhardt, M., & McFadden, G. T. (2006). Predictors of family system functioning after brain injury. *Brain Injury, 20*(6), 587–600.

Garden, R. (2008). Expanding clinical empathy: An activist perspective. *Journal of General Internal Medicine, 24*(1), 122–125.

Ghosh, S., & Greenberg, J. (2009). Aging fathers of adult children with schizophrenia: The toll of caregiving on their mental and physical health. *Psychiatric Services, 60*(7), 982–984.

Hartman, A., DePoy, E., Francis, C., & Gilmer, D. (2000). Adolescents with special health care needs in transition: Three life histories. *Social Work in Health Care, 31*(4), 43–57.

Hirst, M. (2001). Trends in informal care in Great Britain during the 1990s. *Health and Social Care in the Community, 9*(6), 348–357.

Hoffman, R. L., & Mitchell, A. M. (1998). Caregiver burden: Historical development. *Nursing Forum, 33*(4), 5–10.

Honea, J. J., Brintnall, R., Given, B., Sherwood, P., Colao, D. B., Somers, S. C., & Northouse, L .L. (2008). Putting evidence into practice: Nursing assessment and interventions to reduce family caregiver strain and burden. *Clinical Journal of Oncology Nursing, 12*(3), 507–516.

Institute of Medicine. Crossing the Quality Chasm: A New Health System for the 21st Century. Washington, DC, National Academies Press, 2001.

Jacobson, S., & Wood, F. (2004). Contributions of children to the care of adults with diabetes. *The Diabetic Educator, 30*, 820–826.

Keeling, M. L., Dolbin-Macnab, M. L., Hudgins, C., & Ford, J. (2008). Caregiving in family systems: Exploring the potential for systemic therapies. *Journal of Systemic Therapies, 27*(3), 45–63.

Laditka, J. N., & Laditka, S. B. (2000). Aging children and their older parents: The coming generation of caregiving. *Journal of Women and Aging, 12*(1/2), 189–204.

Lawton, M. P., Brody, E. M., & Saperstein, A. R. (1989). A controlled study of respite service for caregivers of Alzheimer's patients. *Gerontologist, 29*, 8–16.

Levine, C., & Zuckerman, C. (2000). Hands on/hands off: Why health care professionals depend on families but keep them at arm's length. *Journal of Law, Medicine and Ethics, 28*(1), 5–18.

Martin, S. L., Gibbs, D. A., Johnson, R. E., Rentz, E. D., Clinton-Sherrod, M., & Hardison, J. (2007). Spouse abuse and child abuse by army soldiers. *Journal of Family Violence, 22*, 587–595.

Martine, L., & Stephens, M. (2003). Juggling parent care and employment responsibilities: The dilemmas of adult daughter caregivers in the workforce. *Sex Roles, 48*, 167–173.

Marziali, E,, Damianakis, T., & Donahue, P. (2006). Internet-based clinical services virtual support groups for family caregivers. *Journal of Technology in Human Services, 24*(2/3), 39–54.

McCullagh, E., Brigstocke, G., Donaldson, N., & Kalra, L. (2005). Determinants of caregiving burden and quality of life in caregivers of stroke patients. *Stroke, 36*, 2181–2186.

National Alliance for Caregiving & American Association of Retired Persons. (2004). *Caregiving in the U.S.* Washington, DC: Authors.

O'Brien, J. (2000). Caring for caregivers. *American Family Physician, 62*(12), 2584–2587.

Ostwald, S. K., Hepburn, K. W., Caron, W., Burns, T. B., & Mantell, R. (1999). Reducing caregiver burden: A randomized psychoeducational intervention for caregivers of persons with dementia. *The Gerontologist, 39*(3), 299–309.

Parks, M. S., & Novielli, K. D. (2000). A practical guide to caring for caregivers. *American Family Physician, 62*(12), 2613–2619.

Pasacreta, J. V., Barg, F., Nuamah, I., & McCorkle, R. (2000). Participant characteristics before and 4 months after attendance at a family caregiver cancer education program. *Cancer Nursing, 23*(4), 295–303.

Pavalko, E. K., & Henderson, K. A. (2006). Combining care work and paid work. *Research on Aging, 28*(3), 359–374.

Pinquart, M., & Sorensen, S. (2003). Associations of stressors and uplifts of caregiving with caregiver burden and depressive mood: A meta-analysis. *Journal of Gerontology, 588*(2), 112–128.

Poole, J. L., Willer, K., & Mendelson, C. (2009). Occupation of motherhood: Challenges for women with scleroderma. *American Journal of Occupational Therapy, 63*(2), 214–219.

Qualls, S. H. (2000). Therapy with aging families: Rationale, opportunities, and challenges. *Aging & Mental Health, 43*(3), 191–199.

Rabkin, J. G., Wagner, G. J., & DelBene, M. (2000). Resilience and distress among amyotrophic lateral sclerosis patients and caregivers. *Psychosomatic Medicine, 62*, 271–279.

Rabow, M. W., Hauser, J. M., & Adams, J. (2004). Supporting family caregivers at the end of life. "They don't know what they don't know." *Journal of the American Medical Association, 291*(4), 483–491.

Radomski, M. V., Davidson, L., Voydetich, D., & Erickson, M. W. (2009). Occupational therapy for service members with mild traumatic brain injury. *American Journal of Occupational Therapy, 64*, 646–655.

Randall, A. D., & Boonyawiroj, E. B. (1999). Client education and family systems. *Physical Therapy, 13*(3), 18–22.

Reiss, J. G., Gibson, R. W., & Walker, L. R. (2005). Health care transition: Youth, family and provider perspectives. *Pediatrics, 115*, 112–120.

Rentz, E. D., Marshall, S. W., Loomis, D., Casteel, C., Martin, S. L., & Gibbs, D. A. (2007). Effect of deployment on the occurrence of child maltreatment in military and nonmilitary families. *American Journal of Epidemiology, 165*, 1199–1206.

Rolland, J. S., & Williams, J. K. (2005). Toward a biopsychosocial model for 21st century genetics. *Family Process, 44*, 3–24.

Sands, R. G., Goldberg-Glen, R. S., & Shin, H. (2009). The voices of grandchildren of grandparent caregivers: A strengths-resilience perspective. *Child Welfare, 88*(2), 25–46.

Savitsky, L., Illingworth, M., & DuLaney, M. (2009). Civilian social work: Serving the military and veteran populations. *Social Work, 54*(4), 327–339.

Schumacher, K., Beck, C., & Marren, J. M. (2006). Family caregivers: Caring for older adults, working with their families. *American Journal of Nursing, 106*(8), 40–49.

Schumacher, K. L., Stewart, B. J., Archbold, P. G., Dodd, M. J., & Dibble, S. L. (2000). Family caregiving skill: Development of the concept. *Research in Nursing and Health, 23*, 191–203.

Schuster, M. A., Chung, P. J., Elliott, M. N., Garfield, C. F., Vestal, K. D., & Klein, D. J. (2009). Perceived effects of leave from work and the role of paid leave among parents of children with special health care needs. *American Journal of Public Health, 99*(4), 698–705.

Shinan-Altman, S., & Cohen, M. (2009). Nursing aides' attitudes to elder abuse in nursing homes: The effect of work stressors and burnout. *Gerontologist, 49*(5), 674–684.

Smith, J. E., & Smith, D. L. (2000). No map, no guide: Family caregivers' perspectives on their journeys through the system. *Case Management Journal, 2*(1), 27–33.

Snyder, J. R. (2000). Impact of caregiver–receiver relationship quality on burden and satisfaction. *Journal of Women and Aging, 12*(1/2), 147–167.

Sorenson, S., Pinquart, M., & Duberstein, P. (2002). How effective are interventions with caregivers? An updated meta-analysis. *Gerontologist, 42*(3), 356–372.

Spillman, B. C., & Long, S. K. (2009). Does high caregiver stress predict nursing home entry? *Inquiry, 46*, 140–161.

Spillman, B. C., & Pezzin, L. E. (2000). Potential and active family caregivers: Changing networks and the "sandwich generation." *The Millbank Quarterly, 78*(3), 347–374.

Stein, M. D., Crystal, S., Cunningham, W. E., Ananthanarayanan, A., Andersen, R. M., Turner, B. J., . . . Schuster, M. A. (2000). Delays in seeking HIV care due to competing caregiver responsibilities. *American Journal of Public Health, 90*(7), 1138–1140.

Szinovacz, M. E., & Davey, A. (2007). Changes in adult child caregiver networks. *Gerontologist, 47*(3), 280–295.

Toth-Cohen, S. (2000). Role perceptions of occupational therapists providing support and education for caregivers of persons with dementia. *American Journal of Occupational Therapy, 54*(5), 509–515.

Valiakalayil, A., Paulson, L., & Tibbo, P. (2004). Burden in adolescent children of parents with schizophrenia: The Edmonton project. *Social Psychiatry and Psychiatric Epidemiology, 39*, 528–535.

Van Volkon, M. (2006). Sibling relationships in middle and older adulthood: A review of the literature. *Marriage & Family Review, 40*(2–3), 151–170.

Wanzer, M., Booth-Butterfield, M., & Booth-Butterfield, S. (2005). "If we didn't use humor, we'd cry": Humorous coping communication in health care settings. *Journal of Health Communication, 10*, 105–125.

Williams, J. K., Ayres, L., Specht, J., Sparbel, K., & Klimek, M. L. (2009). Caregiving by teens for family members with Huntington disease. *Journal of Family Nursing, 15*(3), 273–294.

Wilson, F. L. (2000). Are patient information materials too difficult to read? *Home Healthcare Nurse, 18*(2), 107–115.

Wolff, J. L., & Kasper, I. D. (2006). Caregivers of frail elders: Updating a national profile. *Gerontologist, 46*(3), 322–356.

Wolff, J. L., Rand-Giovannetti, E., Palmer, S., Wegener, S., Reider, L., Frey, K., . . . Boult, C. (2009). Caregiving and chronic care: The guided care program for families and friends. *Journal of Gerontology, 64A*(7), 785–791.

Wolff, J. L., Roter, D. L., Given, B., & Gitlin, L. N. (2009). Optimizing patient and family involvement in geriatric home care. *Journal of Healthcare Quality, 31*(2), 24–33.

Woodgate, R. L. (2006). Siblings' experiences with childhood cancer. *Cancer Nursing, 29*, 406–414.

Yeh, P. M., & Bull, M. (2009). Influences of spiritual well-being and coping on mental health of family caregivers for elders. *Research in Gerontological Nursing, 2*(3), 173–181.

Zwygart-Stauffacher, M., Lindquist, R., & Savik, K. (2000). Development of health care delivery systems that are sensitive to the needs of stroke survivors and their caregivers. *Nursing Administration Quarterly, 24*(3), 33–42.

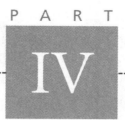

# IV

# Transitions Across the Lifespan

# Disability

> $I$ met the most interesting woman today. As a middle-aged woman with cerebral palsy, she's lived with her disability for a long time. During our session, she was sharing some stories with me about the Independent Living movement that started back in the early 1980s and was eventually responsible for the Americans with Disabilities Act. I guess she was quite the activist. She and a group of her friends participated in a number of demonstrations, including a "sit-in" in front of the State House. She laughed at her own joke as she spoke because apparently they were all in wheelchairs and already sitting down! It was sad listening to her describe the early years of her life, when she was in a state institution and shared a room with 25 other kids. What an eye opening session!
> —*From the journal of Marcy Guttadauro, vocational rehabilitation counseling*

People with disabilities represent the largest minority group in the United States, with the latest estimate standing at 54.4 million (U.S. Census Bureau, 2008). This number is equivalent to 1 in every 19 U.S. citizens. The onset of disability can occur at any point throughout the life span, but the incidence increases with age, when chronic health conditions become common and natural changes associated with death occur (Robine & Michel, 2004). Rapid and significant growth in the population of people with disabilities is anticipated with the aging of the baby boomer generation. Health care officials recognize the need for improving the efficiency and efficacy of health and disability services, to manage the anticipated growth in the number of people who will be straining these systems.

This chapter reviews the social context of disability, a number of challenges associated with meeting the needs of people with disabilities within the current health care system, and existing evidence related to the psychosocial experiences of people with disabilities. A life-span approach to disability is presented to illustrate how changes associated with age increase the complexity of the disability experience, even when the original health condition is a static, nonprogressive one. We will also discuss effects of new-onset disabilities that come with age.

## THE SOCIAL CONTEXT OF DISABILITY

"Nothing about us without us" is the battle cry of disability advocates as they work to infiltrate the existing bureaucracies to improve services that dictate the quality of life experienced by people with disabilities. This mantra communicates the message that people with disabilities want and have the right to be involved in any policy-making decisions that affect their lives. It also reflects a long history of oppression, expressed through the very programs established to "help" them (Charlton, 2000). Consider the traditional problem-oriented medical approach to patient care. It is designed to identify problems (anything that deviates from "normal"), establish treatment goals, and design plans of care to restore health and function to as near "normal" as possible. Does this approach integrate the concerns of clients with permanent functional impairments in a meaningful way? Can people with disabilities ever achieve the goal of "normal"?

The social model of disability is an alternative to the medical model. It is founded in the principle that disability arises not just from impairments, but by society's refusal to accept these impairments and to make accommodations for them. For example, if every building and curb were ramped, Braille signage was prevalent, and entertainment programming was closed captioned, people with disabilities would be able to engage in the same activities and participate in society in the same way that people who do not have disabilities are able to do. "This model locates disability outside of the body or mind and instead grounds it within society and its environmental barriers, discriminatory acts, and socially stigmatizing attitudes" (Taylor, 2005, p. 497). In essence, the social model proposes that impairment alone does not cause disability. It results from a culture that does not accommodate people whose bodies, minds, or senses function differently than the accepted norm. It frames rehabilitation services as valuable only to the extent that they lead to empowerment, access to resources, and social justice. Although physical limitations do affect independence and function outside of social constructs, there is a need to blend the medical and social models to ensure equal access to activity and participation (Taylor, 2005).

The medical model persists because of the infrastructure created by public and private health care policies that view disabilities as medical conditions in need of ongoing treatment. The case of Joseph Connors, a 39-year-old man who sustained a spinal cord injury in a motor vehicle accident, illustrates how this model complicates his ability to achieve his goals. Joseph was unable to return to his job as a car mechanic after the accident because of limitations in strength and sensation that resulted from his spinal cord injury. To qualify for Social Security disability income and vocational rehabilitation services, he needed to undergo a medical examination by a state-appointed physician, who would certify that he had a permanent disability. It did not matter that he already had volumes of documentation related to his injury from his hospital stay. At one point, he was in need of a replacement wheelchair and was looking to obtain an exact replica of the one he had been using successfully since his injury. When he contacted the equipment company to order one, he found out that he would need to undergo a specialty examination at a major medical center, where a physical or occupational therapist and physician would have to certify his need for a wheelchair. He had to wait 3 months for an appointment. Proponents of the medical model might argue that these systems exist to protect consumers, but clients with disabilities often feel frustrated, disempowered, and imprisoned by the policies and procedures that govern their daily lives. Most people with disabilities have few active medical problems yet, like Joseph, they are forced to interact with an overburdened health care system on a regular basis, in order to acquire the services and supplies they need to live safely and independently in the community.

Although progress has been slow, health and human services policy makers have finally realized the value of including the views of people who rely on disability services in the policy-making process (Franitis, 2005). Perhaps the best indication of this accomplishment is demonstrated by two international documents, the World Health Organization's International Classification of Functioning, Disability, and Health (ICF) (World Health Organization [WHO], 2001) and the United Nations Convention on the Rights of Persons with Disabilities (UN High Commissioner for Human Rights, 2006). The ICF and the Convention on the Rights of Persons with Disabilities both integrate the perspectives of people with disabilities, and this is evident in the portrayal of disability as the result of complex interactions that occur among the individual, environment, and society that either enhance or restrict activity and participation. This framework reflects the reality of daily life for people with disabilities and differs significantly from the medical model. Although disability remains highly stigmatized in most cultures around the world, and the medical model persists in most Western societies, these documents provide the guidance needed to bring about important changes to improve the quality of life for people with disabilities. What is needed now is a concerted effort on the part of advocates and practitioners in health and public policy to test, refine, and populate the centralized database at the WHO (Groce & Trani, 2009).

As we review the literature that exists about the psychosocial experiences of people with disabilities, it is important to realize that some topics related to the disability experience have not been studied at all. Others have received attention in past decades but not recently, and very little has been viewed through the lens of the social model of disability. Hastings and Taunt (2002) remind us of the importance of asking positive questions about the experiences of people who have developmental disabilities. The medical model, which is steeped in the tradition of problem identification, has trained us to focus on negative experiences. Shifting the focus to all that is good may help clients, their families, and health professionals to recognize potential resources that can be helpful in improving independence and participation of clients in their own environments.

## DEVELOPMENTAL DISABILITIES

I am so excited about this clinical experience in early intervention. I've wanted to work with babies since I started school, and the time has finally come. My supervisor and I visited our first family today. Their newborn baby has cerebral palsy and a cleft lip and palate. We're helping mom work on feeding and educating her about ways to minimize the risk of ear infections and other complications through positioning. Mom cried a little and confessed that she has some difficulty looking at her baby's face. My supervisor explained the importance of early bonding and reminded her that corrective surgery could be done soon. She seemed more comfortable with the feeding issues by the time we left, but I'm concerned about how she seems to feel about her baby. We'll go back tomorrow—I hope things seem better then.

*—From the journal of Anna Zimmerman, speech and language pathology student*

## Birth to Age Three

More than 6 million individuals in the United States have developmental disabilities. According to the Developmental Disabilities Assistance and Bill of Rights Act of 2000, a developmental disability is defined as a severe, chronic disability that originated at birth or during childhood and is expected to continue indefinitely. It substantially restricts an individual's functioning in three or more of the following areas of major life activity: self-care, receptive and expressive language, learning, mobility, self-direction, capacity for independent living, and economic self-sufficiency. Examples of developmental disabilities include autism, behavior disorders, brain injury, cerebral palsy, Down syndrome, fetal alcohol syndrome, intellectual disability, and spina bifida. The Developmental Disabilities Assistance and Bill of Rights Act recognizes that people with developmental disabilities benefit from comprehensive long-term services through which they are often able to be more active, productive, and independent, to their own benefit and the benefit of their communities.

Each diagnosis that falls within the developmental disabilities umbrella has its own set of symptoms, which can range from mild to severe, and it is not uncommon for clients to have multiple diagnoses, such as cerebral palsy with intellectual disability and a seizure disorder. Although each person's experience varies, some commonalities exist with regard to clients' psychosocial experiences. Within the social model of disability, practitioners are encouraged to engage clients as equal partners in their health care. This is sometimes called relationship-centered care, as described elsewhere in this book. This approach works well within the context of early intervention. Clients are children between the ages of birth and 3 and their families. Practitioners focus on facilitating positive relationships between children and their parents, as described in the journal entry above, using a variety of strategies to maximize developmental and relationship outcomes. For example, Mahoney and Perales (2005) examined one method of intervention that was designed to teach parents how to use responsive teaching strategies to help their children achieve pivotal developmental behaviors. The responsiveness of both parents and children improved for multiple measures of progress over this 1-year study.

Some studies have found that children who have disabilities are at risk for developing unhealthy relationships with their parents. Schaller and De La Garza (1999) questioned children about their sense of belonging, which is a necessary prerequisite for developing self-esteem and achieving self-worth. They found that some children who perceived themselves as being different also felt unsupported and unaccepted from a very young age. One particular child summarized his parents' reaction to his diagnosis and said they told him they love him "in spite of his disability." In this very mixed message, this boy's parents made it clear that he was different from everyone else, and it seemed that their love was anything but unconditional.

It can be overwhelming for parents to adjust to having a child with a disability. Evidence shows that health-related quality of life among mothers of children who have developmental disabilities may be negatively impacted by the stress associated with caregiving, when compared to mothers of children who do not have disabilities (Lee et al., 2009). In addition, Plant and Sanders (2007) found that multiple factors contribute to parental stress, including the difficulty of providing the required caregiving tasks, behavioral problems of the child during caregiving, and the level of dependence of the child. However, they also found that parental stress could be moderated by the parents' cognitive appraisal of caregiving responsibilities and availability of social support. This suggests that intervention strategies aimed at bolstering parents' coping behaviors may be a helpful adjunct to treatment. As discussed in Chapter 8, coping refers to the cognitive and behavioral efforts that people make to manage stressful circumstances. Internal mechanisms include emotion-focused, problem-focused, or appraisal-focused strategies.

Paster, Brandwein, and Walsh (2009) compared the use of coping strategies among parents of children who have disabilities and parents of children who do not have disabilities. The authors asked parents to respond to their use of eight coping strategies: (1) planful problem solving, (2) seeking social support, (3) confrontive coping, (4) distancing, (5) self-control, (6) escape/avoidance, (7) accepting responsibility, and (8) positive reappraisal. Parents who have children with disabilities used all eight strategies more often than parents whose children do not have disabilities and were significantly more likely to use three strategies in particular: seeking social support, escape/avoidance, and positive reappraisal. These results support the findings of a related study which found that parents of children with disabilities do have more stressors in their lives than parents who do not have children with disabilities. The need to cope with these stressors causes them to call more actively on coping mechanisms (Lessenberry & Rehfeldt, 2004).

Evidence also shows that raising a child who has a disability can be exceptionally rewarding (Naseef, 2001). Once effective coping mechanisms are in place, parents can adapt to their circumstances and enjoy the extraordinary rewards of affection and devotion that can accompany the role of parenting a child with a disability (Brinchmann, 1999; Ehrenkrantz, Miller, Vernberg, & Fox, 2001). For example, one study used a sociocultural context to examine nine mothers' experiences of having children with Down syndrome. Mothers discussed responses to their child's diagnosis as positive, in spite of negative attitudes toward disability that had been expressed by their children's health care providers. They pointed to the importance of coping with their circumstance through a process of meaning making and found they needed to maintain a resistance toward negative attitudes about disability. This eventually led to positive transformations in perceptions about disability in general and being mothers of children who have Down syndrome (Lalvani & Taylor, 2008).

Siblings of children who have disabilities are at risk for developing a range of problems. These include lower social competence and self-esteem, shyness, somatic complaints, poor peer relations, delinquency, loneliness and isolation, anxiety and depression, anger, excessive worry, and poor or failing grades in school. However, some children escape these problems. Protective factors include higher socioeconomic status, communication between the parents and children about disability concerns, older age at the time when the child with the disability enters the family, cohesion of the family, positive maternal mood, and absence of maternal depression (Findler, Vardi, & Taylor, 2009; Williams, 1997).

## School-Age Children

School-age children with disabilities spend a significant amount of their time outside of the home interacting with issues related to their education. Once they reach age 3, they are entitled to receive services through the public school system. Since the enactment of the Education for All Handicapped Children Act (1975), public schools have been required to provide educational services in the least restrictive environment possible. These rights were further expanded in 1997 through the Individuals with Disabilities Education Act (IDEA) and the reauthorization of IDEA as the Individuals with Disabilities Education Improvement Act of 2004. These and related federal, state, and local laws protect the rights of students with disabilities by ensuring that everyone receives a free appropriate public education regardless of ability. Special educational instruction may go beyond what is offered in the regular classroom to include individual or small-group instruction, curriculum or teaching modifications, assistive technology, and specialized services, such as physical, occupational, and speech and language therapy, provided in accordance with an individualized education program (IEP) specifically tailored to the unique needs of each student.

Unfortunately, there is a chronic and persistent shortage of special educators and a shortage of university faculty who can generate new knowledge about effective practices that can be translated into teacher preparation programs (Smith, Robb, West, & Tyler, 2010). These shortages are evident in the essential void of current information in academic journals to address the educational needs of children with disabilities. Little work has been generated since the decade spanning the late 1980s to 1990s, and the data that are available hint to little progress being made in special education since that time. For example, even though students entering postsecondary education programs will have to assume nearly full responsibility to ensure that their educational needs are met, few high school–age children are included in the process of establishing IEPs. This fails to empower students to become self-advocates and can lead to student disenchantment, discouragement, and reluctance to perform well (Miller, Garriott, & Mershon, 2005). These findings corroborate with those found in earlier studies.

Schaller and De La Garza (1999) studied children with cerebral palsy. The children reported feeling resentful that their parents were in frequent conflict with school personnel over issues of placement and educational plans. They also reported a sense of separation, few friendships, and frequent taunting from classmates without disabilities. Their most significant positive relationships were those with teachers who made them feel important or recognized. One girl reported spending most of her school experience in a segregated classroom, located in a separate wing of the school. This precluded any interaction with peers without disabilities. When she was mainstreamed into high school, she experienced a very difficult transition, and reported feeling anxious, self-conscious, and fearful that her classmates, who were able bodied, were constantly judging her.

A major portion of time and effort in school may be spent learning methods to compensate or accommodate for the effects of disability. Identification of the cognitive abilities of children who have severe physical disabilities can be very difficult, complicated by speech or language impairment and the limitations of existing screening and intelligence tests. Most tools assume all children have similar physical abilities and social experiences. As a result of these factors, cognitive abilities often go underrecognized and underdeveloped (Willard-Holt, 1998).

Children who have developmental disabilities often have very different life experiences than those who do not. They may be routinely excluded from many social events, such as clubs, sports, and birthday parties, because of mobility impairments or the need for therapies, doctors' visits, or hospitalizations. Wheelchairs or other assistive technologies are visible reminders of being different, are sources of stigmatization, and can limit accessibility (Cahill & Eggleston, 1995; Voll, Krumm, & Fichtner, 1999). For example, wheelchairs cannot traverse stairs, uneven terrain, and narrow spaces, making it difficult or impossible to casually or spontaneously seek out friendships in gathering spots that are inaccessible.

It can be especially difficult to meet the therapeutic needs of adults who have developmental disabilities. Until the 1970s, institutional placement was common for all people with significant disabilities. Consider Steven, a young man who was born in 1974 and diagnosed with Down syndrome just after birth. The pediatrician sternly advised his parents to place Steven in an institution because it was unlikely that he would ever walk or speak and would be a burden to the family. The doctor implied that it would be in the best interest of the child, leaving the parents feeling guilty and confused. Fortunately for this child, his parents did not follow the physician's recommendation. That does not mean that there were no challenges in keeping him at home, but it is likely that his developmental experience was more positive than it would have been had his parents followed the advice of their doctor.

## Adults with Developmental Disabilities

The medical literature has little to report about the needs and concerns of adults with developmental disabilities (Rapp & Torres, 2000; Robinson & Harris, 1997). Formal education of health care professionals also appears to be quite limited (Walsh, Hammerman, Josephson, & Krupka, 2000). Existing literature is based primarily on clinical experiences of the authors, rather than controlled studies or structured observations. Likewise, our review is also based primarily on our own experiences, with supporting references made when available. It is important to address the topic of adults with developmental disabilities separately from children. Because many of today's adults were raised in residential institutions, there are vast differences between their developmental experiences and those of children raised in their parents' homes. It is important for clinicians to be sensitive to the unique psychosocial needs of this population (Robinson & Harris, 1997).

Clients often present with many predictable and unfortunate problems related to living in an institutional setting. Specific problems requiring intervention vary from client to client, but the most common fall into three broad categories: physical, cognitive, and psychosocial. Consider the experience reported in this journal entry:

> Rachael grew up in a state school, which was closed many years ago. All of the residents were discharged. Because she could be taught to manage her own care, she was one of the lucky ones who could be sent to a group home. Many of her friends were sent to nursing homes because they were "not smart enough" to make it in the community. She described her life at the state school as "okay but boring." Each day was pretty much the same. Whoever was assigned to her that day—man or woman—would come in and get her dressed and up into her wheelchair, where she'd spend the day. The process was reversed at night. Some of the attendants would actually talk to her, but most seemed pretty busy and just assumed that she was "deaf, dumb, and blind." Although she experienced "funny feelings" and embarrassment when she had male attendants, there was nothing she could do about it. She recalled one attendant, Mary, whom she especially preferred. When I asked why she was a favorite, Rachael replied, "Mary was the only one who would clean up the food that I spilled on myself as I ate."
>
> *—From the journal of Katia Corbett, counseling psychology student*

**PHYSICAL PROBLEMS**    Physical problems can be due to a specific diagnosis, for example, spastic paraparesis related to brain injury in cerebral palsy. However, because of the relative immobility and limited personal care provided in institutions, various secondary complications are frequently seen (Robinson & Harris, 1997). Relative immobility can lead to limited strength, motor control, and perceptual motor development. Severe contractures can result from difficulty managing spasticity and poor positioning. Cardiopulmonary problems are also common, due to inactivity or scoliosis. Overuse of functional body parts can lead to degenerative joint disease and subluxed or dislocated joints. Finally, skin integrity may be altered by chronic skin breakdown. Cognitive and psychosocial issues can complicate all of these physical problems.

**COGNITION/COMMUNICATION**    Like physical concerns, cognitive problems may have a primary source, such as intellectual disability associated with Down syndrome. However, a phenomenon known as institutional retardation may also be present. This is the result of understimulation during the developmental process. Although residents of institutions were once typically assumed to be retarded, many were not. This was particularly true for clients with communication problems. Difficulties in communication can stem from physical impairment, such as the lack of motor control or breath support needed for verbal communication. Visual or hearing impairments can further complicate communication. There might also be auditory processing problems—that is, clients can hear what is being said but cannot process it effectively or quickly enough for functional communication.

The subtleties of communication make a big difference in how we perceive each other. As outlined in Chapter 5, body language and facial expressions influence how others interpret our messages. People who lack control of their motor skills, such as those with athetoid cerebral palsy, have difficulty with communication because of involuntary movements, grunts, and other distracting behaviors that can be overwhelming to most observers.

Many adults with developmental disabilities have poor communication skills. It can be difficult to extract and interpret information appropriately during the examination process (Robinson & Harris, 1997). It may be tempting, and at times helpful, to augment the client's reported history by speaking with care providers, but this requires particular caution. Just because personal care attendants accompany clients to the clinic, health care providers cannot assume that they can accurately report clients' hopes and dreams. They may be primarily concerned with one aspect of a client's life, such as finding an easier method of transfer. This may not be representative of the client's own goals, but because of learned passivity, difficulty with communication, or fear of repercussions, the client may not feel comfortable contradicting the attendant's report.

**PSYCHOSOCIAL CONCERNS**    Adults with significant developmental disability have complicated psychosocial concerns (Robinson & Harris, 1997). Those raised in an institutional environment face additional difficulties. As infants, children, and adolescents, they lacked the daily nurturing love of family that is required to develop a sense of trust and security. Early experiences may have taught them to develop passive relationship roles. This can result in poor adult life-management skills, such as finding employment, managing personal care attendants, and being effective advocates for themselves. They may have little concept of how to plan for the future, including setting and reaching goals. Social skills are often extremely limited, and confusion about sexuality, dating, and friendships is common, with limited understanding and management of emotions (Konstantareas & Lunsky, 1997; Sulpizi, 1996).

Wellness is a concept that has not typically been addressed with this group of clients. For the general population, health is defined as the absence of illness, injury, and disability. Using this definition, people who have developmental disabilities cannot be considered healthy. Rather, society tends to categorize people in this group based on their cognitive, emotional, or physical limitations. When addressing the needs of people with developmental disabilities, Zajicek-Farber (1998) proposed that we change our concept of health and wellness to incorporate a broad range of social criteria. Proposed criteria include level of satisfaction with personal relationships, education, work, standard of living, community interactions, creative expression, and future prospects for growth and development. This approach focuses attention on clients' capacity for self-direction and helps target interventions appropriately. Similarly, the ICF takes into account physical and social criteria and their impact on activity and participation. The ICF may be a useful framework for meaningful future studies of this population (WHO, 2001).

## SUDDEN-ONSET DISABILITY

The circumstances surrounding some of my patients' lives are so overwhelming. I received a referral to examine Mr. Byers, a 48-year-old man who was admitted for renal bypass surgery last Friday. He expected to go home on Monday morning, but something went terribly wrong during the surgery. The ventilator malfunctioned, and Mr. Byers was without oxygen for an extended period of time. Now, he presents with spastic quadriplegia, and he may not even make it! His wife reminds me so much of my mother, and his daughter is exactly my age. Life can change so quickly. I can't begin to imagine how they will cope with this.
—*From the journal of Althea Gerakas, physician assistant student*

The sudden onset of disability disrupts virtually every aspect of a person's life—self-concept, relationships, vocational and avocational pursuits, independence, and future plans. Trauma, such as spinal cord injury, stroke, or amputation, can be devastating from both physical and psychosocial perspectives. Acceptance and adjustment depend on many factors, including the diagnosis and degree of disability, perception of reality, flexibility in thinking, cognitive adjustment of self-image, awareness of situational demands, and availability of coping strategies (Florian, Katz, & Lahov, 1991). Equally important are the responses of family, friends, and clinicians. Clients are often acutely aware of observers' shock, fear, disgust, curiosity, or pity (Park, Faulkner, & Schaller, 2003).

People who sustain acute-onset disability undergo a traumatic experience. They often fear for their lives and may face the persistence of significant restrictions in activity and participation for many years to come. The latter depends on their physical and psychosocial responses to the traumatic event (WHO, 2001). To account for all aspects of post-traumatic health, it is important to address psychosocial and physical factors during the acute and long-term rehabilitation processes (Sobert, Bautz-Holter, Roise, & Finset, 2010).

Utilization of a team approach to rehabilitation of people with sudden-onset disabilities is of paramount importance to ensure that the full range of client needs is met. Health care has become unnecessarily complicated for clients to manage due to the specialization of the services that are needed. For example, the care of clients who have had amputations requires an integrated approach by specialists from physiatry, surgery, medicine, physical therapy, occupational therapy, nursing, mental health, social work, and prosthetics. Teamwork that involves all services has been shown to improve short- and long-term outcomes. Additionally, incorporating peer support, vocational rehabilitation, community reintegration, and sports and recreational activities greatly enhances a comprehensive program and improves quality of life and the ability to reintegrate into the community. Most importantly, for a program to be successful, team members must recognize the significant role of clients and their families in the rehabilitation process, especially when establishing meaningful short- and long-term goals (Pasquina et al., 2006).

### Adjustment

Contrary to popular belief, people have an amazing ability to adapt to difficult circumstances (Albrecht & Devlieger, 1999; Smith, Loewenstein, Rozin, Sherriff, & Ubel, 2006). Discrepancies exist between quality-of-life estimates from clients and the general public, indicating that the public does not understand how valuable life can be for people with disabilities. Public attitudes can influence the opinions of the policy makers and health care providers who make decisions that impact the services available to people with disabilities. Discrepancies may be due to different perspectives, with clients viewing their illness in terms of the benefits that would result from regaining health, whereas the public views the illness in terms of the costs associated with loss of good health (Ubel, Loewenstein, & Jepson, 2003). Albrecht and Devlieger conducted interviews with 153 people with disabilities, and 54.3 percent of the respondents who had moderate to severe disabilities reported having a good to excellent quality of life. All participants identified the key to achieving satisfaction with life as having the ability to establish a balance between body, mind, and spirit, as well as establishing good relationships with other people and managing the challenges associated with the external environment.

Other studies show the best predictors of greater life satisfaction include optimism, higher levels of perceived health and social support, and an internal locus of control. The use of problem-focused versus emotion-focused coping behaviors was also a significant factor (Chan, Lee, & Lieh-Mak, 2000; Gill, 1999; Lou, Dai, & Catanzaro, 1997). Problem-focused strategies are action oriented and aimed at making changes within the self or in the environment. An example of this is a client who arranges for architectural modifications to the home to ensure wheelchair accessibility. Emotion-focused strategies are best suited for short-term or acute episodes over which the client has little control. Avoidance is one example. Although it may not be particularly damaging for a client to avoid looking at and touching a surgical amputation site in the short term, long-term use of avoidance as a coping strategy would be harmful and detrimental to successful adaptation.

### Return-to-Work Issues

Significant social, emotional, physical, and financial barriers face those trying to enter or reenter the workforce after an acute-onset disability. As discussed earlier, stigma and discrimination are barriers to including people with disabilities as full members of society. The Americans with Disabilities Act (ADA) was passed in 1990 and went into effect in 1992 as a remedy for some of these discriminatory practices. It provides comprehensive civil rights protection to people with disabilities in the areas of employment, transportation, telecommunications, and government services.

The language of the ADA was intentionally designed to be vague to allow for interpretation on an individual basis (Rothstein, 1995). Under the ADA, an individual is considered to have a disability if he or she has a physical or mental impairment that substantially limits one or more of the major life activities. Until the passage of this legislation, people with disabilities had little protection against discrimination on the basis of disability. Now, Title I of the ADA states that employers may not discriminate against otherwise qualified applicants on the basis of disability. However, implementation of the ADA has been difficult.

A key feature of this legislation provides that the employee must be able to perform *essential functions* of the job with *reasonable accommodations*. An accommodation is any modification to the work site or job responsibilities. This may include physical adaptations to the workplace, retraining the employee for a new job, changing the work location, or allowing flexible hours (Seigel & Gaylord-Ross, 1991). The question of what constitutes a reasonable accommodation varies at each work site. For example, it might be reasonable for a large corporation to purchase computer modifications or programs to help an employee with a disability, but that same modification might not be reasonable for a small "mom-and-pop" operation. It may also not be feasible for the company's only receptionist to have flexible hours.

Research indicates that most accommodations are not unduly costly. Twenty-eight percent of accommodations cost less than $1,000, and 69 percent are achieved at no cost. This includes flexible work schedules, moving the employee to a more quiet work environment, or changing the duties of the job (Rothstein, 1995). "Reasonable accommodations facilitate participation in meaningful occupations and enable the integration of persons with disabilities into the mainstream of society with maximal functional independence" (American Occupational Therapy Association, 2000, p. 625).

Difficulty obtaining health insurance prevents many people with disabilities from working (Batavia, 1993). Most public health insurance coverage that is available for people with disabilities, such as Medicaid, requires that the individual also have a low income. Paid employment may raise income too high to be eligible for this public insurance. Many private insurance plans restrict coverage for people with preexisting conditions or charge extremely high premiums. This long-standing problem may become an artifact of history once the anticipated changes associated with health care reform are realized. Signed into law by President Obama on March 23, 2010, this new legislation promises to prohibit denial of health care coverage based on the presence of preexisting conditions and provide coverage for all Americans, regardless of their ability to pay for it.

Work also plays an important role in our culture. Some individuals work without pay as homemakers, parents, or caregivers; others engage in satisfying volunteer activities. Most people, however, define work as a job that pays wages. Unemployment following a disability is a significant financial stressor for the client and his or her family (Krause, Sternberg, Maides, & Lottes, 1998). In addition, employment serves as a primary marker for successful rehabilitation outcomes (Krause & Anson, 1996). Research indicates that people with disabilities who are employed feel better about their quality of life and that employment status is directly related to prolonged survival (Hess, Ripley, McKinley, & Tewksbury, 2000).

Several factors have been identified that are important for successful post-disability employment. Approximately 60 percent of spinal cord injuries occur in people between the ages of 16 and 30, prime years for gaining an education, attaining work skills, and establishing a work history. However, research indicates that only 10 to 50 percent of people with spinal cord injuries are able to return to work following their injury (Hess et al., 2000). Many factors affect this return rate, including the level of lesion and residual motor function, race, age, marital status, the type of work they do, and education (Hess et al., 2000; Krause & Anson, 1996; Krause et al., 1998). Clients who sustain incomplete lesions or lower level lesions typically have higher levels of motor function and are more likely to be employed than those with complete or higher level lesions.

Education is an extremely important variable for employment. Clients who have less than a high school education have the lowest employment rates. Completion of college is predictive of the highest level of employment success, with 72 percent of college graduates being employed following their injury (Krause & Anson, 1996). Other factors that are positively associated with employment are being White, married, and younger at the time of injury.

Levels of impairment and functional skills are also predictive of rehabilitation outcome for other injuries. For clients with traumatic brain injuries, burns, and fractures, level of post-injury rehabilitation is correlated with severity of injury (Horn, Yoels, & Bartolucci, 2000; Wehman et al., 1993). In this diverse group of clients, other factors are also important for rehabilitation outcomes. Socioeconomic status, pre-injury employment, and family support, particularly if the client was married, are associated with higher levels of post-injury function. Access to private insurance, which enhances the availability of funds for services, including rehabilitation and vocational counseling, is also coupled with higher levels of function. It appears that medical personnel are more likely to refer clients for rehabilitation who are White, married, employed, and have health insurance (Horn et al., 2000).

Finally, depression is significantly linked to high rates of disability and unemployment (Broadhead, Blazer, George, & Tse, 1990). An indirect measure of depression is suicidality. Clients whose injuries occur as a result of intentional self-harm have a lower rate of referral to rehabilitation services and, therefore, a lower rate of successful employment (Horn et al., 2000). Depression, phobias, and substance abuse are also highly correlated with disability. The presence of any of these comorbid conditions greatly elevates the probability of unemployment.

## AGE-RELATED DISABILITY

I'm really concerned about one of my favorite clients. My instructor has been treating her on and off for many years. She has diabetes, visual impairment, polyneuropathies, and a fairly recent amputation of her left lower extremity. It seems that every time she's admitted, there's a little more wrong with her and a little less that we can do to help her remain independent. It's very frustrating for us, and it must be even more so for her. What troubled me the most today was her mental status. She seemed very confused and asked for clarification of the same information over and over. Perhaps she's just overwhelmed by this hospitalization, but I called her primary physician, just in case.

—*From the journal of Nicole Jackson, occupational therapy student*

Modern medicine has prolonged life expectancy, but comparable progress has not been made toward wellness and health promotion. Many elders experience chronic conditions, such as arthritis, coronary artery disease, and diabetes, and these conditions may be further complicated by acute episodes of illness or the natural processes of aging.

Because complex patterns of disability are encountered in older clients, treating any condition in isolation is likely to be ineffective (Ferrucci et al., 1996). In younger clients, the effect of minor pathological events on functional status is often counterbalanced by physiological, behavioral, or social compensatory strategies, but these strategies are significantly less common in older clients because resilience generally decreases with age. Therefore, clients who acquire severe disability at an older age are more likely to experience a significant decline in functional status, becoming progressively more disabled over a shorter period of time.

When working with clients who are elderly, it is particularly important to take a careful history in order to identify all of the factors that may be contributing to the medical presentation. In this way, problems can be identified and treated early, and accommodations can be developed to compensate for lost function. Powerful predictors of overall health include the availability of social support, the ability to cope, mental health, and a positive attitude. Above all, it is important to involve the client as a partner in health maintenance in order to identify factors that affect activity and participation (Aldeman, 2001; WHO, 2001).

The plan for health promotion and disease prevention in older clients must be carefully individualized. Healthy older clients, particularly those in the 65- to 75-year-old range, are often enthusiastic about planning for a healthy life. To achieve this, clients need to be educated on the importance of primary and secondary prevention strategies. Vaccines can prevent illnesses, such as influenza and pneumonia. Behavior modification can be implemented to eliminate smoking, limit the use of alcohol, and encourage exercise. Injury prevention is also important because falls, car accidents, fires, and gunshot wounds together represent the fifth leading cause of death among older people. Identification of risk factors, such as difficulty with night driving, also need to be addressed. Secondary prevention, in the form of screening and early detection of problems such as cancer, heart disease, dementia, depression, diabetes, and visual and hearing losses, is also essential (Daly, 2001).

Dementia is a common and perplexing problem among older clients. In 2002, the prevalence of dementia among Americans ages 71 and older was 13.9 percent, comprising about 3.4 million individuals. The corresponding values for Alzheimer's disease were 9.7 percent and 2.4 million individuals. Dementia prevalence increased with age, from 5 percent of those ages 71 to 79 years to 37.4 percent of those ages 90 and older (Plassman et al., 2007). The dementia associated with Alzheimer's disease is typically gradual in its onset and may not be diagnosed until significant deficits appear. Early signs may be dismissed as simple forgetfulness. Even early changes in mental function and personality can cause clients to lose their jobs, cease driving, and surrender financial management to another family member. These losses, coupled with concerns about what is happening to them, can cause clients to become depressed (Logsdon & Teri, 1997). Successful treatment of depression results in an improvement in self-care, reduction in the fears related to progression of the disease, and increased hopefulness (Cotrell & Schulz, 1993). Treating the depression can avoid or minimize mental suffering, early institutionalization, and premature death in the approximately 30 percent of clients with a dual diagnosis of Alzheimer's disease and depression (Lyketsos & Rabins, 1994).

## HEALTH DISPARITIES

As a group, people with disabilities experience poorer physical and mental health when compared to the population without disabilities. One of the major causes of health disparities has been a lack of awareness and responsiveness of the health care system to preventable secondary conditions. For too long, the primary disabling condition has been the focus of care, at the expense of ignoring individual, social, and environmental factors that affect the health and well-being of people with disabilities. The emerging paradigm for examining disability within a social context, as guided by the ICF, holds promise to change this persistent problem (Disability Policy Consortium, 2009).

The existence of a disability presents substantial challenges in achieving access to primary and secondary health care and to preventive services. Physical barriers may prevent a person with a disability from receiving appropriate care. Health providers may not be aware of the specialized needs that accompany disabling conditions, and both health maintenance and promotion services may be unavailable (Sutton & DeJong, 1998). People with disabilities may have no insurance, have to pay high rates for insurance, or need to be in a very low income level to be eligible for public insurance (Batavia, 1993).

Gans, Mann, and Becker (1993) have summarized several specialized health care needs of people with disabilities. Despite the enactment of the Americans with Disabilities Act two decades ago, many public buildings, including hospitals, medical facilities, and doctors' offices, are not physically accessible to people with disabilities. Medical office staff may not be knowledgeable about how to physically handle a client who lacks mobility. They may not know how to transfer a client on or off an examination table, assist with dressing, or gather a urine sample from someone who lacks voluntary bladder control. Examination tables may be too high or too narrow to accommodate a wheelchair transfer. The scale may not be accessible to someone who cannot stand independently, and the bathroom may not accommodate a wheelchair.

Time may also be a barrier to medical office visits. It may take the client who has a disability longer to change into and out of clothing and to move around the office environment. Extra staff time may be needed to assist the person, and the examination itself may take longer to perform. Transportation to the medical office may be unreliable, and the client may arrive late and disrupt the client "flow" (Gans et al., 1993).

Finding providers who understand their specialized needs can be a challenge for people with disabilities. Internists, pediatricians, family practitioners, or gynecologists may be very competent in their specialty area but lack information about the specialized medical needs of people with disabilities (Gans et al., 1993). People with multiple medical conditions may take a "cocktail" of medications, with potentially dangerous drug interactions. Their susceptibility to secondary medical conditions may increase. For example, 67 to 100 percent of people with spinal cord injuries have at least one bladder infection (Sutton & DeJong, 1998). Proper monitoring and care could prevent some of these complications. The functional impact of small changes in health status can be significant for someone with a chronic disability. A fractured wrist due to a fall is an inconvenience to someone who can walk independently. For someone who uses a wheelchair, it may mean the inability to transfer independently and propel the wheelchair until the fracture heals, resulting in immobility and dependence.

Finally, preventive and health maintenance services may not be available for people with disabilities. Osteoporosis, arthritis, balance disorders, obesity, and depression have an increased prevalence in people with disabling conditions (Rimmer, 1999). Although it is important for people with mobility impairments to maintain cardiovascular fitness, few health and fitness centers are accessible and affordable for them (Rimmer, 1999). Routine mammograms, Pap smears, and other cancer screening tests may not be readily available for these same reasons. Clients with disabilities need access to hearing, vision, and dental examinations, yet these health professionals often practice in offices that do not accommodate people in wheelchairs. Access to counseling for personal, marital, or substance abuse problems, stress management, weight management, and smoking cessation programs may also be needed (Gans et al., 1993; Rimmer, 1999).

Daniel Callahan (1993) believed that an ethic of caring should drive our health care system: "Caring means nonabandonment of the sick, rehabilitative care for the injured and disabled, as well as whatever nursing care is needed to relieve immediate pain and suffering" (p. 104). A caring health system would also provide the social and economic support to ensure living a life with dignity. Unfortunately, we are still far from that goal. Collaboration between health care consumers with disabilities and health care providers is needed to improve access and care (Sutton & DeJong, 1998).

## Summary

In this chapter, we addressed psychosocial issues related to people who have disabilities. The social model of disability was considered and contrasted to the medical model. We discussed the integration of impairments and social factors into the ICF and how it promises to provide more insight into the disability experience. The problem of health disparities between people who have disabilities and the general population was presented, along with the need to develop programs of wellness and health promotion to ease the burden of disability on individuals and on society as a whole. It is important for health professionals to promote the use of the ICF in studies and models of care, so that the influences of impairment and the social context of disability can both help to inform strategies to improve activity and participation among people with disabilities.

## Reflective Questions

1. Consider one key experience or activity you have enjoyed since childhood.
   a. How has this influenced the person you have become?
   b. How might you be different if you had been unable to participate in this experience or activity as a result of a developmental disability?
   c. How might your relationships have been different if you had a developmental disability?
2. How might your role in the family have changed if you had a sibling with a significant congenital problem?
3. Consider having a sudden-onset condition versus a progressive disorder.
   a. Which do you think would present a more challenging adjustment for you? Explain why.
   b. What types of coping strategies might you employ?
4. Think about the activities that you do on the weekend. If you needed to use a wheelchair to accomplish these activities, consider how your experience might be different.
   a. What physical barriers might you encounter?
   b. What, if any, attitudinal differences would you expect?
5. Please complete these sentences:
   a. When I think of the future, I am _____.
   b. To achieve life's goals, I have _____.
   c. To me, every day seems to be _____.
   d. My life to this point has been _____.

## Case Study

Michael Carnes is a 16-year-old boy who sustained a spinal cord injury at thoracic level 6 during a skiing accident. He was recently discharged from outpatient rehabilitation services and thinks that he is ready to return to the high school he attended prior to his injury. The rehabilitation team worked with the special educators at Michael's school to help ensure that the transition back to school would go as smoothly as possible.

A number of accommodations were arranged to improve physical accessibility of the school. In addition, all of the sophomore teachers attended a workshop designed to help them understand the physical limitations associated with spinal cord injury. Mrs. McGlathery, Michael's history teacher, asked Michael if he might like to meet John, a student from another school. She explained that John had used a wheelchair for mobility from a very early age because he has cerebral palsy.

Knowing that Michael was still in the process of adjusting to his disability, she thought that meeting another student who uses a wheelchair would be helpful.

1. Based on the developmental experiences of Michael and John up to this point, would you expect such an encounter to be helpful to Michael? Why or why not?
2. What kinds of behaviors might Michael display at school that would suggest adjustment to his new life circumstances?
3. What kinds of behaviors might Michael display at school that would suggest a failure to adjust to his new life circumstances?
4. Contrast Michael's experience of adjustment to that of someone who is experiencing a long, slow decline in function, associated with aging and multiple comorbidities.

## References

Albrecht, G., & Devlieger, P. (1999). The disability paradox: High quality of life against all odds. *Social Science & Medicine, 48,* 977–988.

Aldeman, A. M. (2001). Managing chronic illness. In A. M. Aldeman & M. P. Daly (Eds.), *Twenty common problems in geriatrics* (pp. 3–16), New York, NY: McGraw-Hill.

American Occupational Therapy Association. (2000). Occupational therapy and the Americans with Disabilities Act. *American Journal of Occupational Therapy, 54*(6), 622–625.

Americans with Disabilities Act of 1990, Pub. L. No. 101–336, 104 Stat. 328 (1991).

Batavia, A. I. (1993, Spring). Health care reform and people with disabilities. *Health Affairs, 12*(1), 40–57.

Brinchmann, B. S. (1999). When the home becomes a prison: Living with a severely disabled child. *Nursing Ethics, 6,* 137–143.

Broadhead, W. E., Blazer, D. G., George, L. K., & Tse, C. K. (1990). Depression, disability days, and days lost from work in a prospective epidemiologic survey. *Journal of the American Medical Association, 264,* 2524–2528.

Cahill, S. E., & Eggleston, R. (1995). Reconsidering the stigma of physical disability: Wheelchair use and public kindness. *Sociological Quarterly, 36*(4), 681–698.

Callahan, D. (1993). Allocating health care resources. *American Journal of Physical and Rehabilitation Medicine, 72,* 101–104.

Chan, R. C., Lee, P. W., & Lieh-Mak, F. (2000). The pattern of coping in persons with spinal cord injuries. *Disability and Rehabilitation, 22*(11), 501–507.

Charlton, J. I. (2000). *Nothing about us without us: Disability oppression and empowerment.* Berkeley: University of California Press.

Cotrell, V., & Schulz, R. (1993). The perspective of the patient with Alzheimer's disease: A neglected dimension of dementia research. *Gerontologist, 33,* 205–210.

Daly, M. P. (2001). Health promotion and disease prevention. In A. M. Aldeman & M. P. Daly (Eds.), *Twenty common problems in geriatrics* (pp. 39–52). New York, NY: McGraw-Hill.

Developmental Disabilities Assistance and Bill of Rights Act of 2000, Pub. L. No. 106-402, 114 Stat. 1677 (2000).

Disability Policy Consortium. (2009). *Disability and disparities.* Boston, MA: Author. Retrieved from http://www.dpcma.org/Publications/tabid/423/Default.aspx

Education for All Handicapped Children Act of 1975, Pub. L. No. 94-142, 20 *U.S. Code* § 1401 (1975).

Ehrenkrantz, D., Miller, C., Vernberg, D. K., & Fox, M. H. (2001). Measuring prevalence of childhood disability: Addressing family needs while augmenting prevention. *Journal of Rehabilitation, 67*(2), 48–60.

Ferrucci, L., Guralnik, J. M., Simonsick, E., Salive, M. E., Corti, C., & Langlois, J. (1996). Progressive versus catastrophic disability: A longitudinal view of the disablement process. *Journal of Gerontology, 51A*(3), M123–M130.

Findler, L., Vardi, A., & Taylor, S. J. (2009). Psychological growth among siblings of children with and without intellectual disabilities. *Intellectual and Developmental Disabilities, 47*(1), 1–12.

Florian, V., Katz, S., & Lahov, V. (1991). Impact of traumatic brain damage on family dynamics and functioning: A review. *International Disability Studies, 13,* 150–157.

Franitis, L. E. (2005). Nothing about us without us: Searching for the narrative of disability. *Journal of the American Occupational Therapy Association, 59*(5), 577–579.

Gans, B. M., Mann, N. R., & Becker, B. F. (1993). Delivery of health care to the physically challenged. *Archives of Physical Medicine and Rehabilitation, 74,* S15–S19.

Gill, M. (1999). Psychosocial implications of spinal cord injury. *Critical Care Nursing Quarterly, 22*(2), 1–7.

Groce, N. E., & Trani, J. F. (2009). Millennium development goals and people with disabilities. *Lancet, 374*(9704), 1800–1801.

Hastings, R. P., & Taunt, H. M. (2002). Positive perceptions in families of children with developmental disabilities. *American Journal on Mental Retardation, 107*(2), 116–127.

Hess, D. W., Ripley, D. L., McKinley, W. O., & Tewksbury, M. (2000). Predictors for return to work after spinal cord injury: A 3 year multicenter analysis. *Archives of Physical Medicine and Rehabilitation, 81,* 359–362.

Horn, W., Yoels, W., & Bartolucci, A. (2000). Factors associated with patients' participation in rehabilitation services: A comparative injury analysis 12 months post-discharge. *Disability and Rehabilitation, 22*(8), 358–362.

Individuals with Disabilities Education Act of 1997, Pub. L. No. 105-17, 111 Stat. 37 (1997).

Individuals with Disabilities Education Improvement Act of 2004, Pub. L. No. 108-446, 118 Stat. 2647 (2004).

Konstantareas, M. K., & Lunsky, Y. J. (1997). Sociosexual knowledge, experience, attitudes, and interests of individuals with autistic disorder and developmental delay. *Journal of Autism and Developmental Disorders, 27*(4), 397–413.

Krause, J. S., & Anson, S. A. (1996). Employment after spinal cord injury: Relation to selected participant characteristics. *Archives of Physical Medicine and Rehabilitation, 77,* 737–743.

Krause, J. S., Sternberg, M., Maides, J., & Lottes, S. (1998). Employment after spinal cord injury: Differences related to geographic region, gender, and race. *Archives of Physical Medicine and Rehabilitation, 79,* 615–624.

Lalvani, P., & Taylor, S. J. (2008). Mothers of children with Down syndrome: Constructing the sociocultural meaning of disability. *Intellectual and Developmental Disabilities, 46*(6), 436–445.

Lee, G. K., Lopata, C., Volker, M. A., Thomeer, M. L., Nida, R. E., Toomey, J. A., . . . Smerbeck, A. M. (2009). Health-related quality of life of parents of children with high-functioning autism spectrum disorders. *Focus on Autism and Other Developmental Disabilities, 24*(4), 227–239.

Lessenberry, B. M., & Rehfeldt, R. A. (2004). Evaluating stress levels of parents of children with disabilities. *Exceptional Children, 70*(2), 231–244.

Logsdon, R. G., & Teri, L. (1997). The pleasant events schedule—Alzheimer's disease: Psychometric properties and relationship to depression and cognition in Alzheimer's disease patients. *Gerontologist, 37,* 40–45.

Lou, M. F., Dai, Y. T., & Catanzaro, M. (1997). A pilot study to assess the relationships among coping, self-efficacy, and functional improvement in men with paraplegia. *International Journal of Rehabilitation Research, 20,* 99–105.

Lyketsos, C. G., & Rabins, P. V. (1994). Psychopathology in dementia. *Current Opinions in Psychiatry, 7,* 343–346.

Mahoney, G., & Perales, F. (2005). Relationship-focused early intervention with children with pervasive developmental disorders and other disabilities: A comparative study. *Journal of Developmental & Behavioral Pediatrics, 26*(2), 77–85.

Miller, M., Garriott, P., & Mershon, D. (2005). Special education students' placement preferences, as shown in special education journals. *Electronic Journal of Inclusive Education.* Retrieved from http://www.ed.wright.edu/~prenick/Fall_Winter_05/7_Miller.htm

Naseef, R. A. (2001). *Special children, challenged parents: The struggles and rewards of raising a child with a disability.* Baltimore, MD: Paul H. Brooks.

Park, J. H., Faulkner, J., & Schaller, M. (2003). Evolved disease-avoidance processes and contemporary antisocial behavior: Prejudicial attitudes and avoidance of people with physical disabilities. *Journal of Nonverbal Behavior, 27*(2), 65–87.

Pasquina, P. F., Bryant, P. R., Huang, M. E., Roberts, T. L., Nelson, V. S., & Flood, K. M. (2006). Advances in amputee care. *Archives of Physical Medicine and Rehabilitation, 87*(3), 34–43.

Paster, A., Brandwein, D., & Walsh, J. (2007). A comparison of coping strategies used by parents of children with disabilities and parents of children without

disabilities. *Research in Developmental Disabilities, 30,* 1337–1342.

Plant, K. M., & Sanders, M. R. (2007). Predictors of caregiver stress in families of preschool-aged children with developmental disabilities. *Journal of Intellectual Disability Research, 51*(2), 109–124.

Plassman, B. L., Langa, K. M., Fisher, G. G., Heeringa, S. G., Weir, D. R., Ofstedal, M. B., . . . Wallace, R. B. (2007). Prevalence of dementia in the United States: The aging, demographics, and memory study. *Neuroepidemiology, 29*(1–2), 125–132.

Rapp, C. E., & Torres, M. M. (2000). The adult with cerebral palsy. *Archives of Family Medicine, 9*(5), 466–472.

Rimmer, J. (1999). Health promotion for people with disabilities: The emerging paradigm shift from disability prevention to prevention of secondary conditions. *Physical Therapy, 79*(5), 495–502.

Robine, J. M., & Michel, J. P. (2004). Looking forward to a general theory on populations aging. *Journal of Gerontology, 59,* 590–597.

Robinson, D., & Harris, M. H. (1997). An overview of age-related problems in people with developmental disabilities. *Orthopaedic Physical Therapy Clinics of North America, 6*(3), 369–381.

Rothstein, L. F. (1995). *Disability law.* Charlottesville, VA: LRP Publications.

Schaller, J., & De La Garza, D. (1999). It's about relationships: Perspectives of people with cerebral palsy on belonging in their families, schools, and rehabilitation counseling. *Journal of Applied Rehabilitation Counseling, 30*(2), 7–18.

Seigel, S., & Gaylord-Ross, R. (1991). Factors associated with employment success among youths with learning disabilities. *Journal of Learning Disabilities, 24*(1), 39–47.

Smith, D. M., Loewenstein, G., Rozin, P., Sherriff, R. L., & Ubel, P. A. (2006). Sensitivity to disgust, stigma, and adjustment to life with a colostomy. *Journal of Research in Personality, 41*(4), 787–803.

Smith, D. D., Robb, S. M., West, J., & Tyler, N. C. (2010). The changing education landscape: How special education leadership preparation can make a difference for teachers and their students with disabilities. *Teacher Education & Special Education, 33*(1), 25–43.

Sobert, H. L., Bautz-Holter, E., Roise, O., & Finset, A. (2010). Mental health and posttraumatic stress symptoms 2 years after severe multiple trauma: Self-reported disability and psychosocial functioning. *Archives of Physical Medicine and Rehabilitation, 91,* 481–488.

Sulpizi, L. K. (1996). Issues in sexuality and gynecologic care of women with developmental disabilities. *Journal of Gynecologic and Neonatal Nursing, 25,* 609–614.

Sutton, J. P., & DeJong, G. (1998). Managed care and people with disabilities: Framing the issues. *Archives of Physical Medicine and Rehabilitation, 79,* 1312–1316.

Taylor, R. R. (2005). Can the social model explain all of the disability experience? Perspectives of persons with chronic fatigue syndrome. *American Journal of Occupational Therapy, 59*(5), 497–506.

Ubel, P. A., Loewenstein, G., & Jepson, C. (2003). Whose quality of life? A commentary exploring discrepancies between health state evaluations of patients and the general public. *Quality of Life Research, 12*(6), 599–607.

UN High Commissioner for Human Rights. (2006). *Convention on the rights of persons with disabilities.* Retrieved from http://www.un.org/disabilities/default.asp?id=259

U.S. Census Bureau. (2008). Number of Americans with disability reaches 54.4 million. *U.S. Census Bureau News.* Retrieved from http://www.census.gov/Press-Release/www/releases/archives/income_wealth/013041.html

Voll, R., Krumm, B., & Fichtner, H. J. (1999). Demand for psychosocial counseling of young wheelchair users. *International Journal of Rehabilitation Research, 22,* 119–122.

Walsh, K. K., Hammerman, S., Josephson, F., & Krupka, P. (2000). Caring for people with developmental disabilities: Survey of nurses about their education and experience. *Mental Retardation, 38*(1), 33–41.

Wehman, P., Sherron, P., Kregel, J., Kreutzer, J., Tran, S., & Chu, D. (1993). Return to work for persons following severe traumatic brain injury. *American Journal of Physical Medicine and Rehabilitation, 72,* 355–362.

Willard-Holt, C. (1998). Academic and personality characteristics of gifted students with cerebral palsy: A multiple case study. *Exceptional Children, 65*(1), 37–50.

Williams, P. D. (1997). Siblings and pediatric chronic illness: A review of the literature. *International Journal of Nursing Studies, 34,* 312–323.

World Health Organization. (2001). *International classification of functioning, disability and health (ICF).* Retrieved from http://www.who.int/classifications/icf/en

Zajicek-Farber, M. L. (1998). Promoting good health in adolescents with developmental disabilities. *Health and Social Work, 23*(3), 203–213.

# Chronic Conditions

I'm working with clients who have chronic illnesses during this clinical experience, and I can really relate to what they're going through. When I was diagnosed with asthma, it took me a long time to get my head around the fact that it was a chronic disease. It isn't going to go away. It can be life threatening, if I don't take care of it. It's very different from being diagnosed with my chronic low back pain or the eye problems, for which I've been wearing glasses since I was very young. I had an episode of laryngeal spasm, and I couldn't breathe. I was never so scared in my life! I know that lots of people have asthma, but for me, it's something I have to manage all the time. I rarely know when I won't be able to get any air moving.

I'm tired of coughing. I'm tired of not being able to breathe. I don't always know what will trigger an episode. I know that I've got to manage this and breathe humidified air and get a jump on it. Otherwise, there could be dire consequences. I've learned how to read my body and handle it accordingly. I just can't ignore it. There are times when my life is interrupted, and I can't do what I had planned. I disappoint people, cancel plans, and stay behind. I had to learn to accept the uncertainty and ups-and-downs of a health problem that won't go away, but I think it's going to help me be a more empathetic physical therapist.

—*From the journal of Judy Woodward, physical therapist student*

The goal of the health care system is to treat disease and maintain good health. We perform physical examinations and tests to detect signs of disease, prescribe medication, surgery, or therapy when a problem is detected, and often expect that the client's problem will be cured. However, many people receive treatment for illnesses, survive devastating accidents, or develop chronic disorders that must be managed rather than cured. For these clients, medical problems become a way of life. Some lose hope of ever feeling "well" again.

In this chapter, we discuss what happens when health problems become chronic. We explore the effects of chronic illness and chronic pain on clients' function and psychosocial well-being. Strategies for supporting clients' long-term needs and improving their quality of life are suggested.

## DISEASE VERSUS ILLNESS

Historically, some health care providers have been concerned with disease, which is seen as a biological process gone awry, an alteration in the structure or function of the body. In contrast, clients are also concerned about the illness and its disruption on their lives. Arthur Kleinman (1988) describes this frame of reference in his classic text, *The Illness Narratives*. "By invoking the term illness, I mean to conjure up the innately human experience of symptoms and suffering. Illness refers to how the sick person and members of the family or wider social network perceive, live with, and respond to symptoms and disability" (p. 3). For clients, illness is far more than just a cluster of symptoms or a treatment protocol; it is a lived experience.

The illness experience is the sum total of all life experiences that result from having a disease or injury. This includes the client's and family's belief system about what the disease means to them and how they choose to cope with its practical problems (Kleinman, 1988). Illness does not occur in a vacuum, but rather in a system of social, cultural, and spiritual values. Substantial research indicates that psychological and social factors affect clients' physical improvement or decline. Thoughts and emotions are entwined with physiological processes. The onset of depression or anxiety or loss of significant social support can lead to symptom exacerbation or amplification. Conversely, a strengthened support system, an increased sense of self-efficacy, or renewal of hope are often associated with symptom remission.

People live complex lives that are affected in multiple ways by the chronicity of some health conditions. An expanded scope of reference is important for each client. If health care providers neglect to consider the personal and lifestyle factors that are important to clients, they may unwittingly limit their clients' quality of life. Consider the case of Bronnie, a 35-year-old psychologist, who had a thriving practice in wellness and health promotion until she injured her mid-thoracic spine in a car accident. She had surgery after the accident. During the last follow-up post-surgical appointment, the surgeon instructed her to avoid extremes of movement in her thoracic spine or she would run the risk of undoing the benefits of the surgery. Bronnie followed these instructions faithfully for the next 6 years until she could no longer bear the chronic pain she had in that area of her spine. The rest of her story is captured in this student's journal entry:

I can't believe what my patient, Bronnie, has endured for the past 6 years! The surgeon who repaired the bulging disc in her thoracic spine 6 years ago advised her to limit extremes of movement and to "never allow a physical therapist to touch her spine." I doubt that he meant forever, but that is how Bronnie interpreted these post-surgical instructions. It's difficult to believe, but she's splinting in this area since her surgery and displays extreme hypomobility of the thoracic region, which is compensated by hypermobility above and below. The poor woman has not had a pain-free day since the surgery but thought that was to be expected. When I told her she could and should be moving now, she was shocked and afraid. We started out slowly but after just two sessions, she told me she is now hopeful that "it just might be possible to have a pain-free future."

—*From the journal of Kathleen McDonough, physical therapist student*

Our society and physical world are designed for people who are healthy and fit. Without realizing it, we can place barriers to independence and a good quality of life in the path of people who have illnesses or impairments, often rendering them unable to do the things they want and would otherwise be able to do (Jette, 2009). Short-sighted health providers, social prejudice and stigma, lack of flexible jobs and work schedules, and architectural obstacles all create barriers. The goal of medical treatment and rehabilitation is to restore the ability of clients to live the lifestyles they choose. It is our responsibility to find the meaning of living well for each of our clients and to collaborate with them to attain that goal.

Disease and physical impairments can be diagnosed and assessed using clinical signs, medical symptoms, and degree of variation from normative values. In contrast, illness is unique to each individual, and each client will have his or her own experiences. The presence of illness is assessed by looking at the client's presentation of *illness behaviors.* Illness behaviors are "observable and potentially measurable actions and conduct which express and communicate the individual's own perception of disturbed health" (Waddell, 1991, p. 663). These behaviors may be adaptive, by signaling the need for intervention, or, at times, out of proportion to the level of clinically measurable pathology or dysfunction (Waddell, 1991). Illness behaviors take many forms, such as verbalizing distress or hopelessness, insomnia, fatigue, lying down, sighing, grimacing, moaning, and irritability, cues that perceptive health providers will recognize as those requiring further investigation.

## CHRONIC CONDITIONS

Our current health care system was developed to identify and treat acute diseases, not to support the needs of clients whose lives are affected by chronic conditions. Health care professionals have been trained to provide focused short-term interventions that are effective in eliminating health problems. Both clients and professionals often expect medical problems to be cured so the client can return to his or her premorbid state without ongoing difficulties. However, the explosion of scientific discoveries and advances in medical care that occurred in the past century has enabled many clients with previously fatal conditions to live for many years. The goal of treatment for chronic diseases is to decrease the incidence or severity of symptoms, improve function, and prevent or lessen the occurrence of secondary conditions or disability.

According to the National Center for Health Statistics (2010), a condition is considered to be chronic if it lasts for at least 3 months. Chronic conditions take many forms and affect all age groups. Many are invisible, such as systemic lupus erythematosus, fibromyalgia, myasthenia gravis, bipolar disorder, and the debilitating side effects of cancer treatment. Cardiovascular disease, hypertension, diabetes, and asthma are also invisible and may cause few symptoms in the early stages. The individual might not "*look* sick" and, at any given time, might not "*be* sick." You may not see wheelchairs, canes, or crutches. Yet, pain and fatigue are quite real and debilitating. Living with chronic conditions can be lonely and isolating.

Some conditions are constant with little change in acuity or severity, such as a congenital hearing loss secondary to a nonprogressive condition. Other disorders, such as asthma, diabetes, arthritis, and coronary disease, may have acute exacerbations. Management of these medical problems may involve considerable client time, energy, and lifestyle modifications. Consider the college student who spends up to 5 hours every day managing his cystic fibrosis, which has a significant impact on all aspects of his life. Still other diagnoses may be terminal, such as some kinds of cancer, or progressive, like a type of multiple sclerosis. They can all result in significant loss and grief for the client and his or her family.

## Incidence

Chronic diseases, such as heart disease, stroke, cancer, diabetes, and arthritis, are the primary cause of death and disability in the United States (Centers for Disease Control and Prevention [CDC], 2009). Seven out of 10 deaths in the United States each year are from chronic conditions, with cardiac disease, cancer, and stroke responsible for more than half of the deaths (Kung, Hoyert, Xu, Murphy, 2008). Diabetes is still the major reason for nontraumatic leg amputations, kidney failure, and blindness in people ages 20 to 74 (CDC, 2008). Approximately 25 percent of people with chronic health conditions have at least one limitation in their activities of daily living (CDC, 2007), with almost 19 million Americans who have arthritis reporting such limitations (CDC, 2006).

Chronic conditions are common. More than half of Americans have at least one, that is, one out of two people; unfortunately, the prevalence of these conditions is escalating (Milken Institute, 2010). Chronic health conditions (i.e., obesity, asthma, and behavior/learning problems) among children in the United States have more than doubled from 12.8 percent in 1994 to 26.6 percent in 2006 (Van Cleave, Gortmaker, & Perrin, 2010). Although chronic conditions occur in all age groups, the incidence rises significantly with age. In addition, clients with severe mental illness are more likely to have chronic medical conditions than individuals without mental illness (Dixon, Goldberg, Lehman, & McNary, 2001). Increased rates of cardiovascular disease; lung, kidney, and digestive disorders; and cancer have been found in people with mental illness. Mental illness also affects the outcome of physical disorders, resulting in increased duration, severity, and morbidity and mortality rates for clients with both mental and physical disorders (van Hemert, Hengeveld, Bolk, Rooijmans, & van den Broucke, 1993).

## Chronic Conditions and Income

Chronic medical conditions are linked to poverty, with a well-established connection between low income and poor health. Lynch, Kaplan, and Shema (1997) retrospectively evaluated the records of clients from 1965 to 1994. They found that clients who lived in poverty were more likely to have chronic health problems than clients who earned more than twice the poverty level. In 2009, the poverty level for a family of four was $22,000 per year. There is a significant relationship between sustained economic hardship and ability to function in the physical, psychological, and cognitive arenas. This is important because those who had a low income for a prolonged time had the highest incidence of health-related problems. Rates of depression were particularly high in the people in the study sample who had a low income. Researchers anticipated that poor health might lead to an inability to work and a lower income; however, study data did not support that poor health caused the economic hardship. Rather, it is likely that poverty caused depression (Lynch et al., 1997). See Chapter 3 for a discussion of health disparities in people from different cultures and varying income levels.

It is not surprising that poor health and reduced income are linked. People with low incomes are more likely to be exposed to conditions that would cause health problems or psychological distress. Inadequate housing or homelessness, lack of access to health care, poor nutrition, extended exposure to environmental pollutants, and increased exposure to infectious diseases all amplify risk of disease. Psychosocial stressors, such as exposure to violence and drugs, single-parent households, and overburdened social support systems, also may contribute to the development of psychological difficulties (Lynch et al., 1997; Philipp & Black, 1998).

## Cost of Chronic Conditions

Chronic conditions are costly in many ways. There are the direct costs of medical care, including doctors' visits, hospitalizations, prescriptions, surgery, therapies, supportive personnel, transportation to health care visits, and assistive technologies. Indirect costs include lost wages, decreased productivity, and an inability to manage household responsibilities or child care. Chronic conditions are associated with many types of disorders, even those that do not produce visible disability. For instance, worldwide, migraine headaches are listed as 19th among all causes of years lived with disability (YLD) (World Health Organization, 2004):

> Headache disorders impose recognizable burden on [people who have them], including sometimes substantial personal suffering, impaired quality of life, and financial cost. Repeated headache attacks, and often the constant fear of the next one, damage family life, social life, and employment. For example, social activity and work capacity are reduced in almost all migraine sufferers and in 60% of Tension Type Headache sufferers. (World Health Organization, 2004, web page)

Many chronic conditions affecting older people influence their life expectancy and health costs. Not surprisingly, those in good health live longer than those who are not, but overall life health care costs, even though they are living longer, are not significantly different (Lubitz, Cai, Kramarow, & Lentzner, 2003).

The impact of chronic conditions on the U.S. economy is $1.3 trillion each year (Milken Institute, 2010). This accounts for $1.1 trillion in lost productivity, including sick days and diminished performance, and $277 billion in treatment costs. Many people go to work when they are not feeling well and "cut back" or curtail their performance. In one survey, 17.5 percent of workers reported at least one work-loss day in the past month, and 22 percent reported at least one "cut back" day, which accounts for an estimated 1.5 work-impairment days *per capita, per month*. The most prevalent disorder leading to work-impairment days was cancer, primarily due to fatigue, followed by depression, asthma, arthritis, and high blood pressure (Kessler, Greenberg, Mickelson, Meneades, & Wong, 2001).

Cost issues of chronic conditions are very complex. Consider Cindy, who works for a large university that arranged flexible hours and specialized computer equipment to accommodate the rheumatoid arthritic changes in her hands. When she is feeling well, she is able to work a full day, performing her responsibilities competently and efficiently. Many days, however, she does not feel well or has pain and cannot work to her full potential. The impact of these financial costs is heightened by the social costs that affect her home life. When she experiences pain, she is unable to care for her two children as she would like, and her husband bears the extra burden. Although Cindy would like to be able to coach the soccer team or be a Cub Scout leader, her condition is unpredictable. She often feels badly about all the people she has "failed." She says that she is not the "same person anymore."

Chronic conditions present significant costs to the individual, family, employer, general public, and public agencies that pay for services. Better management of health care resources and services could promote improved health and prevent secondary disability. Corporate America is responding, with the number of companies working on preventive care increasing each year, focusing largely on cardiovascular diseases, diabetes, asthma, and depression (Hewitt Associates, 2010). They are designing condition management programs, promoting healthy lifestyle choices, and assisting employees who are at risk. Some employers are even acting as "health coaches," encouraging participation at on-site weight loss programs and gyms and fostering adherence to prescribed medical treatments (Okie, 2007).

A major cause of the current crisis in providing and financing health care is linked to the failure to change the health care paradigm. Many health plans exclude clients with preexisting conditions, set arbitrary limits for types and costs of services they provide, put more restrictive caps on psychiatric illnesses than on medical diagnoses, and limit reimbursement for rehabilitation services. News reports chronicle clients and families who forgo needed health care visits or avoid filling expensive prescriptions due to their inability to pay. Although the focus of health care has changed significantly, attempts are now afoot to restructure the focus of the delivery system and insurance industry. Health care reform legislation, signed in March 2010 by President Obama, provides a beginning to the necessary change.

## EFFECT OF CHRONIC CONDITIONS ON BODY IMAGE AND SELF-CONCEPT

Psychosocial aspects of body image form a complex framework by which a person understands the self and perceives how other people understand him or her. Body image, self-concept, identity, and ego are so closely entwined that a change in one of these elements will most likely affect the others. When a person becomes ill or has an injury, he or she experiences change and loss. There may be changes in physical or mental function, independence, self-image or identity, and body image. Clients may refer to themselves as "the me before I had . . ." versus "the new me."

In the first half of the 20th century, it was believed that self-image was represented neurologically in the brain. The concept of body image was defined by postural and bodily movements (Head, 1920). Later, psychological constructs (Schilder, 1950) were added to the mix, a mental representation of the physical body. The more contemporary perspective recognizes that body image includes how people *look* and how they *think* they look (Laufer, 1991). It reflects familiar visual and sensory perceptions and incorporates personal, interpersonal, environmental, and temporal criteria (Livneh & Antonak, 1997).

Social, cultural, and personal attitudes and beliefs, plus an individual's internal history relating to the body, help form part of the self-concept. Elements of this aspect of the self-concept include physical strength, endurance, abilities, and perceptions of masculinity, femininity, and physical attractiveness. Body image affects how people relate to themselves, to other people, and to the external environment (Bramble, 1995). Although it can be modified by psychological defense mechanisms, such as denial, body image is thought to remain fairly constant.

Consider a woman whose mother said to her, "Mildred, I don't care what anyone says, I think you're beautiful." What a message to give to someone! In trying to be supportive and complimentary, her mother was simultaneously embedding a negative message that was to stay with this woman—*always!* We have a lifetime of receiving these messages and putting them into our gunnysack, incorporating them into our own body image. Successful psychosocial adaptation is characterized by an integration of disability-related characteristics into a new body image and self-concept (Livneh & Antonak, 1997).

That could be me, sitting in a wheelchair with right hemiplegia and aphasia, waiting for speech therapy to begin. I take the same birth control pills that caused Lisa's stroke. I also have two young kids at home. Most of my clients who have had strokes are in their

60s, 70s, and 80s, not 35! This one's too close for comfort. I'm not used to working with a client whose life parallels mine.

When I brought Lisa into the treatment room and placed her in front of a mirror, she began to cry. I wondered if she was emotionally labile or if she's justifiably upset about how much her life has changed. Can she be both? To think, only last week she was juggling a career as an executive in this hospital, and a home, husband, and two preschool-age kids! I don't think I can handle this.

*—From the journal of Alma Jackson, speech-language pathology student*

Society strongly influences our view of ourselves and others (Monteath & McCabe, 1997). Many people, including Lisa in the journal entry, tend to regard someone who has an illness or impairment as not being "normal." Because Lisa's body image is intermingled with her personality, self-image, identity, ego, and sense of worth (Norris, 1970), alterations in the body and its function have the potential to damage more than her physical being (Bronheim, Strain, & Biller, 1991). Bodily changes and her altered self-image disrupt her social and vocational roles, compounding her situation (Drench, 1995).

## Sudden Onset Versus Chronic or Progressive Course

Although Lisa's problems had a sudden onset, a stroke is often the beginning of a chronic health condition. Might there be any differences in her situation if it were slowly developing or chronic? The Body-Cathexis Scale and the Self-Cathexis Scale, developed by Secord and Jourard, and Kurtzke's Status Disability Scale were used to study perceptions of body image in men with multiple sclerosis (Samonds & Cammermeyer, 1989). Those who had the disease longer had more physical problems, were older, and were more satisfied with themselves and their bodies than other people in the study. Using the Body-Cathexis Scale, years later, physical disability was still shown to have an impact on body image (Taleporos & McCabe, 2001).

The sudden onset of health problems, such as those caused by trauma, can have a "shock value," leaving the person unprepared for the abrupt disruption in body image, self-concept, and lifestyle. Consider a client who was changing a car tire on the shoulder of the road when another car sped by him, amputating his right leg below the knee. Unlike other clients with severe vascular disease who faced surgical amputation, this man had no time to psychologically prepare for the traumatic loss of his limb and subsequent changes in his life. This "shock" hampered both his adjustment to the loss and his progress in rehabilitation. Traumatic amputation may result in a higher incidence of post-traumatic stress syndrome than surgical amputation due to chronic health problems, largely because of the emotional stress of the accident (Cavanagh, Shin, Karamouz, & Rauch, 2006).

Whether the injury or illness is acute, chronic, or progressive, visible or invisible, changes in health have an impact on a person. In one study, adolescents with cancer described their body image in themes that showed the vulnerability they were feeling, for example, "I don't look normal," "I look sick," "People look at me" (Larouche & Chin-Peuckert, 2006). Similar to other psychosocial aspects of health care, no single generic assessment, intervention, or answer applies to everyone. This is why effective communication, comprehensive evaluation, and a host of possible strategies are so crucial to the quality of client care.

## Factors That Influence How a Person Responds to Changes

How a person responds to changes associated with illness depends on numerous factors. We need to consider what *previous loss* the client has experienced, because this will shape his or her response to the current loss. Exploring the *nature of the current loss* will help us understand what else may be going on and if the client has issues that are more urgent than the current loss. The *prognosis for treatment and recovery* is also a factor in how the presence of illness may hinder or enhance the person's quality of life and functional activities. Whether this will be a problem only in the immediate future or something a person will have to "live with" for the next 20 years will also have an impact.

*Patterns of development* also have an impact on how a person responds to these changes. What has the person's lifestyle been so far? Has he or she had other problems with which to deal? What coping strategies were used? *Family and cultural values, beliefs, and attitudes* similarly have an impact. Are the changes associated with an illness the beginning of a new identity?

*Locus of control* is an additional factor influencing how a person responds to changes in health. How strongly does the person believe that he or she has control of his or her health and circumstances? Does the person quickly abdicate control, responsibility, and decision making, turning it over to health care providers? Does the client have a strong need to take responsibility for his or her well-being and exercise control over what is happening to him or her?

The client's concept of *sin and stigma*, viewed in the context of blame, fault, and shame, can be very telling. Does the client feel that the illness is punishment for something real or imagined, perhaps some "sin" he or she may have committed? That can create a rift between what is real and what one hopes for or fantasizes about (Cohen, Krahn, Wise, Epstein, & Ross, 1991). Does the client perceive that the illness or injury was his or her "fault?" Other factors to consider are stigmas of visible (i.e., paraplegia), invisible (i.e., diabetes), and both visible and invisible (i.e., multiple sclerosis) chronic conditions (Joachim & Acorn, 2000). Having a condition that not only sets one apart from others but is also sustained over time can result in being stigmatized by others. Although people's perceptions are changing as society's attitudes toward impairments, functional limitations, and disabilities are becoming more enlightened, people with functional limitations still face negative attitudes and perceptions.

*Social support* is yet another influencing factor. Is the client losing the social support and satisfaction inherent in the usual life endeavors because of an inability to participate in them? Does the client perceive that he or she has been abandoned by friends and family? It is important to note that people without visible signs of their conditions, including those with chronic pain who have no physical manifestations, face the particularly difficult challenge of others' perceptions of "but you look healthy." Because they "look healthy," they often have difficulty getting others to believe that they truly have a problem.

## Concerns About Value and Normalcy

What would a hand condition mean to *you?* A facial disfigurement? Radical neck surgery? What would be your "straw" that would break the proverbial "camel's back"? Using a wheelchair? Losing your sight? How would it affect you professionally? In functional daily living? Socially? Would you be angry at something being taken away from you? Would you wonder, "Why me?"

People with chronic conditions have a strong desire to just feel "normal." For example, adolescents with cancer who participated in a study related to altered body images expressed concerns about the loss of normalcy around their appearance, capabilities, and relationships with others (Larouche & Chin-Peuckert, 2006). Billboards, magazines, television, and movies remind us how highly our society values physical beauty and ability. Think about what a visible physical impairment, with its psychosocial issues, may mean to a person. Think, too, about how disempowering value-laden descriptors are, for example, "suffered" a spinal cord injury rather than "sustained," stroke "victim," "confined" to a wheelchair, and "the" blind. (Refer to Chapter 5 for a discussion of person-first language.)

The psychological impact of facial disfigurement can be traumatic. Disfigurement and dysfunction can severely and adversely affect quality of life (Sainsbury, 2009; Thompson & Kent, 2001). Adjusting to being visibly different as a result of the effects of stroke, Bell's palsy, burns, and dermatological diseases can result in profound distress for clients (Thompson & Kent, 2001). Facial deformities may be more difficult to cope with than deformities in other parts of the body because the face symbolically represents the self-concept (Wright, 1983). Consider a woman with a prior history of breast carcinoma who developed squamous cell cancer of the gum and osteoradionecrosis of the jaw. Surgeons removed her teeth and progressively more of her jaw. She has undergone major reconstruction for functional purposes, such as speaking and eating, as well as cosmesis. At 49 years of age, she is the object of staring wherever she goes. This bright, engaging woman recently took a job that entails going into "rough" neighborhoods in housing projects. She says, "I'll be safe—who would want to bother with *me*?"

"Invisible" changes can be equally devastating. A colostomy and ileostomy are hidden underneath clothing, but they can elicit feelings of being dirty and repulsive. Adjustment may be hampered in people who pride themselves on cleanliness and grooming. For verbally expressive people, a laryngectomy might cause them to retreat from others. With a distorted or lost mode of communication, there may be fears of losing not just the *expression* of their inner core but *part* of their inner core.

Having a mastectomy, hysterectomy, orchidectomy, or prostatectomy can affect one's self-esteem and sexual identity (Drench & Losee, 1996; Wess, 2007). The fear may heighten if the person strongly associates his or her sense of masculinity or femininity with the lost body part. According to responses on a body image index, women with total mastectomies were more afraid of losing their sexual attractiveness than were women with partial mastectomies (Lasry et al., 1987). Women who had total mastectomies were more depressed and dissatisfied with their body image than women who had lumpectomies. Negative body image was directly proportional to the extent of the surgery.

Physical appearance is not always intricately related to self-esteem. One woman who has worn breast prostheses since she had bilateral mastectomies appears "normal" to others. On hot summer days, though, she's more comfortable going without the prostheses, but not everyone around her is ready for that. For her, appearance is not *who* she is. In contrast, an illness or injury that alters the body may be the worst-case scenario to a person whose physical appearance is tightly linked with self-esteem. Accepting the impairment might injure the sense of self. What if that person premorbidly believed that disease or injury meant uselessness or ugliness? How do you think this belief system would affect the person's ability to realistically evaluate the situation and find solutions?

Our physical appearance is an expression of ourselves to others. Even early research on body image showed that appearance can bias impressions and serve to identify a person based on his or her loss (White, Wright, & Dembo, 1948). How many people think of Beethoven as a "deaf" composer, identifying him based on this one characteristic? Do you consider him as a person who was able to do something great even though he had an impairment or someone who was an accomplished, talented person who happened to have an impairment?

The fear of loss can drive the need to remain physically and emotionally intact. Consider a client who had gas gangrene of his lower extremities and absolutely refused surgery to have his legs surgically amputated, even though the physicians explained that the spread of toxins from his legs to the rest of his body would kill him. Was he gambling with his life by keeping his body "whole"? He understood the situation and adamantly maintained control of his destiny, to the chagrin of his health care providers. Remaining "whole" was more important to him than remaining alive.

When we work with clients who have chronic conditions, we need to be aware of our own beliefs, values, prejudices, and biases. Consider the following journal entry:

> Today at noon, I attended an in-service about psychiatric disorders. When I arrived, I saw two women standing together at the front of the room. One of them, who I assumed was a psychiatrist, was very well groomed, wearing a suit jacket and skirt. I figured the other woman was a person with a psychiatric illness. She was really disheveled and was wearing a dirty sweat suit and sneakers. I was shocked when they introduced themselves because, as it turned out, they *both* had psychiatric diagnoses. As someone who plans to work with this population, I can't believe that I made such an assumption!
> —*From the journal of Esther Williams, occupational therapy student*

### Achieving "Success"

In spite of the difficulty involved, most people are able to adapt to a greater or lesser extent to the changes associated with chronic conditions. Overcoming obstacles, acquiring new skills, and achieving a level of success that they had not thought possible may enhance self-concept. Many clients and their families have said they consider the experience to be positive. Some have even considered it a gift.

We must not fall prey, however, to the common myth that adversity always makes you stronger. After 2 years of rehabilitation for a near-fatal war injury that resulted in the loss of both legs and parts of his hands, Lewis B. Puller, Jr., seemed to accept the changes in his life (Puller, 1993). He used a wheelchair to regain mobility and independence; reclaimed his family roles as husband, father, and breadwinner; and served as senior attorney in the Office of the General Counsel at the Department of Defense. Yet, less than 1 year after his inspiring keynote address to an audience of physical therapists and physical therapist assistants at their annual conference, he ended his life. "Personal demons may be more complex and pervasive than we realize. Even 'success' stories carry scars" (Drench, 1994, p. 14).

## CHRONIC PAIN

> The Chronic Pain Clinic is a very difficult place to work. All of the clients are there because no one else has been able to "fix" their problems. Many clients have been sick for years. All of them are in severe distress. It is especially hard for me to work with Alejandro, a very proud man who emigrated from Guatemala when he was in his teens. Working his way through college washing dishes in a restaurant, he became a certified public accountant and landed a really good job in an accounting firm. Everything was going well until five years

ago, when his car was rear ended, and he sustained a severe whiplash injury. Ever since the accident, he's had headaches and pain in his neck, radiating down his right arm. Because of the pain, he can't concentrate or sit at a desk longer than an hour. He had to give up his job and is collecting disability payments. His wife now works to help support their family of three children, but this doesn't feel "right" to Alejandro. In addition to his physical pain, he feels like a failure as a husband, a provider, and man. I hope that we'll be able to help him.
*—From the journal of Melissa Chan, occupational therapy student*

Everyone experiences pain. Physical pain can result from a fall on the stairs or an acute illness. Emotional pain follows a death, the loss of a job, or the beginning of a psychiatric or physical disorder. It serves a positive, protective function, indicating significant changes or injuries that demand attention and may require medical care.

According to the International Association for the Study of Pain (IASP Task Force on Taxonomy, 1994b), pain is defined as "an unpleasant sensory and emotional experience associated with actual or potential tissue damage" (p. 209). The IASP recognizes that:

> Many people report pain in the absence of tissue damage or any likely pathophysiological cause; usually this happens for psychological reasons. There is usually no way to distinguish their experience from that due to tissue damage if we take the subjective report. If they regard their experience as pain and if they report it in the same ways as pain caused by tissue damage, it should be accepted as pain. This definition avoids tying pain to the stimulus. Activity induced in the nociceptor and nociceptive pathways by a noxious stimulus is not pain, which is always a psychological state, even though we may well appreciate that pain most often has a proximate physical cause. (IASP, 2007, web page)

Pain has been defined as localized physical suffering associated with bodily disorder (disease or injury) or acute mental or emotional distress (Apkarian et al., 2004; Robinson & Apkarian, 2009). Acute pain is caused by a noxious peripheral stimulus or tissue damage. The amount of discomfort or distress is typically in direct proportion to the level of injury or disease (Waddell, 1991). Once lacerations, burns, fractures, or other tissue injuries heal, the pain generally subsides. Conversely, in some instances, the pain does not abate, even after the tissue heals. This condition is recognized as chronic or persistent pain and may or may not have an obvious physical relationship to current pathology (Anderson, 2004; Law, 2002; Truchon, 2001). "In this case, the individual may experience one or more of the following: spontaneous pain (pain for no apparent reason), hyperpathia (more pain than would be expected after a painful event), hyperalgesia (increased intensity of pain to a further noxious stimulus), secondary hyperalgesia (spreading of sensitivity or pain to nearby, uninjured tissue), and allodynia (sensation of pain from a normally innocuous stimulus)" (Henry, 2008, p. 59).

For some clients, an acute medical event becomes a chronic, often unremitting, condition. Chronic pain is defined as a subjective physical and emotional phenomenon that the patient has experienced for at least several months (Anderson, 2004; Frischenschlager & Pucher, 2002). Although the former temporal "rule of thumb" of chronic pain was experiencing it for greater than 6 months, it is now recognized that chronic pain can be described as less than 1 month, 1 to 6 months, and longer than 6 months (IASP Task Force on Taxonomy, 1994a). The time variable can be of questionable value as a distinction, though. For example, there is a difference between recurring acute pain or prolonged pain, which may last for months or years, and chronic pain syndrome, which has psychological and neurophysiological factors extending over time.

Pain specialists estimate that more than one quarter of Americans suffer daily from chronic pain, making it the leading cause of disability (Jackson, 2000), and resulting in about $60 billion each year in the United States in lost productivity (Krueger & Stone, 2008). Many factors affect people with pain:

- *Economics.* In the United States, those with annual household incomes less than $30,000 report moderate to severe pain 20 percent of their overall time versus less than 8 percent of those with incomes around $100,000.
- *Years of formal education.* People who were not high school graduates described 2 times the pain as those who graduated from college.
- *Age.* The rating of pain climbed with age, leveling off between ages 45 and 75.
- *Health status.* The better the overall health status, the fewer reports of pain.
- *Life satisfaction.* The greater the satisfaction with life, the fewer reports of pain (Krueger & Stone, 2008).

Chronic pain syndrome is multifactorial and not well understood. Some investigators propose that it is learned behavior that occurs in response to a noxious stimulus that results in pain (Singh, Patel, & Gallagher, 2010). Pain behavior can be reinforced by internal factors, such as respite from emotions of guilt, fear of work, or freedom from other responsibilities. It can also have external secondary rewards, such as attention from others, leave time from work, and financial compensation. Clients with certain psychological disorders, such as depression, anxiety, somatization disorder, hypochondriasis, and conversion disorder, are at greater risk for developing chronic pain syndrome (Singh et al., 2010).

Because pain is multidimensional, merely asking the client to rate his or her pain on a 0-to-10-point pain scale is limited in its assessment value. Many different types of pain assessment scales are available from which to choose (Sluka, 2009). For example, the McGill Pain Questionnaire (Melzack, 1975) explores the subjective pain experience by asking the client, "What does your pain feel like?" "How does your pain change with time?" and "How strong is your pain?" To address what the pain feels like, the client chooses the one best word in each category that describes the current pain; for incisive pressure, for instance, the client could circle whether the pain is sharp, cutting, or lacerating. The more information that team members have, the better they can determine what treatment would have the best outcome.

Duration is not the only determinant of pain's chronicity. Cultural and historical factors, such as previous experience, cultural beliefs, and sensory input, can also influence a client's response to pain (Geiser, Robinson, Miller, & Bade, 2003). Because of this, even clients with similar underlying pathology can have different pain presentations and experiences. As a multidimensional phenomenon, chronic pain can affect overall quality of life (Friedrich, Hahne, & Wepner, 2009), as seen in Box 11–1.

## Progression From Acute to Chronic Pain

For a small percentage of clients, acute pain will develop into a subacute or chronic condition. A common response to pain is to become passive and physically inactive. This leads to weakness, tight muscles, and deconditioning, which can result in more pain when the client attempts to resume activity. Pain may also be accompanied by insomnia, fatigue, loss of appetite,

---

**BOX 11–1    Areas of Impact of Chronic Pain**

- Sleep (Marty et al., 2008; O'Donoghue, Fox, Heneghan, & Hurley, 2009)
- Functional capacity, social functions, and finances (Ericsson et al., 2002; Geiser et al., 2003; Saastamoinen, Leino-Arjas, Laaksonen, & Lahelma, 2005; Truchon, 2001)
- Employment absenteeism and job loss (Anderson, 2004; Kääriä et al., 2005; Keough & Fisher, 2001; Newth & Delongis, 2004)
- Depression (Ericsson et al., 2002; Henderson, Kidd, Pearson, & White, 2005)
- In extreme cases, depression can result in suicide (Braden & Sullivan, 2008; Fishbain, Bruns, Disorbio, & Lewis, 2009; Ilgen, Zivin, McCammon, & Valenstein, 2008)

---

and disturbances in family or social life. Anger, depression, and anxiety are frequently seen in clients with chronic pain. This emotional distress is often somaticized, turned into physical distress, which triggers a cycle of more physical pain, leading to more emotional distress. The relationship between emotional distress and increased pain is physiological. It is important to understand that physiological manifestations of psychological issues are legitimate problems, which need to be addressed. The pain is just as "real" as the pain that results from tissue damage. In addition, prolonged absence from work and social roles is detrimental to physical, social, and mental well-being (McGrail, Lohman, & Gorman, 2001). Although physical impairments may have subsided, the client may genuinely feel too ill to return to work or assume other life responsibilities (de Buck et al., 2005).

Researchers have proposed that chronic and acute pain are entirely different disorders (Apkarian et al., 2004; Robinson & Apkarian, 2009). Acute pain has a direct relationship to pathology and impairment, whereas chronic pain, chronic disability, and chronic illness behavior may be dissociated from the original source, with little evidence of the original physical condition. Magnetic resonance imaging studies reveal that acute pain activates the sensory part of the thalamus, and chronic pain is more evident in the prefrontal cortex, areas of emotion and learning (Apkarian et al., 2004; Apkarian, Baliki, & Geha, 2009). Apkarian and colleagues say that cognitive memory and emotional elements are involved.

Chronic pain progressively becomes a self-sustaining condition or "pain syndrome," which is resistant to traditional medical treatment (Apkarian et al., 2009). The initial response to pain is triggered by a nociceptive stimulus. Nerve endings called nociceptors react to unpleasant stimuli and alert the body that something is amiss. Pain messages pass upward through the spinal cord to the thalamus, where they are interpreted, and terminate at the cortex, where pain is perceived. Although once considered to be a "passive relay station" for sensory information traveling to the brain, we now know that much of the processing of the nociceptive signal takes place in the dorsal horn of the spinal cord (Henry, 2008). There is a particular pain pathway from nociceptors to the brain (Craig, 2003; Craig, Krout, & Andrew, 2001; Henry, 2008; Romanelli & Esposito, 2004; Vanderah, 2007). Researchers have hypothesized that the memory of the pain is retained in the cortex where neurons become sensitized to future stimuli. In the absence of noxious stimuli, small, non-noxious events can trigger the reactivation of the cycle. Even though an injury may be the cause of the initial pain, the pain may be chronically triggered after the resulting damage has healed, perhaps due to changes caused in the brain (Wu, Xu, Ren, Cao, & Zhuo, 2007).

Nonmalignant musculoskeletal pain is one of the leading causes for consulting primary care providers, missing work days, and losing wages. Neck, back, and shoulder pain account for many of these complaints (Karjalainen et al., 2001). Low back pain has been well studied and presents a model for explaining the progression from acute to chronic pain. A high percentage of clients with low back pain improve, regardless of treatment; the remainder develop chronic pain (Robinson & Apkarian, 2009). The decision to seek health care for low back pain appears dependent on the client's perception and interpretation of the pain, which may be enhanced by the presence of anxiety or emotional distress. Other premorbid risk factors for the onset of chronic pain include personal or family history of disability, dysfunctional family dynamics or abuse, history of substance abuse, and comorbid medical conditions (McGrail et al., 2001).

Prolonged pain causes difficulties in physical, psychological, and social areas of function. For example, people with chronic pain can be impaired in emotional decision making (Apkarian et al., 2004). It is estimated that half of all clients with chronic pain also have depression (Kleinman, 1988). Manifestations of chronic pain may be frequent complaints, irritability, and inability to participate in "normal" activities. This can exhaust family and friends, driving the client into social isolation. The most difficult aspect of chronic pain may be that, after a time, other people no longer believe the pain is real.

The wise clinician avoids believing that the client's pain has no basis in reality. Making assumptions, negatively labeling clients, and, perhaps, disregarding their complaints are barriers to good practice. Consider Elizabeth, a postal worker who injured her back as a result of carrying large sacks of mail. In the 8 years following her back injury, she has been placed on bedrest several times, received physical therapy, consumed large amounts of nonsteroidal pain medications, and, for the past 3 years, has been taking steroids. Yet, she is still disabled by her pain and only works sporadically. She is unable to participate in family social activities, go out with her friends, or fully enjoy the company of her husband. Her life revolves around the pain and her attempts to find relief.

## Pain and the Mind–Body Connection

Perhaps nowhere in medicine are the mind and body more closely linked than in chronic pain. The sympathetic nervous system responds to physical pain with emotional distress. Pain creates fear that releases catecholamines and stress hormones that can disrupt bodily functions, causing muscle tension and more pain. The linkages are powerful, and pain cannot be distinctly dichotomized into physical and psychological realms. Physical and psychological pain are both regulated through central nervous system mechanisms at several levels, leading to the pain–stress–fear cycle (Yocum, Castro, & Cornett, 2000). Refer to Chapter 4 for a detailed discussion of the mind–body connection.

What matters most about pain may well be the personal and social meaning that we attach to it. Religion, culture, gender, age, socioeconomic status, past experiences, and psychological traits all converge to affect our perception and response to pain. For example, the person who has pain as a result of bone cancer is generally afforded sympathy and care. In contrast, the person with perhaps equally severe pain secondary to a migraine headache may be perceived as exaggerating pain for secondary gain; after all, it is "*just* a headache."

The gate control theory of pain, developed by Melzack and Wall (1965) and elucidated by Melzack and Casey (1968), has been useful for decades because it explains how the direct physical stimuli that cause pain impulses are affected by ascending and descending neurological input at the level of the spinal cord. It also acknowledges the role of emotional and cognitive factors in mediating the perception of pain. This theory provides the framework for a holistic approach to medical care and is frequently employed in centers that treat clients with chronic pain (Karjalainen et al., 2001). It enables clinicians to add psychological, behavioral, and educational interventions to physical rehabilitation techniques (Karjalainen et al., 2001).

Although Melzack's and Casey's pain theory (1968) is still highly valued, researchers now realize the greater complexities involved in these mechanisms. Scientists have discovered that many of the dorsal horn interneurons can be excitatory or inhibitory, rather than the earlier belief that they were inhibitory; these dorsal horn interneurons also get information from both higher brain centers and other interneurons, as well as the periphery (Henry, 2008; Woolf, 2007). In addition, scientists now know that reduction of pain to certain sensory input can take place mostly in the cerebral cortex, with little happening at the spinal level (Inui, Tsuji, & Kakigi, 2006).

## Symptom Magnification

According to Matheson (1988), symptom magnification can be a conscious or unconscious self-destructive learned behavior pattern, reinforced by the social environment in which the person demonstrates or reports symptoms that exaggerate the seriousness of a medical condition.

Waddell, McCulloch, Kummel, and Venner (1980) developed test items to be used in the assessment of clients with low back pain—tenderness, regional disturbances, overreaction, simulation tests, and distraction tests—to identify the presence of psychosocial factors that may have an impact on a client's recovery. Responses to the tests, referred to as Waddell's nonorganic signs, include disproportionate signs of duress, unexplained sensory or muscular patterns, nonanatomical signs, and unexplained abilities or inabilities to perform certain functions, to name a few. Three or more positive nonorganic signs *suggest* nonmechanical, pain-focused behavior. That is to say, the nonorganic signs are not congruent with physical findings of organic pathologies. That being said, the presence of these kinds of behavioral signs does not conclusively indicate the absence of pathology (Thimineur, Kaliszewski, & Sood, 2000). Health providers need to further investigate the pain.

The identification of nonorganic signs was designed to be used only as a screening tool for clients who might benefit from psychological intervention and indicated the need for referral to a mental health professional. After many years of use, the nonorganic signs have been shown to be valid as a clinical measure of distress and illness behavior. However, these signs have often been misused by health care providers as a diagnostic test for malingering, even though no relationship has been found between nonorganic physical findings (Waddell signs) and secondary gain/malingering (Fishbain, Cutler, Rosomoff, & Rosomoff, 2004). In addition, the presence of these nonorganic signs is not an effective screening tool for return-to-work in clients with acute low back pain (Fritz, Wainner, & Hicks, 2000). As a result of this misinterpretation, Main and Waddell (1998) have renamed their test items *behavioral signs,* rather than nonorganic signs, to help clarify their significance.

The Tampa Scale for Kinesiophobia (TSK) and the Fear Avoidance Beliefs Questionnaire (FABQ) measure physical and work activity. They assess fear of movement or reinjury in clients with chronic pain and are validated instruments to assess fear-avoidance behavior (Bunketorp, Carlsson, Kowalski, & Stener-Victorin, 2005; French, France, Vigneau, French, & Evans, 2007; Swinkels-Meewisse, Swinkels, Verbeek, Vlaeyen, & Oostendorp, 2004). Kinesiophobia is defined as "an irrational and debilitating fear of physical movement and activity resulting from a feeling of vulnerability to painful injury or (re)injury" (Kori, Miller, & Todd, 1990, p. 35).

Fear-avoidance beliefs and pain amplification have an impact on self-ratings of disability in people with whiplash-associated disorders (Vernon, Guerriero, Kavanaugh, Soave, & Moreton, 2010). Higher scores of kinesiophobia are associated with depression and anxiety (French et al., 2007). Futher, Pfingsten and associates (2001) found that anticipation of pain and fear-avoidance beliefs strongly heighten the fear-avoidance behavior of clients with low back pain. They stress that clinicians need to understand the influence of cognitive processes, which can lead to pain-related fear and, therefore, avoidance behavior.

Although pain is a neurophysiological process, pain behavior is influenced by a number of factors, including culture, environment, race, ethnicity, verbal reinforcement, relationship with one's spouse (Edwards, Doleys, Fillingim, & Lowery, 2001; Kleinman, 1988; Lechner, Bradbury, & Bradley, 1998; Morris, 1991), personality, situation, and emotional state (Henry, 2008). Clinicians need to distinguish between people who deliberately exaggerate symptoms and those who have central sensitization syndrome, in which neural responses are amplified, and clients' behavioral responses may appear exaggerated. For example, typically nonpainful stimuli (i.e., brushing the hair, shaving, showering, and donning glasses or earrings) can elicit pain in clients with allodynia. Clients with hyperalgesia have an increased sensitivity to pain that may be triggered by a painful stimulus or a lowered pain threshold. Clients with allodynia, hyperalgesia, and multiple symptom involvement may appear to be histrionic or "faking," when, in fact, there is a true physiological response, consistent with central sensitization.

## THERAPEUTIC INTERVENTIONS

In Chapter 8, we discussed adaptation to long-term health problems, disabilities, and terminal illness. Strategies were recommended for appropriate therapeutic responses to support clients in their journey from loss to adjustment. These responses are also applicable for clients with chronic conditions. Clients and care providers may need to work together for a significant period of time, perhaps for many years; therefore, the client–provider relationship is particularly significant and is the foundation on which healing is built. The health care provider's ability to ask questions, listen, and interpret the client's needs creates a powerful therapeutic intervention. Clients with chronic conditions can have complex problems and histories, and multiple treatment strategies are often necessary. It is imperative that health care providers consider prior treatments, clients' beliefs and goals, and medical and personal priorities.

Screening clients with outcome measures like the TSK and FABQ, as discussed earlier, can help inform more effective interventions. Health care professionals may be able to help prevent the progression from pain and acute problems to disability. Successful disability prevention relies on appropriate diagnosis and management of the illness and its symptoms, as well as on open communication and trust between the client and health care provider. For example, a client who asks for documentation of a disability to avoid returning to work may actually be communicating difficulty coping with other life demands. Sensitive listening and counseling may identify a manageable condition, such as family problems, anxiety, depression, or substance abuse. Early assessment and intervention can ease the client's journey and should be everyone's responsibility within the scope of their discipline. Can you appropriately evaluate which clients need reassurance and which may need psychiatric intervention? The assessment may be beyond your scope of practice, but you can identify red warning flags that will compel you to seek assistance.

Careful client education and instruction can convey the message that chronic conditions are not necessarily disabling and may be self-limiting. They can also address the impairments and barriers to participation that can benefit from intervention or accommodation. If pain, for example, cannot be eliminated, health care providers can work with the client, employer, and family to adjust work and home demands or make reasonable accommodations for the residual impairments (McGrail et al., 2001). A multidisciplinary team approach to chronic pain involves many different providers, such as physical therapists, physicians, nurses, and psychologists, and all may participate in this process. The client is also a functional member of the team, whose broad goal is to assess the effect of treatment on his or her pain and increase independence (Sluka, 2009).

Client education and support are critical to quality of life. Learning self-care reduces client anxiety and promotes body image reintegration. Practitioners can assist clients in developing these skills by scheduling small-group educational or training classes (Gutiérrez Vilaplana, Zampieron, Craver, & Buja, 2009). As a result of feeling anxious and fearful, clients may be reluctant to do dressing changes, look at and touch altered areas, or try new skills, such as using a prosthetic device in the presence of others. Helping clients confront their fears and deal with practical challenges, such as those from social encounters, can ease those difficulties (Larouche & Chin-Peuckert, 2006; Thompson & Kent, 2001).

Support from health care providers, friends, and family is very meaningful if it is positive. In a study among adults, ages 65 and older, with arthritis, diabetes, and/or cardiac disease, friends had more positive influences than family on their self-management in key areas: managing the disease, making decisions about it, and coping with its psychosocial aspects (Gallant, Spitze, & Prohaska, 2007).

Consistent and congruent verbal and behavioral messages can help a client adapt to chronic health conditions (Cohen, 1991; French & Phillips, 1991). This is a critical time to make sure your actions match your words. Emotional honesty is also important. If you want the client to trust you, you cannot say that everything is fine, that nothing has changed. Alterations in the body and life have occurred that necessitate the client's attention (Drench, 1996). The client needs to integrate the changes that have occurred to his or her body into a new self-concept. As health providers, we need to listen to the clients' concerns, acknowledge the difficulty of their situations, and help them realize they will be able to do this. Our role as change agents is to help the client understand and appreciate the value he or she continues to have as a person.

During the first four years after she was diagnosed with systemic lupus erythematosus, 29-year-old Brittany had severe joint pain and swelling, debilitating fatigue, mouth ulcers, skin rashes, recurrent infections of pneumonia and meningitis, reduced kidney function, and hair loss. She says that she was "sick and tired of feeling tired and achy." She has learned how to listen to her body's signals to help prevent flare-ups. To better control the lupus, Brittany exercises daily, including yoga, stretching, and weight-bearing activities, to improve her bone density, diminished secondary to her taking steroid medication for years. She also eats a well-balanced diet and gets plenty of rest. Because lupus is invisible, and she doesn't use a cane or a wheelchair, she says that people just "don't get it that I'm working so hard to control my illness."

—*From the journal of Pat Thompson, occupational therapy student*

We can also help clients emphasize their capabilities rather than their deficiencies. Understanding their own inherent strengths and values, what Wright in her classic works (1960, 1983) calls "asset values," can be motivating and promote a greater appreciation for "what is." In contrast, comparing themselves to other people (Wright's "comparative values") who have no or different disabilities can place obstacles in the path of recovery. In the acceptance of loss theory, these are among the value changes associated with acceptance of disability (Keany & Glueckauf, 1993).

If health providers and clients are aiming for a return to the premorbid state, anything short of that gold standard will be perceived as failure and cause frustration. Through the phenomenon of spread, a concept that an individual's perception of one characteristic can spread to color other attributes, the person may see other areas, besides the physical, as being inferior and unacceptable (Dembo, Leviton, & Wright, 1956). Wright (1983) held that negative thoughts and feelings, including one's own, toward people with chronic illness and disability trigger negative perceptions. The outcome of this thinking is biased stereotypes of people with chronic illness and disability (Chou, Lee, Catalano, Ditchman, & Wilson, 2009). Success in recovery, improving function, and overcoming obstacles are dependent on the person's feeling effective and capable.

We can help clients use an asset rather than comparative value system to place greater weight on nonphysical attributes. Sixteen-year-old Jim Langevin had spent his summer vacation working as a police cadet, dreaming of becoming a police officer or an agent of the Federal Bureau of Investigation. As two members of the SWAT team were examining a handgun in the police department locker room, it inadvertently discharged, sending a bullet ricocheting off a metal locker and ripping through the teenager's neck. A gunshot wound to the cervical spine caused a complete cervical spinal cord injury. Not only did Langevin survive, he ultimately thrived, later becoming Secretary of State of Rhode Island. Twenty years after the accident, he became the first person with quadriplegia elected to the U.S. House of Representatives. Instead of enforcing the law, he is part of creating it.

Although initially Langevin reacted with disbelief, anger, and frustration, he was able to see possibilities and work toward them. He also hopes that his actions will inspire others to follow their dreams and not yield to their limitations (personal communication, April 4, 2002). Emphasizing a client's assets and sharing stories with "successful" outcomes, parts of which a client might be able to achieve, can also be motivating.

Becoming involved in life's activities and developing a sense of mastery and pride in one's abilities may minimize, prevent, or replace grieving and self-pity. A valuable lesson to share with clients is that they are people with chronic conditions rather than "sick" people. Maintaining a healthy level of fitness within one's limitations is important, and playing sports adapted for people with different abilities can improve socialization, self-esteem, cognition, and have many other benefits (Moberg-Wolff & Kiesling, 2008). Health care professionals may want to consider attending or volunteering to assist with adaptive sports programs, such as wheelchair basketball, rugby, surfing, horseback riding, baseball, or other activities. Interacting with people with chronic conditions or disabilities outside of the clinic, and seeing them in a very different environment, may help providers develop a new perspective, which can assist them in providing more comprehensive care to future clients.

## Summary

In this chapter, we explained the effects of chronic health conditions. Some conditions allow the client to live a "normal" life with minimal disruption. Others, like chronic pain, may affect every waking moment and cause the client significant distress. Certain conditions result in functional limitations and, ultimately, permanent disabilities, requiring accommodations in lifestyle, work, physical environments, and relationships to maximize social access and participation. The health care needs of clients with chronic conditions may be more complex than for those with acute conditions and will require different types of interventions.

We also explored the relationship between body image and self-concept, how clients respond to changes in body image, and strategies that health professionals can employ to help clients adjust to these changes. Because body image is so closely associated with self-concept and personal identity, a change of one aspect can affect the whole person. Health care providers are instrumental in fostering clients' adjustment and acceptance by recognizing and helping them work through their losses and emphasizing their strengths.

## Reflective Questions

1. Consider what is important to your body image and self-concept.
   a. What attributes do you most value?
   b. What impairments or deficits would you find most difficult to accept?
   c. How do you think your beliefs and values affect the way you feel about clients? Do you think clients can sense this? Explain.
   d. How do you think your values and beliefs affect your ability to set goals for clients?
   e. How do you think your values and beliefs affect your ability to support clients' goals?
2. Consider your own experiences interacting with your health care providers.
   a. Describe how you were treated. Was a biomedical, biopsychosocial, or other model used?
   b. What impact did this have on your outcome?

3. a. What are your personal health care beliefs?
   b. How have your personal health care beliefs been shaped by your social, family, religious, and cultural values?
4. There is a strong link between low income and poor health. Describe strategies that could minimize this problem
   a. on a personal level.
   b. at the government level.
   c. in the workplace.
5. a. Do you think people with a sudden onset of illness or impairment respond differently than those with a progressive condition?
   b. In what ways might they be similar or different?

## Case Study

Marguerite Finley is a 36-year-old executive of an investment firm. Diagnosed with rheumatoid arthritis when she was 28, she has been progressively hampered by pain, deformity, and loss of functional mobility in her hands. She is now seeking surgery to improve function, pain, and appearance.

Marguerite enjoys a happy marriage, a wide circle of friends, and a highly satisfying career. However, she has become increasingly troubled by the appearance of her hands, seeing them as unattractive compared to her memory of her hands as they once were. Although she grooms her nails and wears nail polish, she is no longer able to wear rings. She now tends to hide her hands when she is with friends, as well as strangers, and is very sensitive to "looks of pity" from others.

1. What factors may influence how Marguerite responds to changes in body image?
2. What impact might Marguerite's physical changes have on her self-concept and on her self-esteem?
3. Discuss the relationship between stigma, perceptions of negative changes, and impairment for Marguerite.
4. a. What can you do to foster Marguerite's adjustment and acceptance of the changes in her body image?
   b. Knowing that rheumatoid arthritis is a progressive disease that will continue even after this surgery, how will you address Marguerite's chronic pain?

# References

Anderson, I. H. (2004). The course of non-malignant chronic pain: A 12-year follow-up of a cohort from the general population. *European Journal of Pain, 8,* 47–53.

Apkarian, A. V., Baliki, M. N., & Geha, P. Y. (2009). Towards a theory of chronic pain. *Progress in Neurobiology, 87*(2), 81–97.

Apkarian, A. V., Sosa, Y., Krauss, B. R., Thomas, P. S., Fredrickson, B. E., Levy, R. E., . . . Chialvo, D. R. (2004). Chronic pain patients are impaired on an emotional decision-making task. *Journal of the International Association for the Study of Pain, 108*(1), 129–136.

Braden, J. B., & Sullivan, M. D. (2008). Suicidal thoughts and behavior among adults with self-reported pain conditions in the national comorbidity survey replication. *Journal of Pain, 9*(12), 1106–1115.

Bramble, K. (1995). Body image. In I. M. Lubkin (Ed.), *Chronic illness: Impact and interventions* (3rd ed., pp. 285–299). Boston, MA: Jones and Bartlett.

Bronheim, H., Strain, J. J., & Biller, H. F. (1991). Psychiatric aspects of head and neck surgery. Part II: Body image and psychiatric intervention. *General Hospital Psychiatry, 13*(4), 225–232.

Bunketorp, L., Carlsson, J., Kowalski, J., & Stener-Victorin, E. (2005). Evaluating the reliability of multi-item scales: A non-parametric approach to the ordered categorical structure of data collected with the Swedish version of the Tampa Scale for Kinesiophobia and the self-efficacy scale. *Journal of Rehabilitation Medicine, 37,* 330–334.

Cavanagh, S. R., Shin, L. M., Karamouz, N., & Rauch, S. L. (2006). Psychiatric and emotional sequelae of surgical amputation. *Psychosomatics, 47,* 459–464.

Centers for Disease Control and Prevention. (2006). Prevalence of doctor-diagnosed arthritis and arthritis-attributable activity limitation—United States, 2003–2005. *Morbidity and Mortality Weekly Report, 55,* 1089–1092.

Centers for Disease Control and Prevention. (2007). Prevalence of self-reported physically active adults—United States. *Morbidity and Mortality Weekly Report, 57,* 1297–1300.

Centers for Disease Control and Prevention. (2008). *National diabetes fact sheet, 2007.* Atlanta, GA: U.S. Department of Health and Human Services. Retrieved from http://www.cdc.gov/Diabetes/pubs/factsheet07.htm

Centers for Disease Control and Prevention. (2009). *Chronic diseases and health promotion.* Atlanta, GA: U.S. Department of Health and Human Services. Retrieved from http://www.cdc.gov/chronicdisease/overview/index.htm

Chou, C.-.C, Lee, E.-J., Catalano, D. E., Ditchman, N., & Wilson, L. M. (2009). Positive psychology and psychosocial adjustment to chronic illness and disability. In F. Chan, E. da Silva Cardoso, & J. A. Chronister (Eds.), *Understanding psychosocial adjustment to chronic illness and disability: A handbook for evidence-based practitioners in rehabilitation* (pp. 207–233). New York, NY: Springer.

Cohen, A. (1991). Body image in the person with a stoma. *Journal of Enterostomal Therapy, 18*(2), 68–71.

Cohen, C. G., Krahn, L., Wise, T. N., Epstein, S., & Ross, R. (1991). Delusions of disfigurement in a woman with acne rosacea. *General Hospital Psychiatry, 13*(4), 273–277.

Craig, A. D. (2003). Pain mechanisms: Labeled lines versus convergence in central processing. *Annual Review of Neuroscience, 26,* 1–30.

Craig, A. D., Krout, K., & Andrew, D. (2001). Quantitative response characteristics of thermoreceptive and nociceptive lamina I spinothalamic neurons in the cat. *Journal of Neurophysiology, 86*(3), 1459–1480.

de Buck, P. D., le Cessie, S., van den Hout, W. B., Peeters, A. J., Ronday, H. K., Westedt, M. L., . . . Vliet Vlieland, T. P. (2005). Randomized comparison of a multidisciplinary job-retention vocational rehabilitation program with usual outpatient care in patients with chronic arthritis at risk for job loss. *Arthritis and Rheumatism, 53*(5), 682–690.

Dembo, T., Leviton, G. L., & Wright, B. A. (1956). Adjustment to misfortune: A problem of social-psychological rehabilitation. *Artificial Limbs, 3*(2), 4–62.

Dixon, L., Goldberg, R., Lehman, A., & McNary, S. (2001). The impact of health status on work, symptoms, and functional outcomes in severe mental illness. *Journal of Nervous and Mental Disease, 189*(1), 17–23.

Drench, M. (1994). Lewis B. Puller, Jr. [Letter to the Editors]. *PT—Magazine of Physical Therapy, 2*(10), 14.

Drench, M. (1995). Coping with loss—Adjusting to change. *International Society for Behavioral Science in Physical Therapy, 7*(2), 1–3.

Drench, M. E. (1996). Changes in body image secondary to disease and injury. In *Nursing focus: Psychosocial adaptation to disability and chronic illness* (pp. 15–19). Glenview, IL: Association of Rehabilitation Nurses.

Drench, M. E., & Losee, R. H. (1996). Sexuality and sexual capacities of elderly people. *Rehabilitation Nursing, 21*(3), 118–123.

Edwards, R. R., Doleys, D. M., Fillingim, R. B., & Lowery, D. (2001). Ethnic differences in pain tolerance: Clinical implications in a chronic pain population. *Psychosomatic Medicine, 63,* 316–323.

Ericsson, M., Poston, W. S. C., Linder, J., Taylor, J. E., Haddock, C. K., & Foreyt, J. P. (2002). Depression predicts disability in long-term chronic pain patients. *Disability and Rehabilitation, 24,* 334–340.

Fishbain, D. A., Bruns, D., Disorbio, J. M, & Lewis, J. E. (2009). Risk for five forms of suicidality in acute pain patients and chronic pain patients vs. pain-free community controls. *Pain Medicine, 10*(6), 1095–1105.

Fishbain, D. A., Cutler, R. B., Rosomoff, H. L., & Rosomoff, R. S. (2004). Is there a relationship between nonorganic physical findings (Waddell signs) and secondary gain/malingering? *Clinical Journal of Pain, 20*(6), 399–408.

French, D. J., France, C., Vigneau, F., French, J., & Evans, R. (2007). Fear of movement/(re)injury in chronic pain: A psychometric assessment of the original English version of the Tampa Scale for kinesiophobia (TSK). *Pain, 127*(1–2), 42–51.

French, J. K., & Phillips, J. A. (1991). Shattered images: Recovery for the SCI client. *Rehabilitation Nursing, 16*(3), 134–136.

Friedrich, M., Hahne, J., & Wepner, F. (2009). A controlled examination of medical and psychosocial factors associated with low back pain in combination with widespread musculoskeletal pain. *Physical Therapy, 89*(8), 786–803.

Frischenschlager, O. & Pucher, I. (2002). Psychological management of pain. *Disability and Rehabilitation, 8,* 416–422.

Fritz, J. M., Wainner, R. S., & Hicks, G. E. (2000). The use of nonorganic signs and symptoms as a screening tool for return-to-work in patients with acute low back pain. *Spine, 25*(15), 1925–1931.

Gallant, M. P., Spitze, G. D., & Prohaska, T. R. (2007). Help or hindrance? How family and friends influence chronic illness self-management among older adults. *Aging, 29*(5), 375–409.

Geiser, M. E., Robinson, M. E., Miller, Q. L., & Bade, S. M. (2003). Psychosocial factors and functional capacity evaluation among persons with chronic pain. *Journal of Occupational Rehabilitation, 4,* 259–276.

Gutiérrez Vilaplana, J. M., Zampieron, A., Craver, L., & Buja, A. (2009). Evaluation of psychological outcomes following the intervention "teaching group": Study on predialysis patients. *Journal of Renal Care, 35*(3), 159–164.

Head, H. (1920). *Studies of neurology* (Vol. 1). London, United Kingdom: Hodder & Stoughton.

Henderson, M., Kidd, B. L., Pearson, R. M., & White, P. D. (2005). Chronic upper limb pain: An exploration of the biopsychosocial model. *Journal of Rheumatology, 32,* 118–122.

Henry, J. L. (2008). Pathophysiology of chronic pain. In S. Rashiq, D. Schlopflocher, P. Taenzer, & E. Jonsson (Eds.), *Chronic pain: A health policy perspective* (pp. 59–66). Weinheim, Germany: Wiley-Blackwell.

Hewitt Associates. (2010). *Cardiovascular disease and diabetes are the most frequently targeted conditions among employers.* Retrieved from http://www. hewittassociates.com/Intl/NA/en-US/AboutHewitt/ Newsroom/PressRelease

Ilgen, M. A., Zivin, K., McCammon, R. J., & Valenstein, M. (2008). Pain and suicidal thoughts, plans and attempts in the United States. *General Hospital Psychiatry, 30*(6), 521–527.

International Association for the Study of Pain. (2007). *IASP pain terminology.* Retrieved from http://www. iasp-pain.org/AM/Template.cfm?Section=Home& Template=/CM/HTMLDisplay.cfm&ContentID=17 28#Pain

International Association for the Study of Pain Task Force on Taxonomy. (1994a). *Classification of chronic pain: Descriptions of chronic pain syndromes and definitions of pain terms.* Seattle, WA: IASP Press.

International Association for the Study of Pain Task Force on Taxonomy. (1994b). Part III: Pain terms, a current list with definitions and notes on usage. In H. Merskey & N. Bogduk (Eds.), *Classification of chronic pain* (2nd ed., pp. 209–214). Seattle, WA: IASP Press.

Inui, K., Tsuji, T., & Kakigi, R. (2006). Temporal analysis of cortical mechanisms for pain relief by tactile stimuli in humans. *Cerebral Cortex, 16*(3), 355–365.

Jackson, J. E. (2000). *"Camp Pain": Talking with chronic pain patients.* Philadelphia: University of Pennsylvania Press.

Jette, A. M. (2009). Toward a common language of disablement. *Journals of Gerontology, Series A, Biological Sciences and Medical Sciences, 64A*(11), 1165–1168.

Joachim, G., & Acorn, S. (2000). Stigma of visible and invisible chronic conditions. *Journal of Advanced Nursing, 32*(1), 243–248.

Käariä, S., Kaila-Kangas, L., Kirjonen, J., Riihimäki, H., Luukkonen, R. K., & Leino-Arjas, P. (2005). Low back pain, work absenteeism, chronic back disorders, and clinical findings in the low back as predictors of hospitalization due to low back disorders: A 28-year follow-up of industrial employees. *Spine, 30*(10), 1211–1218.

Karjalainen, K., Melmivivaara, A., Tuldar, M., Roine, R., Jauhiainen, M., Hurri, H., & Koes, B. (2001). Multidisciplinary biopsychosocial rehabilitation for subacute low back pain in working-age adults. *Spine, 26*, 262–269.

Keany, K. C., & Glueckauf, R. L. (1993). Disability and value change: An overview and reanalysis of acceptance of loss theory. *Rehabilitation Psychology, 38*(3), 199–210.

Keough, J. L., & Fisher, T. F. (2001). Occupational-psychological perceptions influencing return to work and functional performance of injured workers. *Work, 16*, 101–110.

Kessler, R. C., Greenberg, P. E., Mickelson, K. D., Meneades, L. M., & Wong, P. S. (2001). The effects of chronic medical conditions on work loss and work cutback. *Journal of Occupational and Environmental Medicine, 43*, 218–225.

Kleinman, A. (1988). *The illness narratives.* New York, NY: Basic Books.

Kori, S., Miller, R., & Todd, D. (1990). *Kinesiophobia: A new view of chronic pain behavior.* New York, NY: International Universities Press.

Krueger, A. B., & Stone, A. A. (2008). Assessment of pain: A community-based diary survey in the USA. *The Lancet, 371*(9623), 1519–1525.

Kung, H. C., Hoyert, D. L., Xu, J. Q., & Murphy, S. L. (2008). Deaths: Final data for 2005. *National Vital Statistics Reports, 56*(10). Retrieved from http://www.cdc.gov/nchs/data/nvsr/nvsr56/nvsr56_10.pdf

Larouche, S. S., & Chin-Peuckert, L. (2006). Changes in body image experienced by adolescents with cancer. *Journal of Pediatric Oncology Nursing, 23*(4), 200–209.

Lasry, J. C., Margolese, R. G., Poisson, R., Shibata, H., Fleischer, D., LaFleur, D., . . . Taillefer, S. (1987). Depression and body image following mastectomy and lumpectomy. *Journal of Chronic Diseases, 40*(6), 529–534.

Laufer, M. E. (1991). Body image, sexuality and the psychotic core. *International Journal of Psychoanalysis, 72*(Pt. 1), 63–71.

Law, M. (2002). Participation in the occupations of everyday life. *American Journal of Occupational Therapy, 56*, 640–649.

Lechner, D. E., Bradbury, S. A., & Bradley, L. A. (1998). Detecting sincerity of effort: A summary of methods and approaches. *Physical Therapy, 78*, 867–888.

Livneh, H., & Antonak, R. (1997). *Psychosocial adaptation to chronic illness and disability.* Gaithersburg, MD: Aspen.

Lubitz, J., Cai, L., Kramarow, E., & Lentzner, H. (2003). Health, life expectancy, and health care spending among the elderly. *New England Journal of Medicine, 349*(11), 1048–1055.

Lynch, J. W., Kaplan, G. A., & Shema, S. J. (1997). Cumulative impact of sustained economic hardship on physical, cognitive, psychological, and social functioning. *Massachusetts Medical Society, 337*(26), 1889–1895.

Main, C. J., & Waddell, G. (1998). Behavioral responses: A reappraisal of the interpretation of nonorganic signs. *Spine, 23*(21), 2367–2371.

Marty, M., Rozenberg, S., Duplan, B., Thomas, P. Duquesnoy, B., & Allaert, F. (2008). Quality of sleep in patients with chronic low back pain: A case-control study. *European Spine Journal, 17*(6), 839–844.

Matheson, L. N. (1988). How do you know he tried his best? *Journal of Industrial Rehabilitation Quarterly, 1*, 10–12.

McGrail, M. P., Lohman, W., & Gorman, R. (2001). Disability prevention principles in the primary care office. *American Family Physician, 63*(4), 679–684.

Melzack, R. (1975). The McGill Pain Questionnaire: Major properties and scoring methods. *Pain, 1*, 277–299.

Melzack, R., & Casey, K. L. (1968). Sensory, motivational, and central control determinants of chronic pain: A new conceptual model. In D. Kenshalo (Ed.), *The skin senses* (pp. 423–443). Springfield, IL: Thomas.

Melzack, R., & Wall, P. (1965). Pain mechanisms: A new theory. *Science, 150*, 971–979.

Milken Institute. (2010). *An unhealthy America: The economic burden of chronic disease.* Retrieved from http://www.milkeninstitute.org/publications/publications.taf?function=detail&ID=38801018

Moberg-Wolff, E., & Kiesling, S. (2008). Adapted recreational and sports programs for children with disabilities: Then and now. *Journal of Pediatric Rehabilitation Medicine, 1*(2), 155–161.

Monteath, S. A., & McCabe, M. P. (1997). The influence of societal factors on female body image. *Journal of Social Psychology, 137*(6), 708–727.

Morris, D. B. (1991). *The culture of pain.* Berkeley: University of California Press.

National Center for Health Statistics. (2010). *Health, United States, 2009: With special feature on medical technology.* Hyattsville, MD: Author.

Newth, S., & Delongis, A. (2004). Individual differences, mood, and coping with chronic pain in rheumatoid arthritis: A daily process analysis. *Psychology and Health, 3,* 283–305.

Norris, C. (1970). The professional nurse and body image. In C. E. Carlson (Ed.), *Behavioral concepts and nursing intervention* (p.43). Philadelphia: J. B. Lippincott.

O'Donoghue, G. M., Fox, N., Heneghan, C., & Hurley, D. A. (2009). Objective and subjective assessment of sleep in chronic low back pain patients compared with healthy age and gender matched controls: A pilot study. *BMC Musculoskeletal Disorders, 10,* 122–127.

Okie, S. (2007). The employer as coach. *New England Journal of Medicine, 357*(15), 1465–1469.

Pfingsten, M., Leibing, E., Harter, W., Kröner-Herwig, B., Hempel, D., Kronshage, U., & Hildebrandt, J. (2001). Fear-avoidance behavior and anticipation of pain in patients with chronic low back pain: A randomized controlled study. *Pain Medicine, 2*(4), 259–266.

Philipp, T., & Black, L. (1998). Financial impact. In I. M. Lubkin & P. D. Larsen (Eds.), *Chronic illness* (pp. 501–527). Sudbury, MA: Jones and Bartlett.

Puller, L. B., Jr. (1993). *Fortunate son: The autobiography of Lewis B. Puller, Jr.* New York, NY: Bantam Books.

Robinson, J. P., & Apkarian, A. V. (2009). Low back pain. In E. A. Mayer & M. C. Bushnell (Eds.), *Functional pain syndromes: Presentation and pathophysiology* (pp. 23–53). Seattle, WA: IASP Press.

Romanelli, P., & Esposito, V. (2004). The functional anatomy of neuropathic pain. *Neurosurgical Clinics of North America, 15*(3), 257–268.

Saastamoinen, P., Leino-Arjas, P., Laaksonen, M., & Lahelma, E. (2005). Socio-economic differences in the prevalence of acute, chronic and disabling chronic pain among aging employees. *Pain, 3,* 364–371.

Sainsbury, D. C. (2009). Body image and facial burns. *Advances in Skin and Wound Care, 22*(1), 39–44.

Samonds, R. J., & Cammermeyer, M. (1989). Perceptions of body image in subjects with multiple sclerosis: A pilot study. *Journal of Neuroscience Nursing, 21*(3), 190–194.

Schilder, P. (1950). *The image and appearance of the human body: Studies in the constructive energies of the psyche.* New York, NY: International Universities Press.

Singh, M. K., Patel, J., & Gallagher, R. M. (2010). *Chronic pain syndrome.* Retrieved from http://emedicine. medscape.com/article/310834-overview

Sluka, K. A. (Ed.). (2009). *Mechanisms and management of pain for the physical therapist.* Seattle, WA: IASP Press.

Swinkels-Meewisse, E. J., Swinkels, R. A., Verbeek, A. L., Vlaeyen, J. W., & Oostendorp, R. A. (2004). Psychometric properties of the Tampa Scale for Kinesiophobia and the fear-avoidance beliefs questionnaire in acute low back pain. *Manual Therapy, 8*(1), 29–36.

Taleporos, G., & McCabe, M. P. (2001). The impact of physical disability on body esteem. *Sexuality and Disability, 19*(4), 293–308.

Thimineur, M., Kaliszewski, T., & Sood, P. (2000). Malingering and symptom magnification: A case report illustrating the limitations of clinical judgment. *Connecticut Medicine, 64*(7), 399–401.

Thompson, A., & Kent, G. (2001). Adjusting to disfigurement: Processes involved in dealing with being visibly different. *Clinical Psychology Review, 21*(5), 663–682.

Truchon, M. (2001). Determinants of chronic disability related to low back pain: Towards an integrative biopsychosocial model. *Disability and Rehabilitation, 23,* 758–767.

Van Cleave, J., Gortmaker, S. L., & Perrin, J. M. (2010). Dynamics of obesity and chronic health conditions among children and youth. *Journal of the American Medical Association, 303*(7), 623–630.

Vanderah, T. W. (2007). Pathophysiology of pain. *Medical Clinics of North America, 91*(1), 1–12.

van Hemert, A. M., Hengeveld, M. W., Bolk, J. H., Rooijmans, H. G., & van den Broucke, J. P. (1993). Psychiatric disorder in relation to medical illness among patients of a general medical outpatient clinic. *Psychological Medicine, 23,* 167–173.

Vernon, H., Guerriero, R., Kavanaugh, S., Soave, D., & Moreton, J. (2010). Psychological factors in the use of the neck disability index in chronic whiplash patients. *Spine, 35*(1), E16–E21.

Waddell, G. (1991). Occupational low-back pain, illness behavior, and disability. *Spine, 16*(6), 663–664.

Waddell G., McCulloch, J. A., Kummel, E., & Venner, R. M. (1980). Nonorganic physical signs in low back pain. *Spine, 5,* 117–125.

Wess, M. (2007). Bringing hope and healing to grieving patients with cancer. *Journal of the American Osteopathic Association, 107*(12), ES41–ES47.

White, R. K., Wright, B. A., & Dembo, T. (1948). Studies in adjustment to visible injuries: Evaluation of curiosity by the injured. *Journal of Abnormal Social Psychology, 43,* 13–28.

Woolf, C. J. (2007). Deconstructing pain: A deterministic dissection of the molecular basis of pain. In S. Coakley & K. Kaufman Shelemay (Eds.), *Pain and its transformations: The interface of biology and culture* (pp. 27–31). Cambridge, MA: Harvard University Press.

World Health Organization (2004). *Headache disorders.* Retrieved from http://www.who.int/mediacentre/factsheets/fs277/en

Wright, B. A. (1960). *Physical disability: A psychological approach.* New York, NY: Harper & Row.

Wright, B. A. (1983). *Physical disability: A psychosocial approach* (2nd ed.). New York, NY: Harper & Row.

Wu, L. J., Xu, H., Ren, M., Cao, X., & Zhuo, M. (2007). Pharmacological isolation of postsynaptic currents mediated by NR2A- and NR2B-containing NMDA receptors in the anterior cingulated cortex. *Molecular Pain, 3,* 11–16.

Yocum, D. F., Castro, W., & Cornett, L. (2000). Exercise, education, and behavioral modification as alternative therapy for pain and stress in rheumatic disease. *Rheumatic Disease Clinics of North America, 26*(1), 145–159.

## 12

# Sexuality

Poor Mr. Michaels was so distressed today. He can't imagine how he can possibly resume a sexual relationship with his wife now that he has lost sensation below his chest, cannot maintain an erection, cannot ejaculate, and must wear an external condom catheter to manage urinary incontinence. It's difficult for him to even bring up the topic with her. Although he expects that Mrs. Michaels will be as disgusted as he is about the whole thing, he fears that she'll deny it "out of pity and embarrassment." After a very emotional session, Mr. Michaels finally agreed to ask his wife to meet with us next time to begin to talk about their options for resuming a sexual relationship.

*—From the journal of Teresa Dumont, counseling psychology student*

Sexuality is an important aspect of life and is strongly linked to many biological, psychological, familial, social, cultural, and religious factors. It is an important determinant in all interpersonal relationships and encompasses gender identity, attractiveness, and sexual attitudes, beliefs, and practices. Perceptions about sexuality are strongly affected by parents and society in general.

The sexual development of young children begins in the home, but as their experiences expand to include school and the greater society, views are more widely impacted by educators, peers, the media, and other influences. For example, consider the stereotypical concepts of masculinity and femininity, which assume that men are primarily interested in emotionally detached sexual acts, whereas women prefer the emotional connectedness associated with intimacy. These stereotypes persist in American culture despite evidence that the personal concepts of masculinity and femininity reflect significantly more latitude and openness across the sexes (Hoffman, Hattie, & Borders, 2005; Sand, Fisher, Rosen, Heiman, & Eardley, 2008). Unfortunately, the influence of these erroneous societal standards can be harmful to people who adopt them as truths. In the journal entry above, Mr. Michaels fails to see how he can continue to relate sexually with his wife now that he has lost the ability to perform physically.

Sexual health is influenced by a number of factors, including, but not limited to, changes in mental and physical health, sexual abuse and other forms of violence, sexually transmitted diseases, unintended pregnancy, abortion, and medications that alter libido. Our ability to adequately address sexual health with clients is complicated by social mores and the persistent view of sexuality as a taboo subject. It takes a well-trained team of human services personnel that is comfortable with sexuality to successfully address clients' sexual health (World Health Organization, 2010).

In this chapter, we explore sexuality across the life span, identify some common problems that impact sexual health, and provide concrete examples for raising this sensitive subject during client–provider interactions.

## SEXUAL DEVELOPMENT

### Prenatal

Sexual development begins *in utero*. During the prenatal period, biological influences determine whether the embryo develops as male or female. This differentiation involves the genitals, internal reproductive organs (gonads), and the central nervous system. Sexual reflexes are all present at birth, except the male's ability to ejaculate, which depends on heightened levels of sex hormones that emerge during puberty. Following birth, psychological, social, and cultural factors become more significant than biological factors as sexual development continues (Masters, Johnson, & Kolodny, 1992). Fetal development is sometimes complicated by disorders of sexual development (DSD), a term that denotes atypical sexual differentiation. Some children have disorders of testicular development, characterized by the presence of XY chromosomes, the usual number of 46 autosomes, but ambiguous external genitalia. Others have disorders of ovarian development with the presence of XX chromosomes and 46 autosomes, and ambiguous external genitalia. Although it is rare, some children can have both ovarian and testicular tissue, a condition known as ovotesticular DSD. Until recently, health professionals counseled parents into early surgical genital reconstruction, but better outcomes in sexual function and psychosocial health seem to be associated with a delay in gender assignment until children are mature enough to determine which gender best fits their concept of sexual identity (Johansen, Ripa, Mortensen, & Main, 2006; Lee, Houk, Ahmed, & Hughes, 2006).

The role of most health professionals who encounter persons with DSD is to recognize it as a variation of human development, provide psychosocial support as needed, answer questions that might arise in conjunction with treatment, and facilitate referral to a specialist in sexual and reproductive health, if indicated.

### Early Childhood

The major sexual task of early childhood is to develop gender identity. This is the perceived sense of being male or female and is primarily shaped by psychosocial factors. Kohlberg (1966) proposes that gender development parallels intellectual development. He identifies three tasks that are involved in the process of developing gender identity:

1. Accurate identification of self and others as male or female (labeling)
2. The realization that boys become men and girls become women (stability)
3. The realization that gender is permanent and not changed by cultural gender cues, such as hairstyle or clothing (constancy).

Very young children understand gender in simplistic terms that match their views of the world. For example, preschool-age girls may believe that they can grow up to be fathers. By the age of 5 or 6, children understand that gender is constant. Through observation and imitation, they learn which behaviors are socially and culturally appropriate for each gender. Cognitive theorists, such as Kohlberg, believe that children mimic the behaviors of same-sex parents because it helps them achieve self-identity. In contrast, learning theorists believe that children are motivated to imitate same-sex parents simply because parents reward this behavior (Masters et al., 1992).

Healthy sexual development depends on the availability of appropriate same-sex role models. Parental attitudes, behaviors, beliefs, and values first influence a child's sexual identity. Children receive verbal and nonverbal messages about how their parents view themselves and their own bodies. As children mature, use of proper vocabulary to describe body parts and functions may help to ensure ongoing effective communication about sexual issues between parents, children, and health providers (American Academy of Child & Adolescent Psychiatry, 2005; Masters et al., 1992).

During early childhood, sexual exploration takes the form of genital play. Parents' negative reactions to self-exploration can lead to feelings of guilt, shame, and a negative self-image. Rather than discouraging such behaviors, parents can instruct children to seek privacy for such exploration. The concept of appropriate versus inappropriate touching by others also needs to be clarified. Parents' general level of comfort with physical affection, the way they wash their children's genitals, and their responses to their children's genital exploration all provide signals to children about how they should feel about their own sexuality (American Academy of Child & Adolescent Psychiatry, 2005).

## Children with Disabilities

Sexual development of children who have congenital or early childhood–onset disabilities may be impacted by competing interests. The time and attention that typically developing children spend understanding the physical, emotional, and social aspects of sexual development may be consumed by more pressing issues related to medical and functional concerns in children with disabilities (Murphy & Elias, 2006). It also may be difficult or impossible for children with mobility problems to imitate the behaviors of the same-sex parent. Sensory impairment, bowel and bladder incontinence, and abnormal muscle tone may interfere with normal self-exploration, making it difficult for children to gain an early understanding of the anatomical and physiological functions of their bodies. The presence of cognitive impairment can further impact sexual development because it may alter interactions between the child and significant others.

Parents are often pessimistic regarding the potential of their children with disabilities to enjoy sexual intimacy in their relationships. They may believe their children will always be childlike, asexual, and in need of protection (Murphy & Elias, 2006). Pediatric health care providers can help parents understand the potential of their children by raising questions about sexuality and modeling appropriate sex education. Consider the approach taken by the Smiths' pediatrician. During their baby's recent visit to the Cerebral Palsy Clinic at a local teaching hospital, he offered the following:

> *Some parents who have a child with cerebral palsy wonder what it will be like when their child grows up. Do you ever wonder if he'll be able to have a sexual relationship or a family of his own? Would you like to spend some time talking about this? Perhaps I can help you identify some appropriate reference materials that you might find helpful.*

Murphy and Elias (2006) encourage pediatric specialists to help parents understand their children's unique needs. Parental concerns will vary, depending on their views of the impact of disability, as well as their own children's physical and cognitive abilities. An explicit plan to discuss development, maturity, and sexuality on a regular basis with parents (and eventually with the child) will help ease fears and dispel myths that children with developmental disabilities are not sexual beings. Parents need to understand the importance of encouraging their children to gain independence in self-care and effective social skills as early as possible to ensure safe and healthy sexual development that is in sync with that of peers.

Parents of children with disabilities may feel overwhelmed by the day-to-day responsibilities of caring for a child who has a disability. Health professionals can help by providing the support and resources parents need to manage all aspects of daily living, as well as helping them assume the role of their child's primary "sex ed." teacher. Family values, cultural traditions, and religious beliefs are important to healthy sexual development, and that information is most appropriately provided by family members.

## Child Sexual Abuse

Sexual abuse is a form of child abuse that involves interactions of a sexual nature between a child and an adult or older child, most commonly male. Overt sexual abuse may take the form of physical contact with genitalia, pressure to perform sexual acts, or use of the child as a subject in pornographic pictures or movies. Other abusers use more covert methods, such as cuddling for the purpose of sexual arousal, staring, glaring, or engaging the child in inappropriate dialogue about sexual matters. Most children who are abused know the person who has abused them, with one third of reported cases committed by family members (National Library of Medicine, 2010).

The long-term health effects on people who do not receive interventions for a history of childhood sexual abuse are significant and can include autoimmune disorders, such as fibromyalgia, irritable bowel syndrome, and asthma; disordered eating, such as anorexia nervosa, bulimia nervosa, and obesity; depression and other mood disorders; post-traumatic stress disorder; substance abuse or addictions; and other forms of maladaptive coping (Wilson, 2010).

Very few screening tools for assessing the risk of childhood sexual abuse have been published in the literature. However, Salvagni and Wagner (2006) developed a questionnaire that can be administered to parents of children ages 2 to 12. It is a 5-item survey of behavioral symptoms, including any abnormal curiosity about the genitals, fear of being left with a specific person, sudden emotional or behavioral changes, abandonment of previous play habits, and any history of injury to the anal or genital areas. This tool has significant limitations, including testing with a small sample size and the risk that the parent answering the questions is the actual abuser. Unfortunately, other potential indicators of abuse have not been able to distinguish differences between children who have a history of sexual abuse and those who do not. In spite of the limitations of standardized tools, health professionals are obligated to act on suspicions of child sexual abuse, making appropriate referrals to have suspected problems investigated for the good of the child. Details and resources are discussed in Chapter 15.

Children with disabilities are 3.4 times more likely to be sexually abused than their typically developing peers (Skarbek, Hahn, & Parrish, 2009). Pedophiles tend to seek vulnerable targets that are least likely to disclose the abuse. Therefore, it is particularly important to help parents understand the need to carefully screen child care providers, including personal care attendants, educational aides, and others who have close personal contact with their children and the opportunity to interact with them in private places. Parents also need to help their children learn to trust their instincts about any discomfort they feel toward particular care providers. Parents of children who use alternative or augmentative methods of communication, such as word boards or electronic devices, can be assisted in developing a warning system that is understood by parents and other trusted allies in the event that inappropriate sexual interactions have occurred.

## Later Childhood and Adolescence

Adolescence represents the most dramatic period in sexual development. Milestones of this period include achieving independence in thinking and problem solving, managing a wide range of emotions, and attaining the physical qualities necessary for reproduction (Murphy & Elias, 2006). The onset of puberty is brought about by a significant increase in sex hormones. Exciting physical and psychological changes occur as children of both genders experience rapid physical growth, maturation of the gonads and genitals, and the development of secondary sexual characteristics. Girls develop breasts and grow pubic and axillary hair. Boys experience increased muscle mass, growth of facial, pubic, and axillary hair, and deepening of the voice. Girls begin menstruation, and boys develop the ability to ejaculate, marking the onset of fertility. Hormonal changes are responsible for new sexual sensations and erotic thoughts and dreams in both boys and girls (Masters et al., 1992).

Sexual self-exploration continues, but more intimate interactions with partners emerge, including hand-holding, kissing, and other forms of physical closeness. These are early expressions of personal sexual identity and independent decision making. The extent to which adolescents experiment with sexual behavior varies according to the individual's personal readiness, moral reasoning, fear of consequences, level of romantic attachment to the partner, and peer pressure. It is also strongly affected by religious and cultural norms and prohibitions. Those who seek complete personal independence from parental influences are more likely to engage in early sexual intercourse. Interestingly, these teens are also more likely to experiment with drugs and alcohol, whereas adolescents who have learned about sex at an early age from well-informed parents are more likely to abstain until they are more mature (Masters et al., 1992).

Socially, adolescents experience many challenges, including developing progressive independence from parents, struggling to fit in with peers, and forming their own sets of values. While doing so, they must also cope with the rapid physical changes and enhanced sexual feelings previously described. Many adolescents have incomplete or inaccurate information about sex that may cause them to feel anxious about how normal they are. The changes associated with puberty are closely linked to the development of body image and self-concept. Adolescents are particularly concerned about physical attractiveness, and any perception of being different threatens their self-image (Masters et al., 1992). The influence of the media can be damaging, especially television, movies, and popular magazines, which place a premium on the young and beautiful, the strong and conspicuously muscled.

Discussions with adolescents should not assume heterosexuality. Sexual orientation of teens with disabilities and other chronic conditions is believed to be comparable to the general population. Therefore, any information made available should reference gay, lesbian, bisexual, or transgender information because clients who are in the midst of gay identity formation may be reluctant to ask questions directly. Individuals with disabilities who are wondering if they may have gay, lesbian, bisexual, or transgender orientations also have the challenge of negotiating the formation of two identities simultaneously. Little study of dual-identity formation of this type has been done, but Schulz (2009) discovered one study while conducting a comprehensive review of theories related to disability and sexuality. Conducted by Whitney (2006), the study utilized a multidimensional, nonlinear model to explain the process of dual-identity formation in lesbians with disabilities. The author used a conceptual framework introduced by Eliason (1996) to capture the stages of developing a lesbian identity. Based on four stages, individuals are seen as progressing or regressing as needed until identity is redefined and eventually developed. The four stages include (1) pre-identity, (2) emerging identities, (3) experiences and recognition of oppression and reevaluation, and (4) evolution of identities. Whitney found that the model worked well in the assessment of identity formation for lesbians with disabilities, but noted that the identity to develop earliest in life was the stronger, more positive identity than the one that emerged later (Schulz, 2009).

Adolescents who have chronic health conditions may need additional support and encouragement to develop a positive sense of self as a sexual person (Murphy & Elias, 2006). They face the same developmental tasks as their peers, but often have fewer opportunities to learn, practice, and perfect social skills. Body image and self-concept are often impaired, particularly if the disability is visible or if a wheelchair or other assistive technology is required (Anderson & Kitchin, 2000). Finding peer groups where they can fit in is extremely important because it is through group interactions that adolescents acquire sexual language, discuss sexual ideals, and form important relationships (Kelton, 1999).

Consider Tom, a 14-year-old boy with a diagnosis of Duchenne's muscular dystrophy. Until last year, he was able to walk around school independently. Now that he is in middle school, he requires the use of a wheelchair and occasional physical assistance from a personal aide. Although his classmates have been asked to "treat Tom like any other kid," this is not always practical. He is the only student in the school who uses a wheelchair. He is unable to pass through the busy halls during class changes without the assistance of his aide. In a recent conversation with his occupational therapist, Tom asked for ideas about how he could use his wheelchair to dance with a girl during the next school social. Without a peer group to model appropriate behavior, he had no idea how to begin to take social risks now that he required a wheelchair.

Adolescents who have disabilities tend to receive less formal sexual education than their peers. When they do receive information, the presented materials may not include disability-specific content. This is unfortunate because adolescents with chronic conditions are at least as sexually involved as their peers and significantly more likely to be sexually abused. It is critical to provide information regarding medically safe and appropriate contraception, reproduction, and genetics, as well as strategies for establishing appropriate personal boundaries (Swango-Wilson, 2009).

Evidence shows that adolescents who have disabilities are interested in discussing sexuality with their health care providers, but practitioners often fail to offer the opportunity because of underestimating clients' sexual concerns, lack of knowledge, embarrassment, or fear that the client will feel embarrassed (Reissing & Giulio, 2010; Zajicek-Farber, 1998). Missed opportunities to discuss and solve adolescents' sexual concerns increase the likelihood of impaired sexuality as development continues.

## Early Adulthood

Early adulthood marks the time when important lifestyle choices are made and increasing responsibilities are assumed with respect to relationships. Major developmental tasks of this period include attaining physical and psychological independence, beginning a career, and finding a lifelong partner. Developing effective interpersonal skills is paramount because the ability to share feelings is essential to developing healthy, intimate relationships. Couples must openly explore topics, including sex outside of marriage, pregnancy, the use of contraceptives, monogamy, sexually transmitted diseases, future plans, and parenthood.

Authors of a 10-year study examined the personal goals of 297 healthy, young adults to see how their personal goals changed from the time they were emerging young adults in college through the period following graduation. Participants completed personal analysis and life-event questionnaires at five points during the course of the study. Early goals, reflecting the time spent in college, were focused on friends, education, and travel. As graduation approached and roles changed, however, goals shifted to family, work, and health. Participants expressing more family-related goals were the most likely to get married and have children or live with their partners (Salmela-Aro, Aunola, & Nurmi, 2007).

Evidence suggests that young adults who choose to live together rather than commit to marriage may be at a higher risk for unhappy relationships. When compared to married couples, people who live together are more likely to have lower quality and unstable relationships (Brown, 2000), are more likely to become depressed (Brown, 2000), and have a higher incidence of alcohol abuse (Horwitz & White, 1998). For these reasons, the choice of cohabitation in lieu of marriage may be particularly dangerous for young adults who have disabilities. The confluence of all potential negative influences could be overwhelming. Young adults who have disabilities are more likely than their counterparts without disabilities to have insecurities related to the unpredictability of their daily lives, their sexuality, and their ability to form intimate relationships (Ostlie, Johansson, & Moller, 2009; Voll, Krumm, & Fichtner, 1999). Consider the case of Mary Ellen, described in the journal entry below:

I have been working with Mary Ellen over the last week. She was admitted to the hospital after she had a significant flare-up of symptoms related to her diagnosis of juvenile rheumatoid arthritis. She's had a really tough time, and I can relate to it to some degree because we are the same age, we both live with our boyfriends, and we even have the same kind of dog! The biggest difference is that she has to deal with all of this pain and the uncertainty of knowing how she'll feel each day. Like me, she's in her last semester of college and trying to keep up with all of the work so she can graduate in June. She wants to move on with her life, but it's hard for her to see where's she's going from here. She worries that no one will hire her because of her diagnosis, that her boyfriend will leave her for someone else, and that she'll have to move back home with her parents. I feel so bad for her!
—*From the journal of Samantha Wong, occupational therapy student*

Mary Ellen's fears are grounded in the reality of living with a chronic illness. The commitment of marriage and the vows "to love and honor, in sickness and in health" are likely to have more significant meaning to her than they will to young adults who enter into lifetime relationships with their health intact.

## Middle Adulthood

The middle-aged adult generally enjoys a time of sexual freedom and comfort. Most adults have established careers and families and can now spend more time and energy focused on themselves and their partners. Previous sexual experiences allow for more open and realistic sexual relationships. However, this is also an age when many adults begin to question their sexual attractiveness because of age-related changes. Reflection on past accomplishments and setting future goals are common themes. Identity and role confusion can occur and may give rise to a midlife crisis (Masters et al., 1992).

Men seem to be more vulnerable to midlife crises than women. When men begin to question their sexual abilities and attractiveness, they are likely to experience sexual performance difficulties, which only adds to the crisis. In contrast, women often experience midlife as a time of self-discovery, enjoying unprecedented sexual openness that they were too inhibited to enjoy when they were younger, especially if they had children to raise or were concerned about getting pregnant. However, women are not immune to the physical changes associated with aging (Masters et al., 1992).

Perimenopause generally begins when women reach their 40s, and menopause is usually completed by age 55. The timing and symptoms vary, but most women will experience at least minor problems related to declining levels of hormones. Vaginal changes have the most significant effect on the sexual relationship at this time. Lower estrogen levels cause a reduction in vaginal elasticity and lubrication, which can cause pain during sexual intercourse. These problems can generally be eliminated with artificial lubricants or estrogen replacement. If a couple enjoys a loving and supportive relationship, they tend to discover means to adjust to age-related changes. Those who are unwilling to commit time or emotional energy to their relationships are more likely to experience waning sexual interest, seek extramarital affairs, or divorce during this time (Masters et al., 1992). The incidence of divorce rises dramatically during this period of life, from approximately 10 percent of people in their 30s to 40 percent of people in their 50s (U.S. Bureau of the Census, 2007).

The onset of an illness or disability during this period may complicate midlife challenges. Rather than enjoying each other's company, the couple must adjust to changes associated with the illness or disability. Sexual changes associated with this phase of development may be exacerbated, along with the emergence of new problems associated with the specific illness or disability encountered, as illustrated by Mr. Michaels in the journal entry at the beginning of this chapter.

## Older Adulthood

I met with the Arnolds today to discuss their discharge plan. As a routine question, I asked if either of them had any concerns about resuming their sexual relationship. Mrs. Arnold became flustered and got red in the face. She sputtered something that sounded like "those days are over." Mr. Arnold simply looked away. Since Mrs. Arnold was clearly upset and embarrassed, I dropped the issue and finished the meeting. As I continued my rounds, Mrs. Arnold's reaction bothered me. I waited until her husband left the room, then returned to talk with her. This time, I started by acknowledging her obvious discomfort with the subject and asked her if she had any questions or concerns that I might be able to address. Although she was still noticeably uncomfortable, she confided that she couldn't imagine how sexual intercourse would be possible in light of all the precautions she has to follow to avoid dislocating her new hip. We spent some time discussing alternative positioning and precautions. As we talked, she appeared more relaxed and at ease. She assured me that Mr. Arnold would be forever in my debt!

*—From the journal of Mitzy Riley, nursing student*

## BOX 12–1  Conditions Affecting Sexual Activity in Older People

**Psychosocial Changes**

- Depression
- Poor self-concept

- Social isolation
- Poverty

**Diabetic Changes**

- Vascular problems
- Erectile dysfunction

- Orgasmic impairment
- Neuropathies

**Hormonal/Medication Effects**

- Reduced testosterone
- Hyperthyroidism
- Hypothyroidism

- Fatigue
- Erectile dysfunction
- Premature or retrograde ejaculation

**Cardiopulmonary/Mobility Impairments**

- Arteriosclerosis
- Decreased cardiac output
- Dyspnea on exertion

- Arthritis
- Postsurgical limitations
- Paralysis

*Source:* Mooradian (1991).

Older adulthood is characterized by numerous physical and mental changes and can also be emotionally difficult. Many older adults retire from their professional positions, which can lead to identity confusion. They are also burdened with the decline of physical and mental functions and are confronted with the real possibility of their own death and the death of their partners and significant others (d'Epinay, Cavalli, & Guillet, 2009).

Declining health is one of the main problems associated with reduced sexual activity among older people. Older adults of both sexes are more likely to take medications, have chronic diseases, and undergo surgery. Box 12–1 outlines the most common problems experienced by older adults. When designing any intervention for sexual dysfunction for this age group—whether educational, functional, or medical—information about common age-related problems should be considered.

Contrary to popular belief, age and declining health do not necessarily eliminate the desire or ability to engage in sexual relationships or activities. In their ground-breaking work on sexuality, Kinsey, Pomeroy, and Martin (1948) concluded that people continue sexual interest and activity well into old age. This finding has been supported by many others (Brecher, 1984; Bretschneider & McCoy, 1988; Langer, 2009; McKinlay & Brambilla, 1993; Wiley & Bortz, 1996). However, age-related changes do call for adaptations to ensure continued enjoyment and satisfaction (Blümel, Del Pino, Aprikian, Vallejo, & Castelo-Branco, 2008; Drench & Losee, 1996).

The physical changes that began earlier during menopause can persist into older age for some women, which can negatively affect physical and psychological aspects of sexuality. Medical treatment can help to abate some of the problems associated with aging. For example, in their study of sexual function and quality of life among postmenopausal women, Blümel and coworkers (2008) found that hormone replacement therapy significantly improved vasomotor, psychological, and physical aspects of sexual functioning, when compared to a control group that did not receive hormone therapy. Like all medications, however, hormone replacement therapy can be accompanied by undesired side effects and should be considered carefully to assess potential risks and benefits, especially if the patient has other medical problems.

Although men also face psychosocial concerns related to aging and sexuality, they tend to focus their attention on the physical aspects of sexual dysfunction. They are more likely to experience more overt physical changes, including the need for longer and more direct stimulation to achieve erection, a reduction in the amount of semen, less intense sensations with ejaculation, and a longer recovery period after ejaculation before repeat ejaculation can occur (McCarthy & Metz, 2008a). Erectile dysfunction can initiate a pattern of negativity involving expectation of failure, avoidance, and withdrawal. This can lead to blaming and anger in relationships, unless the couple is able to communicate freely about needs and desires and consider other sexually satisfying alternatives to intercourse (Melby, 2010).

Irman and colleagues (2009) studied erectile dysfunction (ED), which is one of the most common sexual problems experienced by older men. The prevalence of ED increases with age, affecting 5 to 10 percent of men at age 40 and climbing to 40 to 60 percent by age 70. Although it can occur in the absence of other physical problems, ED is often associated with certain medications and the presence of a number of cardiovascular risk factors, including diabetes, obesity, and smoking. Further, ED appears to be a significant predictor of coronary artery disease, and for this reason, the potential functional benefits of medications like Viagra should be carefully weighed against its known risks and side effects.

Alternatives to medical interventions have begun to emerge in an effort to counteract the social influences that discount the importance of psychosocial factors affecting male sexuality. An example is a 12-step intervention called the "Good Enough Sex" model (McCarthy & Metz, 2008b), which encourages couples to expand the range of activities they associate with sexual intimacy, including cuddling and erotic play. Programs such as this are capable of directly helping participants, but also may help change society's strongly held stereotypes that lead men to devalue other characteristics of masculinity, including being seen as a man of honor, being in control of one's own life, having the respect of friends, having a good job, and coping with problems on one's own. A randomly selected, multinational sample of 27,839 men, ages 20 to 27, consistently rated these characteristics above having an active sex life, being physically attractive, and having success with women (Sand et al., 2008).

## CLINICAL INTERVENTIONS

Today I attended a group therapy session that involved clients and their partners. Of all things, the topic was sexuality. All of the clients had experienced strokes. Some were several years post-stroke, while others had only been living with the consequences of their strokes for a short time. I was a little surprised when I learned what the meeting was going to be about because all of the clients were well over age 65. I didn't expect the kind of discussion that ensued. They were talking about everything from extending the use of foreplay to ensure adequate vaginal lubrication to modifying positions needed to accommodate unilateral extremity weakness. At the end of the session, couples were discussing plans for practicing some of the techniques discussed. I was so impressed with their openness with each other. I never realized that people in this age group had the same sexual needs and desires that I do. I certainly have a new appreciation for my older clients now.

*—From the journal of Stephanie Ducey, social work student*

Clients are extremely sensitive to the perceived and actual attitudes of health care practitioners. For this reason, it is particularly important to become aware of our *own* biases, beliefs, and need for additional education before attempting to help clients with *their* concerns about sexuality (Drench & Losee, 1996). Health care providers are not immune to prejudices and misconceptions. Remember that a particularly common myth is that older adults or people with disabilities either have no sexual needs or desires or have excessive or perverted needs and desires (Anderson & Kitchin, 2000). Even when educated to the contrary, many providers remain influenced by their own experiences and still have difficulty understanding and accepting the needs of their clients (Eliason & Raheim, 2000). In addition, many practitioners fail to discuss sexuality with their clients because of their own embarrassment or lack of knowledge and the fear that their clients will be embarrassed (Reissing & Giulio, 2010).

As illustrated in the journal entry above, accurate practitioner knowledge is associated with more positive attitudes about the sexuality of clients (Kelton, 1999). Practitioners who understand that their clients have sexual needs can help them accommodate to changes of age, illness, and disability. Education can also help providers become more comfortable with sexuality, making it easier to facilitate discussions with clients.

Recognizing that many health professionals are uncomfortable addressing sexual issues with their clients, Kelton (1999) suggests a four-step approach to sexuality education:

1. Initiate a program of self-learning about sexuality by reading books and accessing other resources specific to the needs of the client population being treated.
2. Raise the consciousness of other members of the team by asking questions related to the impact that medications or other proposed treatments may have on sexual function and fertility.
3. Become comfortable discussing issues of sexuality with clients. Begin with topics that are easier for the clients to discuss and move toward more personal, intimate topics as clients invite you into their more private realms. Use correct scientific terms rather than jargon or street language to maintain professional boundaries, but be prepared to offer alternate terminology if confusion is evident.
4. Document the topics discussed and create a written plan for the future. It is not necessary to discuss sexuality during every interaction nor is it appropriate to cover every aspect of sexuality in a single visit.

Resources related to sexuality are included among the additional readings listed in the online student workbook that accompanies this text. Readers may find these resources helpful for their own education. Providers should review sources before recommending them to individual clients. By doing so, resources that respect individual beliefs, values, and preferences can be selected.

Education can help providers develop knowledge, but a true sensitivity and respect for the individual needs of each client is required in order to avoid imposing our own values. By obtaining a thorough history that reflects the client's beliefs, morals, and personal preferences, recommendations can be "tailor-made" to fit each client.

## Taking a Sexual History

Mrs. O'Leary was referred to physical therapy for lymphedema management. As she was reporting her social history to me today, she began to weep. Although she and her husband have always enjoyed an open and satisfying sexual relationship, she has been avoiding any intimate contact with him. She said that Mr. O'Leary is very supportive and has approached her many times just to "cuddle and be close," but she just has no interest. Her left upper extremity is "ugly and swollen," and she still can't bear to look at the mastectomy site. I thought she seemed pretty open to suggestions, and I offered ideas that would help her progress to more intimate contact with her husband. She seemed so relieved when she left. As we talked, she remembered that one of the nurses made some of the same suggestions before the surgery, but at the time, she really didn't think they applied to her. Because of the close relationship she and her husband had always enjoyed, she never expected any of these problems.

*—From the journal of Maria Menendez, physical therapist student*

A sexual history can be taken in conjunction with the medical and social history. It is best to begin with nonthreatening information and move toward more intimate details. This progressive approach to history taking provides an opportunity for clients to share verbal and nonverbal feedback that establishes boundaries based on their comfort level (Drench & Losee, 1996; Shell & Miller, 1999).

Health care practitioners need to remember to remain objective, nonjudgmental, and sensitive throughout the discussion. Clients need to believe that the information they are sharing will remain confidential. Embarrassment is a common barrier. It may be more comfortable for some clients to respond in writing. Many published questionnaires can be used to obtain information about sexual concerns, fears, and preferences (Davis, Yarber, Bauseman, Schreer, & Davis, 1998; McCabe, Cummins, & Deeks, 1999). Written responses can then be used as the basis for discussion.

Practitioners need to refrain from judging clients based on their own beliefs and values about what is normal or abnormal, right or wrong. Each client has his or her own value system, and caution must be taken to respect individual differences. Consider the client's and his or her partner's cultural, social, sexual, and religious orientations. What is perceived to be moral and right varies according to these factors. What one client will find to be an acceptable expression of sexuality, another may find abhorrent (Martin Hilber et al., 2010; Whitehead, 2010).

There may or may not be a need to focus attention on sexuality and sexual function during the examination or treatment session. The subject can be presented along with other functional issues in a matter-of-fact manner. Clients who trust their health care practitioners will be open to counseling and assistance. It is important that they know that this subject can remain open for future discussion. Some clients may be initially reluctant to discuss sexuality and sexual function. However, if given another opportunity, they may decide to accept the invitation to discuss their concerns.

## Summary

Sexuality is an integral component of health. Until recently, health care practitioners have overlooked this component of wellness, particularly for their clients who are older than 60 or those who have chronic health conditions. In this chapter, we discussed the importance of addressing clients' sexuality, regardless of their age or physical abilities. The stages of sexual development were presented, and the impact of disability or illness discussed. Evidence exists that not all health care providers have the knowledge needed to effectively address the sexual needs of their clients. Guidelines for professional development were outlined. A sensitive, progressive approach for obtaining a sexual history was described.

## Reflective Questions

1. Reflect on the cultural, religious, family, and social influences in your life.
   a. How have these shaped your attitudes, beliefs, and values about sexuality?
   b. How have these shaped your beliefs and comfort level when discussing sexuality with clients?
2. What do you believe are your responsibilities for discussing issues of sexuality with clients?
3. Consider gender identity, attractiveness, sexual attitudes and beliefs, and sexual behaviors and practices. How might each of the following conditions affect these aspects of a person's sexuality?
   a. a congenital disability, such as spina bifida
   b. a progressive disorder, such as multiple sclerosis
   c. an acute onset of lower extremity amputation
   d. end-stage renal disease
   e. a painful condition that limits mobility, such as rheumatoid arthritis
4. What strategies might you use to discuss sexuality with someone whose opinions, beliefs, and attitudes are different from your own?
5. a. How do *you* differentiate between sexuality and sexual function?
   b. Provide examples to support your beliefs.

## Case Study

Lucy Bluecreek is a 13-year-old girl with a hearing impairment. She recently received a new hearing aid that markedly improves her ability to hear, but it is significantly larger than her previous one. Lucy feels embarrassed about wearing the new hearing aid, feeling certain that everyone notices it. Her parents made her promise that she would wear it at school, but she often removes it, especially when she's in the company of boys.

1. Discuss the developmental factors that are likely to be influencing Lucy's feelings and behaviors.
2. How and why might Lucy's perspective be changed if a boy that she liked asked her to go out with him?
3. In what ways might Lucy's response to this new device be different if she were a student about to graduate from college? A middle-aged woman who was married with children? Explain the reason(s) for the differences.
4. If you were Lucy's teacher and were aware of her apparent discomfort with this new device, what kind of interventions might you suggest?

## References

American Academy of Child & Adolescent Psychiatry. (2005). Talking to your kids about sex. *Facts for Families*, No. 62. Retrieved from http://www.aacap.org/cs/root/facts_for_families/talking_to_your_kids_about_sex

Anderson, P., & Kitchin, R. (2000). Disability, space, and sexuality: Access to family planning services. *Social Science and Medicine, 51*, 1163–1173.

Blümel, J., Del Pino, M., Aprikian, D., Vallejo, S., Sarrá, S., & Castelo-Branco, C. (2008). Effect of androgens combined with hormone therapy on quality of life in post-menopausal women with sexual dysfunction. *Gynecological Endocrinology, 24*(12), 691–695.

Brecher, E. (1984). *Love, sex, and aging.* Boston, MA: Little, Brown.

Bretschneider, J., & McCoy, N. (1988). Sexual interest and behavior in healthy 80–102 year olds. *Annals of Sex Behavior, 17,* 108–129.

Brown, S. L. (2000). The effect of union type on psychological well-being: Depression of cohabitants versus married. *Journal of Health and Social Behavior, 41,* 241–255.

Davis, C. M., Yarber, W. L., Bauseman, R., Schreer, G., & Davis, S. L. (1998). *Handbook of sexually-related measures.* Thousand Oaks, CA: Sage.

d'Epinay, C., Cavalli, S., & Guillet, L. (2009). Bereavement in very old age: Impact on health and relationships of the loss of a spouse, a child, a sibling, or a close friend. *Omega: Journal of Death & Dying, 60*(4), 301–325.

Drench, M. E., & Losee, R. H. (1996). Sexuality and sexual capacities of elderly people. *Rehabilitation Nursing, 21*(3), 118–122.

Eliason, M. J. (1996). Identify formation for lesbian, bisexual and gay persons: Beyond a "minoritizing" view. *Journal of Homosexuality, 30,* 31–57.

Eliason, M. J., & Raheim, S. (2000). Experiences and comfort with culturally diverse groups in undergraduate pre-nursing students. *Journal of Nursing Education, 39*(4), 161–165.

Hoffman, R. M., Hattie, J. A., & Borders, L. D. (2005). Personal definitions of masculinity and femininity as an aspect of gender self-concept. *Journal of Humanistic Counseling Education and Development, 44*(1), 66–84.

Horwitz, A. V., & White, H. R. (1998). The relationship of cohabitation and mental health: A longitudinal study of a young adult cohort. *Journal of Marriage and the Family, 60,* 505–514.

Irman, B., Sauver, J., Jacobson, D., McGree, M., Nehra, A., & Lieber, M. (2009). A population-based, longitudinal study of erectile dysfunction and future coronary artery disease. *Mayo Clinic Proceedings, 84*(2), 108–113.

Johansen, T. H., Ripa, C. P., Mortensen, E. L., & Main, K. M. (2006). Quality of life in 70 women with disorders of sexual development. *European Journal of Endocrinology, 155,* 877–885.

Kelton, S. (1999). Sexuality education for youth with chronic conditions. *Pediatric Nursing, 25*(5), 491.

Kinsey, A. C., Pomeroy, W. B., & Martin, C. E. (1948). Age and sexual outlet. In A. Kinsey, W. Pomeroy, & C. Martin, *Sexual behavior in the human male* (pp. 218–262). Philadelphia, PA: W. B. Saunders.

Kohlberg, L. (1966). A cognitive-developmental analysis of children's sex-role concepts and attitudes. In E. Maccoby (Ed.), *The development of sex differences* (pp. 82–172). Stanford, CA: Stanford University Press.

Langer, N. (2009). Late life love and intimacy. *Educational Gerontology, 35*(8), 752–764.

Lee, P. A., Houk, C. P., Ahmed, S. F., & Hughes, I. A. (2006). Consensus statement on management of intersex disorders. *Pediatrics, 118,* e488–e500.

Martin Hilber, A., Hull, T., Preston-Whyte, E., Bagnol, B., Smit, J., & Wacharasin, C. (2010). A cross cultural study of vaginal practices and sexuality: Implications for sexual health. *Social Science & Medicine, 70*(3), 392–400.

Masters, W. H., Johnson, V. E., & Kolodny, R. C. (1992). *Human sexuality* (4th ed.). New York, NY: HarperCollins.

McCabe, M. P., Cummins, R. A., & Deeks, A. A. (1999). Construction and psychometric properties of sexuality scales: Sex knowledge, experience and needs scales for people with intellectual disabilities (SexKen-ID), people with physical disabilities (SexKen-PD), and the general population (SexKen-GP). *Research in Developmental Disabilities, 20*(4), 241–254.

McCarthy, B. W., & Metz, M. E. (2008a). *Men's sexual health: Fitness for satisfying sex.* New York, NY: Routledge.

McCarthy, B. W., & Metz, M. E. (2008b). The "Good-Enough Sex" model: A case illustration. *Sexual & Relationship Therapy, 23*(3), 227–234.

McKinlay, J. B., & Brambilla, D. (1993). Where do we go from here? Disentangling aging processes from the processes of aging. In J. Schroots (Ed.), *Aging, health, and competence* (pp. 223–242). New York, NY: Elsevier.

Melby, T. (2010). What's it mean to be a man? *Contemporary Sexuality, 44*(2), 1–5.

Mooradian, A. D. (1991). Geriatric sexuality and chronic diseases. *Geriatric Sexuality, 7*(1), 113–131.

Murphy, N. A., & Elias, E. R. (2006). Sexuality of children and adolescents with developmental disabilities. *Pediatrics, 118*(1), 398–403.

National Library of Medicine. (2010). Child sexual abuse. *Medline Plus.* Retrieved from http://www.nlm.nih.gov/medlineplus/print/childsexualabuse.html

Ostlie, I., Johansson, I., & Moller, A. (2009). Struggle and adjustment to an insecure everyday life and an unpredictable life course. *Disability & Rehabilitation, 31*(8), 666–674.

Reissing, E., & Giulio, G. (2010). Practicing clinical psychologists' provision of sexual health care services. *Professional Psychology: Research and Practice, 41*(1), 57–63.

Salmela-Aro, K., Aunola, K., & Nurmi, J. (2007). Personal goals during emerging adulthood: A 10-year follow up. *Journal of Adolescent Research, 22*(6), 670–715.

Salvagni, E. P., & Wagner, M. B. (2006). Development of a questionnaire for the assessment of sexual abuse in children and estimation of its discriminate validity: A case-control study. *Jornal de Pediatria (Rio J), 6,* 431–436.

Sand, M. S., Fisher, R. C., Rosen, R., Heiman, J., & Eardley, I. (2008). Erectile dysfunction and constructs of masculinity and quality of life in the multinational Men's Attitudes to Life Events and Sexuality (MALES) study. *Journal of Sexual Medicine, 5,* 583–594.

Schulz, S. L. (2009). Psychological theories of disability and sexuality: A literature review. *Journal of Human Behavior in the Social Environment, 19,* 58–69.

Shell, J. A., & Miller, M. E. (1999). The cancer amputee and sexuality. *Orthopedic Nursing, 18*(5), 53.

Skarbek, D., Hahn, K., & Parrish, P. (2009). Stop sexual abuse in special education: An ecological model of prevention and intervention strategies for sexual abuse in special education. *Sexuality & Disability, 27*(3), 155–164.

Swango-Wilson, A. (2009). Perception of sex education for individuals with developmental and cognitive disability: A four cohort study. *Sexuality & Disability, 27*(4), 223–228.

U.S. Bureau of the Census. (2007). *Detailed tables–Number, timing, and duration of marriages and divorces: 2004.* Retrieved from http://www.census.gov/population/www/socdemo/marrdiv/2004detailed_tables.html.

Voll, R., Krumm, B., & Fichtner, H. J. (1999). Demand for psychosocial counseling of young wheelchair users. *International Journal of Rehabilitation Research, 22,* 119–122.

Whitehead, A. (2010). Sacred rites and civil rights: Religion's effect on attitudes toward same-sex unions and the perceived cause of homosexuality. *Social Science Quarterly, 91*(1), 63–79.

Whitney, C. (2006). Intersections in identity—identity development among queer women with disabilities. *Sexuality and Disability, 24*(1), 39–52.

Wiley, D., & Bortz, W. M., II. (1996). Sexuality and aging—usual and successful. *Journal of Gerontology, 51A*(3), M142–M146.

Wilson, D. (2010). Health consequences of childhood sexual abuse. *Perspectives in Psychiatric Care, 46*(1), 56–64.

World Health Organization. (2010). *Gender and human rights.* Retrieved from http://www.who.int/reproductivehealth/topics/gender_rights/sexual_health/en/print.html

Zajicek-Farber, M. (1998). Promoting good health in adolescents with disabilities. *Health and Social Work, 23*(3), 203–213.

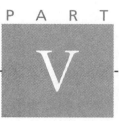

P A R T

V

# Conditions That Challenge Care

CHAPTER

# 13

# Psychiatric Disorders

I am very worried about one of the clients that we have been seeing in the clinic where I am doing my current rotation. She has very low energy and complains that she is always fatigued. Blood work and other physical findings have all come back within normal limits. Although she has a great family who participates in many activities, she no longer has any interest in them. It seems all she wants to do is hang around the house and watch television. When we suggested that she take a daily walk or join the local Y, she agreed but never followed-through.

—*From the journal of Judy Goldstein, nursing student*

Historically, health care providers divided illness into two broad but distinct categories: medical or physical illnesses, which affect the body and its organs, and mental or psychiatric disorders, which affect the mind or emotions. This simplistic division of illness has disappeared because evidence indicates that psychiatric disorders create pain and dysfunction of the body, and medical conditions can affect the brain in ways that create illnesses, such as depression or anxiety. Further, we know from Chapter 4 that the mind and body function as a unified whole. Separating disorders of the body and mind does not recognize the effects that medical and psychiatric illnesses have on the client's course of illness and recovery.

"Mental illness can be defined as a disturbance in an individual's thinking, emotions, behaviors, and physiology" (Glod, 1998, p. 9). It negatively affects mood and feelings, cognition, social interactions, and life-sustaining functions, such as eating, sleeping, focus and attention, and monitoring the environment for safety. There are times when we all experience some of the symptoms of various mental illnesses. For example, some of us may be "compulsive" about keeping our home and workspaces neat. Others may get "nervous" about tests or an important social event. Feeling sad or blue happens to everyone from time to time. However, in order for symptoms to reach a level of pathology, they must significantly impair the individual's ability to function effectively at work and social settings, consistent with cultural norms.

To further complicate things, cultural norms affect how people understand the symptoms of illness and the meanings assigned to them. "Indeed, evidence exists that even the specific symptoms associated with such psychiatric conditions as depression show impressive cultural variability" (Karp & Sisson, 2010, p. 12). Some cultures lack a word for depression, and others, such as the Chinese, express symptoms as physical rather than emotional. For Native Americans, it is considered normal to hear and speak to dead ancestors (Mahan, 2006). To provide optimal care for individuals from ethnocultural minorities who have mental illnesses, we must understand and accommodate their beliefs. For example, 63 percent of African Americans believe that depression is caused by personal weakness, and two thirds believe that the most effective form of treatment is prayer (Mahan, 2006). For ethnic groups with collectivist belief systems, conforming to the norms of the group and including their opinions and desires are essential components of care, even superseding what individuals might think is best for themselves. Unfortunately, this often deters people from seeking care and contributes to higher drop-out rates (Whitley, 2009).

Currently, close to 400 psychiatric conditions are included in the *Diagnostic and Statistical Manual of Mental Disorders, fourth edition, text revision* (*DSM-IV-TR*; American Psychiatric Association [APA], 2000). Although some controversy exists about the accuracy of labeling these conditions, there is no doubt that all cause distress to the affected individual and his or her family and friends. Over the course of each year, approximately 22 percent of Americans will have a diagnosable mental disorder, the most common being anxiety disorders, impulse control disorders, mood disorders, and substance abuse (Williams, Chapman, & Lando, 2005). These disorders affect people of all ages, racial and ethnic groups, and all income levels. However, many affected individuals will have a mild form of an illness or an illness that is not severe enough to cause disablement. When the symptoms of a psychiatric disorder are severe enough to significantly limit participation in functional activities, they are considered Serious and Persistent Mental Illness (McDevitt & Wilbur, 2006). Approximately 6 percent of Americans are diagnosed with these conditions (Kiraly, Gunning, & Leiser, 2008). It is important to recognize and diagnose all mental health conditions because they can be effectively treated. With appropriate care, many clients can manage their illnesses and enjoy a good quality of life. Without proper attention, however, they can be lethal disorders. Psychiatric disorders present an array of symptoms that range from very mild to sufficiently severe to warrant hospitalization for safety.

Our goal in discussing these challenging conditions is to provide an awareness of common diagnostic features and the importance of recognition and treatment. This will enable you to recognize symptoms that may explain your clients' failure to make progress in treatment, lack of motivation, and "odd" or troubling behaviors. In this chapter, we discuss only mood disorders (depression and bipolar disorder) and anxiety disorders, including post-traumatic stress disorder, because these disorders account for the majority of the cases of illness (Kinnier, Hofsess, Pongratz, & Lambert, 2009).

## CAUSES

Mental disorders are now understood to be diseases of the brain. This is a remarkable transformation from the not-so-distant past when people who were seriously ill were believed to be possessed by demons or cursed by gods. In the middle of the 20th century, inadequate parenting was believed to be the cause, and families were routinely blamed for their loved one's illness. Current research indicates that complex interactions take place between inherited genetic vulnerabilities and environmental triggers (Caspi et al., 2003; Glod, 1998; Hariri et al., 2002). For example, researchers have identified an abnormal variation of a gene that controls the production of a serotonin transporter. A study that focused on this gene followed 847 people for a period of 5 years, asking them to record adverse life stresses, such as a breakup of a relationship, loss of a job, loss of a loved one, or prolonged illness. Among the people who experienced four or more life stresses, 17 percent with two normal transporter genes developed depression, whereas 43 percent with two abnormal variations became depressed (Caspi et al., 2003). Other evidence has shown that people who are routinely exposed to high levels of stress, such as those with low socioeconomic status who live in a poor neighborhood or are routinely exposed to violence, also have increased levels of depression. We also know that a clear causal link exists between severe life-threatening events and post-traumatic stress disorder (PTSD). Abnormal gene variations have also been linked to anxiety (Hariri et al., 2002).

## BURDEN OF ILLNESS

"Mental disorders account for approximately 25 percent of disability in the United States, Canada and Western Europe and are a leading cause of premature death" (Williams et al., 2005, p. 2293). These disorders typically emerge in adolescence and early adult life and persist for many years, impacting education, work life, and parenting and causing a tremendous illness burden world-wide (Wells & Miranda, 2007). People with psychiatric disorders typically present with physical, as well as emotional or cognitive, symptoms. For example, they may have neck or back pain, severe headaches, gastrointestinal distress, chest pain, or insomnia. In addition, there is a high rate of co-occurring medical diagnoses (Steer, Cavalieri, Leonard, & Beck, 1999).

These physical and emotional symptoms may create significant barriers to diagnosing these conditions because people generally see their primary care provider (PCP) first when they do not feel well. The diagnostic focus typically turns to the diagnosis of the physical symptoms without consideration of a co-occurring mental health condition. As we mentioned in Chapter 5, an important part of the client interview is learning about how people are doing in all aspects of their lives so that a complete picture of their health can be determined. An accurate assessment and diagnosis of illness depends on the client's truthfulness, ability to communicate, and cooperation, as well as the skill of the health professional. The stigma and shame associated with mental illness often prevent an individual from disclosing suspicious symptoms, even when they cause significant distress. Although depression is a common psychiatric disorder with effective interventions, only one-half of individuals with depression seek care for their illness, and only 42 percent of those who do seek help receive adequate care (Kessler et al., 2003). Therefore, we are likely to see many clients with undiagnosed mental health conditions who come to us for treatment of their somatic symptoms. Unless we are able to identify these and assist the client to get additional care, the symptoms will not fully respond to our intervention.

People with mental illness have poorer health than people without these disorders. They also experience an increased prevalence of asthma, diabetes, arthritis, obesity, and cardiovascular disease (Kiraly et al., 2008). For example, nearly 50 percent of people with asthma or cancer have depression, and it is twice as frequent in people with diabetes, compared with those who do not have it (Chapman, Perry, & Strine, 2005). Forty percent of clients with cardiovascular disease also have depression (Steer et al., 1999). Conversely, medical conditions or disabilities can trigger mental illness and mask symptoms that might herald the need for treatment. An additional factor in the poor health of people with mental illness is that they are more likely to smoke, use drugs or alcohol, be overweight, have a sedentary lifestyle, and are less likely to receive preventive health care (Kiraly et al., 2008).

People with mental illness are also more likely to engage in high-risk behaviors, which can lead to accidents, injuries, and unsafe sex. In a study of youth in juvenile detention, more than 70 percent of the girls and 65 percent of the boys had one or more psychiatric disorders. They were also significantly more likely to have substance abuse disorders (Abram, Teplin, McClelland, & Dulcan, 2003). Another very significant factor in these adverse outcomes may be partly due to clients with mental illness being three times more likely not to adhere to medical interventions and recommendations (DiMatteo, Lepper, & Groghan, 2000).

When mental illness coexists with other medical problems, it can affect the onset, progression, and outcome of those disorders, increasing both morbidity and mortality (Chapman et al., 2005; Williams et al., 2005). Some mental illnesses, such as depression, have been proven to affect multiple organ systems, including the endocrine, cardiovascular, and immune systems (Insel & Charney, 2003). Having a psychiatric disorder with a physical condition can complicate the care of both conditions. Screening for mental illnesses may not occur as routinely as it should. For example, despite evidence of a high correlation between low back pain and depression that results in a poor treatment outcome, many clients are not screened for depression. A study of physical therapists in Australia, who are able to treat clients without physician referral, revealed that they did not recognize the presence of depressive symptoms, even when the symptoms were more distinctive (Haggman, Maher, & Refshauge, 2004). When the researchers screened for depressive symptoms, 40 percent of the clients tested positive, with 23 percent having severe or extremely severe depression. Furthermore, most of these clients' illnesses had gone unnoticed by their primary care providers.

A confounding factor in the assessment and treatment of people with mental illness is that many disorders are episodic. A person may experience significant periods of remission with high levels of function, followed by periods of exacerbation. Personal stress and challenging life events may precipitate or trigger a recurrence of symptoms. This reinforces a belief that the individual is not really "ill" but rather is using the symptoms to avoid work or other responsibilities. For many health care providers, it is easier to feel empathy for a client with arthritis, who has swollen and, apparently, painful joints, than for a client with severe depression whose pain is "invisible." It is even more difficult to feel empathy toward clients who refuse your care or get angry at you for not treating them satisfactorily.

## DEPRESSION

For many years, we have known that depression was common in clients treated in medical and rehabilitation settings. We assumed that the depression was a result of their physical condition or injury. After all, who would not be depressed following a spinal cord injury or heart attack? However, we now know that depression may be present premorbidly, that is, before the current injury, or may occur as a result of the medical condition (Chapman et al., 2005). In addition, secondary to the depression, the clients may behave in ways that put them at risk for injury, such as driving recklessly or abusing substances.

Depression is not synonymous with sadness or grief. As we discussed in Chapter 7, grieving is the normal, but variable, response to a loss. It can be the loss of a loved one, loss of something that is of significant importance to the individual, such as a job or home, or loss of function due to illness or injury. Grief is a normal part of the mourning process, and the individual who is grieving may demonstrate profound sadness and hopelessness (Weisman, 1998). This is often painful for friends or health care providers to witness. Someone who is experiencing "normal" grief, though, does not express a sense of worthlessness, severe guilt, or a desire to die. These are signs of depression. As health care providers, our response to those who are grieving is to listen compassionately and validate their feelings, without trying to mitigate their distress or "cheer them up." Over time, the mourning process usually ends, and the individual will, hopefully, be able to integrate the experience and resume previous life activities.

Psychiatrists use the terms *clinical depression, major depressive disorder* (MDD), or *unipolar depression* to diagnose someone who demonstrates depressive symptoms over a prolonged period of time. Depression is considered a *spectrum disorder*, with symptoms that range from mild to very severe. MDD is at the most serious end of this spectrum. Depression affects 10 percent of the general population and 17 percent of all adults (APA, 2000; Wells & Miranda, 2007). Women are twice as likely to be diagnosed with depression as men.

People who have never experienced major depression often have difficulty understanding or feeling empathy for those affected by this illness. We have all had "the blues" or felt sad or unhappy at various points in our lives. However, the number and severity of symptoms that are experienced by people with depression distinguishes it from these milder mood swings. It is an illness with both high morbidity and mortality. In one study, during a 12-month period, 96 percent of people with depression reported significant role impairments and, on average, reported missing 35 days from work (Kessler et al., 2003). Although many clients attend work while depressed, they perform at suboptimal levels, resulting in lost productive time. This is accounted for by reduced concentration, needing to repeat a job, working more slowly, making errors, and feeling fatigue (Stewart, Ricci, Chee, Hahn, & Morganstein, 2003). In addition, MDD causes role impairment in many aspects of the client's life, including work and social responsibilities, thinking, and self-care. The burden of illness is magnified by the frequent comorbidity of other psychiatric disorders, commonly anxiety and substance abuse (Kessler et al., 2003). It is also a life-threatening illness with high mortality. One in five clients with MDD dies by suicide, the eighth leading cause of death in the United States. For every successful suicide, there are 8 to 10 unsuccessful attempts. Failed suicide attempts account for 10 percent of general hospital admissions each year (Weisman, 1998).

According to the *DSM-IV-TR*, the essential features of a major depressive episode must occur most of the day, every day, for at least 2 weeks. During that time, there is a depressed mood or the loss of interest and pleasure in most activities the person once enjoyed (APA, 2000). The diagnosis of depression is dependent on the presence of at least four additional symptoms as listed in Table 13–1. Note that having a sad or depressed mood is not an essential feature of the diagnosis of depression. If you suspect depression, helpful questions to ask are given in Box 13–1.

Social withdrawal, isolating behaviors, and loss of interest in previously pleasurable activities are equally as significant as a depressed mood. Many clients with depression describe feeling "empty" or lonely, even in the presence of loved ones. This social withdrawal and loss of interest may be striking to friends and family members. It can mistakenly be perceived as lacking motivation or being lazy.

People who are experiencing an episode of major depression have an array of other symptoms in addition to a depressed mood, isolating behaviors, or loss of interest. Some clients act angry or irritable rather than sad. Some clients with depression are short tempered or verbally abusive. Others report loss of energy, fatigue, and a feeling of heaviness in the limbs. Clients sometimes describe feeling like they are moving through molasses or have heavy weights attached to their arms or legs. Many people with depression "self-medicate" with drugs or alcohol, which exacerbates the effects of depression.

| Table 13–1 | Depression Symptoms |
|---|---|
| *Cognitive* | Helpless, hopeless worthless, "life is not worth living" |
| | Poor concentration and memory, inability to make decisions |
| | Suicidal thoughts |
| | Loss of interest in previously enjoyable activities |
| *Physiological* | Inability to sleep or sleeps too much |
| | Loss of appetite or increased hunger, especially for carbohydrates |
| | Joint/muscle pain, gastrointestinal distress, feelings of malaise |
| | Fatigue or loss of energy |
| *Emotional* | Sad, depressed |
| | Excessive guilt |
| | Lack of affect, inability to feel joy or pleasure |
| | Feeling bored or disinterested |
| | Loneliness |

*Note:* It is possible to have depression without having symptoms of sadness or feeling depressed.

| | |
|---|---|
| *Behavioral* | Social withdrawal or isolation |
| | Restlessness or irritability |
| | Lack of initiative or motivation |
| | Irritable, angry, or hostile |
| | Giving up previously pleasurable activities |
| *Appraisal problems* | Unable to access strategies to perform necessary daily tasks |
| | Unable to make a decision and follow through |
| | Unable to accurately assess self-worth |

Significant cognitive changes, such as poor ability to concentrate or focus and loss of memory, are associated with depression. Studies have demonstrated declines in executive functions that are controlled in the prefrontal cortex of the brain (Murphy & Sahakian, 2001). These substantially contribute to a high illness burden by negatively impacting work, learning, and pleasurable activities. Further, the presence of a triad of cognitive signs is a hallmark of depression. These signs include feeling worthless or unworthy, feeling negative or pessimistic about the future, and being unable to make a decision or a plan of action. In other words, the depressed person feels helpless, hopeless, and worthless. In addition to mood and cognition, depression also affects neurovegetative functions. Changes in eating and sleeping patterns are usually seen, with affected individuals doing too much or too little. Other physical symptoms of depression include fatigue

## BOX 13–1    Questions to Ask If You Suspect Depression

- In the past 2 weeks, for most of the day, every day, have you felt down, depressed, or hopeless?
- In the past 2 weeks, for most of the day, every day, have you felt little interest in doing things you used to enjoy?
- Have you ever thought about hurting yourself?

A "yes" answer to either of the first two questions is highly indicative of a diagnosis of MDD. "Yes" to the last question should prompt an immediate referral to the client's doctor.

and physical complaints, such as headaches or backaches. Greater than 90 percent of clients with depression manifest physical symptoms (Stewart et al., 2003). Generally, the more severe the depression, the greater the number and intensity of symptoms. Individuals with depression often "look" depressed, with a slouched posture, unkempt appearance, and slowed movements.

These distressing symptoms interfere with the ability to function at school, work, or in social settings. Surprisingly, some people who are able to perform well, despite feeling depressed, report that it requires enormous energy. Consider Molly, a high school student. She is an excellent student, a member of the swim team, and an officer in two extracurricular groups. Although she appears well, she reports feeling numb and hollow inside. Her thoughts are preoccupied with sadness and loneliness. Fortunately, she was able to communicate her difficulties to her parents who arranged counseling for her. She reports that the interventions of the counselor "saved her life."

It is important to "tune in" when interviewing clients or taking a history. Changes in lifestyle or function may indicate depression. A study of physical therapists who treat outpatients with low back pain found that they are able to identify clients who are experiencing a depressive episode by asking two simple questions: "During the past month, have you been bothered by feeling down, depressed, or hopeless?" and "During the past month, have you been bothered by little interest or pleasure in doing things?" (Haggman et al., 2004). It only takes a little extra time to add these two questions when taking a client's history, and the answers may have a significant impact on the outcome of care.

If left untreated, depression can be life threatening. Listen carefully to clients with suicidal thoughts, and let them know that you are concerned. When clients describe severe feelings of hopelessness, ask if they have ever considered suicide. If the answer is "yes," ask if they have a plan. If the client has intention, a plan, and the means to carry out the plan, an immediate referral to a mental health professional is mandated. You may need to make this referral without the client's consent.

Consider Linda, a young mother with a 3-week-old baby. She was attending a parenting skills class for first-time mothers. She told Doris, the nurse/instructor, that she was crying all the time. Doris followed up on this after class, and Linda admitted that she was so sad that she wanted to die. In fact, she had a plan. Her husband was out of town on a business trip, and she was estranged from her family. She was alone. Doris immediately contacted Linda's doctor, who arranged for a psychiatric evaluation that day.

## Special Populations

As noted above, depression can strike at any age. We typically think of childhood as a happy and carefree time with only fleeting sadness or worry. However, depression can occur in children and adolescents, as well as adults. In fact, half of all adults who have a mental illness reported that their symptoms appeared by age 14 (Kuehn, 2005). Rates of depression for young people vary and have been reported to occur in 9 to 28 percent of the population (Cheung, Ewigman, Zuckerbrot, & Jensen, 2009). Young people have many of the same symptoms of depression as adults, including physical complaints, sleep and appetite disturbances, and changes in mood or thinking. However, because they are developmentally and cognitively different than adults, symptoms may manifest differently. Typically, we see irritability or anger rather than sadness. Children or adolescents may lack the language and cognitive experience to identify depression. For example, one depressed child described himself as feeling "hollow." Isolation and withdrawal from typical activities are as common as they are in adults, but rather than describing loss of interest, the child may refer to being "bored." Unfortunately, moody behavior and some withdrawal from parents and family are normal parts of adolescence. It is not uncommon for many to consider a depressed teen to be just having a typical adolescent experience. It is important to consider the impact of the symptoms on the young person's life and function before assuming this is just a normal part of growing up. For example, Betsey gave up her interest in sports, horseback riding, and her friends. She came home from school every day and stayed in her room, only coming out to eat a little dinner. Her grades also slipped. School and extracurricular activities are the "work" of children, and falling behind in these areas can have long-term consequences.

In addition to being irritable rather than sad, teens may look fine when with their peers and only fall apart when they are alone or with family. There are additional behavioral symptoms that should also cause concern about depression. These include fights with family and peers, skipping school, declining grades, antisocial behaviors, and drug use (Cheung et al., 2009). In the adolescent or young adult population, risk-taking behaviors and a lack of concern for personal safety can be problematic. Depression in teens typically has a more rapid onset than in adults and is more likely to take a severe form (Korczak & Goldstein, 2009). Any suicidal ideation should receive immediate attention.

Elders are another population in which depression may have a less typical presentation. As noted earlier, depression is most common in people with chronic health conditions, which is true of many elders. There is a two-way relationship between depression and illness. Depression increases the impact of the illness or disability, and the illness or disability may contribute to the onset or progression of the depression. In either case, depression creates a large illness burden and diminishes quality of life, while also increasing the symptoms of comorbid conditions.

Elders with depression tend to present with more physical symptoms rather than feeling sad or depressed. For example, fatigue, insomnia, loss of appetite, and pain are frequently reported, as well as a chronic feeling of being in "low" spirits (Butcher & McGonigal-Kenney, 2005). Other frequently reported physical symptoms include headache, low back or generalized pain, and gastrointestinal distress (Mynatt, 2004). In addition, depression can negatively affect adherence to medical regimes, activity levels, memory, cognition, and problem-solving skills (Alexopoulos, Raue, Sirey, & Arean, 2007). Thus, depression can both increase physical symptoms and decrease functional capacity (Mynatt, 2004). The onset of depression also appears to be a significant factor leading to nursing home placement and suicide, further increasing the burden of illness that older people experience (Harris & Cooper, 2006).

Unfortunately, elderly clients may have certain symptoms of various illnesses that make a differential diagnosis difficult. Older individuals are more likely to be uncomfortable talking about their sadness and, therefore, underreport their symptoms. They are also more likely to perceive the stigma of being labeled with a mental illness and refuse medications. Many health care practitioners mistakenly believe that depression is a typical part of aging and, therefore, does not need to be treated. However, this is a treatable condition, and elders do not need to suffer in silence.

### Dysthymia

Dysthymia, low or depressed mood, can last for 2 or more years (APA, 2000). The distinguishing feature between dysthymia and MDD is the degree and number of symptoms. The client has too few symptoms to qualify for a diagnosis of depression, and the severity of the symptoms is not as great. Neurovegetative symptoms, such as changes in eating and sleeping patterns and physical discomfort, are either absent or are present to a lesser degree.

This condition is chronic and may be described as a "depressed personality." Even though the condition does not cause severe distress, clients are affected by the symptoms and do not experience life as fully as they might otherwise. In some cases, dysthymia may progress to MDD. Like MDD, symptoms of dysthymia can have a significant negative impact on other health conditions (Chapman et al., 2005).

## BIPOLAR SPECTRUM DISORDER

Although 10 to 17 percent of the population experiences depressive illness, bipolar disorder occurs in only 1 to 2 percent of the population (Akiskal, 1996). In this disorder, symptoms are episodic with intervals of depression and mania, interspersed with periods of remission when clients may be symptom free. It is a more complex disorder than depression alone and carries a higher morbidity and mortality rate. When ill, the person experiences extreme emotional discomfort as do those around him or her, including family, friends, and coworkers. Typically, many years go by between the onset of bipolar symptoms and a definitive diagnosis. In the meantime, the individuals often present many difficult behaviors to family and friends, spend enormous amounts of money, and may frequently lose jobs and ruin relationships. In addition, they may present many challenging behaviors in the health care setting.

Although the onset of depression can occur at any age, bipolar illness typically begins in young adults. Recent studies indicate that approximately 20 percent of clients with bipolar illness have their first episode between the ages of 15 and 19 (American Academy of Child and Adolescent Psychiatry [AACAP] Official Action, 1997). Children with bipolar illness have a different clinical picture than adults, making diagnosis much more challenging. Irritability, explosive anger, agitation, antisocial activity, and extreme risk-taking behaviors are the most typical signs of bipolar disorder in children and adolescents. Furthermore, the course of the disease in adolescents tends to be chronic rather than episodic, as in adults.

During an episode of mania, a client may be either manic or hypomanic. During a manic episode, the individual has an elevated or extremely high mood that is beyond being happy and is often accompanied by an irritable mood and irrational thoughts (APA, 2000). This elevated mood must last for at least 1 week or be severe enough to warrant hospitalization. Many people mistakenly assume that an "elevated" mood is one of extreme happiness or euphoria. In fact, mania is often anything but a happy event. Someone who is "going high," or moving into a manic state, may have a period of elation or happiness, but this quickly progresses to a state of expansive and chaotic thinking and poor judgment. The behavior of a client in a manic state is often "out of control."

Hypomania is an elevated mood that is not high enough, severe enough, or does not demonstrate sufficient symptoms to be true mania. Some clients pass through a state of hypomania on their way to mania, whereas others do not. Many clients who are in a hypomanic state enjoy this "high" and can be very productive, due to creativity and high energy. This productive state may not last. If the hypomania escalates into a full manic episode, judgment and cognitive ability deteriorate.

In addition to the elevated or irritable mood, an individual must demonstrate at least three additional symptoms to be considered manic (APA, 2000). These may include feelings of inflated importance or grandiosity with delusions. For example, a college student with grandiose ideas thought that she could fly. She decided to soar out her dormitory window to a better place. Fortunately, she believed that she would need to take her clothes with her. Thinking the clothing could also fly, she threw them out the window first. Someone on the ground noticed this and called for help—a call that saved her life.

Other examples of grandiose ideas include making impossible business plans or thinking of oneself as an extremely powerful and important person, such as one with special religious

| **Table 13–2**     Mania | |
|---|---|
| *Cognitive* | Grandiose thinking—I can do anything! |
| | Invulnerability—Nothing can hurt me! |
| | Decreased ability to assess risks—physical, social, financial |
| | Significant lack of concern for safety |
| | In advanced stages, thoughts are chaotic and disorganized, psychotic |
| *Physiological* | Decreased need for sleep |
| | Extremely high energy levels |
| | Loss of perceived need to eat or drink |
| *Mood/emotion* | Elevated, expansive mood, excited |
| | Feeling "high"—I can accomplish anything! |
| | Agitated, irritable, angry |
| *Behavioral* | May be hostile, aggressive, or belligerent |
| | Rapid, incessant talking (pressured speech) |
| | Creative, flight of ideas |
| | Engages in dangerous behaviors, without regard to safety |
| | Hypersexuality |
| | "Out of control" |
| *Appraisal problems* | Unrealistic appraisals of capacities and limitations |
| | Lacks safety awareness—frequently engages in extremely high-risk behaviors |

powers. While in a manic state, clients commonly feel invincible and believe that no harm can come to them. This poor judgment, combined with hyperactivity or psychomotor agitation, can lead to dangerous ideas and serious risk-taking behaviors, without concern for personal safety. For example, people may drive recklessly, get into arguments or fistfights, walk down the middle of a highway, or even commit suicide. Refer to Table 13–2 for a summary of key aspects of mania.

Mania also affects the quality and style of speech. Clients may exhibit "pressured speech" (APA, 2000), talking incessantly about topics of interest only to themselves. It is often impossible to interrupt or redirect them. In addition, their social interactions may be domineering, intrusive, and demanding. One mother described her daughter as being "like a bulldozer" when she is manic. The manic individual often experiences racing thoughts with an uncontrolled flight of ideas. Many of these thoughts are disordered and irrational. Like depression, mania also causes changes in neurovegetative functions. There is increased energy, with a decreased need for sleep, and a loss of appetite.

## ANXIETY DISORDERS

Feelings of anxiety are common, and people often comment that they are "nervous" about such things as facing a difficult test in school or meeting someone's parents for the first time. These anxious feelings do not usually impair our ability to function or make us give up activities we enjoy. However, some people experience feelings of anxiety that are out of proportion to the intensity of the situational threat or persist longer than is typical; they are experiencing some form of anxiety disorder.

Anxiety disorder is an extremely common disorder, with many affected individuals having symptoms of physical distress. It is, in fact, the most common psychiatric disorder worldwide, affecting literally millions of people (Dowbiggin, 2009). Further, 15 percent of primary care visits in America are for symptoms of anxiety (Kinnier et al., 2009). However, many people do not seek care for anxiety because they are unaware that their symptoms are caused by this disorder, or they fear being stigmatized by a psychiatric diagnosis.

Anxiety is a diagnostic category covering a broad range of disorders that share the common feature of feeling excessively fearful. Several cognitive manifestations have been documented with anxiety disorders (APA, 2000). Clients may report irrational beliefs about themselves or their environment. They may have a negative self-concept and self-perception and pessimistically interpret information. Many individuals with anxiety overestimate the risk involved in their daily lives and are hypervigilant for environmental stimuli or cues. Here we discuss symptoms common to anxiety disorders, as well as describe several specific disorders. Refer to Table 13–3 for a summary of key symptoms of anxiety disorders.

Clients with anxiety often fear losing control, feel that the worst is going to happen, or report feeling terrified. These thoughts have been termed *catastrophization*. For example, every headache "becomes" a brain tumor, every joint pain is arthritis, and any social *faux pas* threatens social standing. Clients with anxiety disorders describe being unable to relax or feel calm. There may be too much focus on the "what ifs" of life. Clients report restlessness, fatigue, poor memory or concentration, irritability, and disturbed sleep (AACAP, 1997). Physical symptoms accompany anxiety, such as increased heart rate, sweating, muscle tension, and hyperventilation. In addition, many clients report somatic sensations for which there is no apparent cause, such as headaches, backaches, stomachaches, nausea, or feeling dizzy, shaky, or faint. Many overutilize the health care system and frequently seek emergency department evaluations for symptoms that have no physical basis (Stern, Herman, & Slavin, 1998). Diagnosis may be difficult because even in severe cases of anxiety, the symptoms are usually episodic; during a visit to a physician, they may not be present.

| Table 13–3 | Anxiety Disorders |
|---|---|
| *Cognitive* | Irrational fears, worry, apprehension<br>Impaired memory and concentration<br>Catastrophizing |
| *Physiological* | Somatization—aches, pains, discomforts, without a physical cause<br>Increased sympathetic arousal—increased heart rate and blood pressure, palpitations, sweating, shortness of breath, increased muscle tension<br>Nausea, gastrointestinal distress, dizziness, paresthesias |
| *Mood/emotion* | "Anxious" thoughts and feelings, terror<br>Irrational fears<br>May be constant (generalized anxiety disorder) or transient (panic disorder, social or other phobias) |
| *Behavioral* | Very emotionally "needy" or clingy<br>Avoidance of anxiety-producing situations<br>Constantly asking for reassurance and guidance<br>May repeatedly request help when making simple decisions<br>May exhibit rigid and controlling behaviors<br>Restless, pacing movements, unable to sit still |
| *Appraisal problems* | Catastrophization—every molehill becomes a mountain<br>Somatization—amplification of somatic symptoms |

These cognitive and physical symptoms are unpleasant and troublesome to the client. However, they typically occur in situations or at particular times that trigger their appearance (Alpers, 2009). Therefore, in an attempt to eliminate situations that trigger their anxiety, clients tend to exhibit avoidance behaviors. Because anxiety causes overstimulation of the sympathetic nervous system, we typically see fight-or-flight behaviors. Clients may rigidly structure their schedules or environment to eliminate or avoid fear-producing stimuli or unexpected situations.

### Generalized Anxiety Disorder

Symptoms of anxiety may be present all the time or may be episodic in nature. Generalized anxiety disorder (GAD) is characterized by a persistently high level of tension, with pervasive feelings of anxiety and apprehension, loss of appetite, difficulty concentrating, restlessness, sleep disturbances, and feelings of overarousal.

Some health providers refer to clients with anxiety as "the worried well." Diagnosing the various anxiety disorders is challenging due to their episodic nature and the potential for inaccurate recall and reporting of symptoms. In addition, these clients may stress the resources of the health care provider by making frequent demands for information and assurances that all is well. They may emotionally cling to the provider for support and guidance, repeatedly asking the same questions. These clients may be rigid or manipulative and have difficulty adjusting to the demands of the health care setting because they fear losing control.

### Social and Other Phobias

Many individuals with anxiety have specific phobias that trigger symptoms to appear or worsen. A phobia is an intense fear of an event, object, person, or situation. The fear, which occurs whenever the triggering event is present, is intense and not under voluntary control (APA, 2000). Social phobias include the fear of public speaking or performing one's job in front of others. Some clients fear behaving in a socially awkward manner and causing embarrassment to themselves or their families. Others avoid leaving their homes or familiar settings. Even though adults may recognize that their fears are irrational, many take elaborate steps to avoid an anxiety-producing situation, such as refusing to drive over a bridge or avoiding contact with a dog. Extreme cases can cause severe morbidity that is as significant as that which occurs with Serious and Persistent Mental Illness (SPMI).

Consider a middle-aged woman who did not visit her grandchildren because she would need to drive on the highway to an unfamiliar, larger city 2 hours away. She was also not comfortable having them visit her because her home was "too small," and they disrupted her routines. Furthermore, she was always "sick" with vague ailments, which made it even more difficult to tolerate visits. Sadly, she and her grandchildren were unable to develop a relationship.

### Panic Disorder

A panic attack is defined as a sudden, uncued, and intense feeling of anxiety. There is literally a sympathetic nervous system cascade that causes a sudden and intense "fight-or-flight" response. Symptoms include palpitations, hyperventilation, and shortness of breath. This may be so overwhelming in its intensity that the person feels that he or she is going insane or will die. Although it is of brief duration, usually lasting no more than 10 minutes, the severe intensity of the panic attack can be alarming.

To establish a diagnosis, the individual must experience at least four of the following symptoms during the episode (APA, 2000): pounding heart, sweating, trembling, choking or smothering sensations, chest pain, nausea, dizziness, depersonalization, fear of losing control, fear of dying, numbness or tingling, and hot or cold flashes. Clients may experience anticipatory anxiety, caused by the fear of having a panic attack, as well as specific phobias, such as those related to places or events where panic attacks occurred in the past. Catastrophization of physical symptoms, described earlier, can also occur. In these situations, clients develop a fear of going to places or events where a panic attack could be dangerous or embarrassing. They are diagnosed with panic disorder when they have frequent panic attacks that cause them significant concern and may lead to agoraphobia (Alpers, 2009). In the extreme, a client may become homebound (Alpers, 2009). Health care providers can support the needs of clients with anxiety disorders by understanding the cognitive, physical, and behavioral symptoms they present. Avoiding unnecessary tests and procedures could save health care dollars. In addition, clients would also be spared the discomfort and inconvenience of these procedures.

## Post-Traumatic Stress Disorder

Post-traumatic stress disorder (PTSD) is another type of anxiety disorder. It is unique because it only occurs after clients have experienced a traumatic event that is perceived by the clients to put themselves or a loved one at risk for death or serious injury (APA, 2000). The subjective appraisal of the severity of the event is the crucial element for the triggering event (Bush, 2009). "When catastrophic stress overwhelms individuals' adaptive biological and coping responses, post-traumatic psychiatric disorder results" (Reeves, Parker, & Konkle-Parker, 2005, p. 18). A diagnosis of PTSD in adults is based on the presence of three clusters of symptoms: reexperiencing the traumatic event, hyperarousal and hypervigilant behaviors, and avoidance of stimuli that trigger memories of the event (Gill, Szanton, Taylor, Page, & Campbell, 2009). In contrast, children may express their emotions as agitation or disorganized behavior.

Various types of events can cause this disorder, including rape, domestic violence, war experiences, surviving a natural disaster, or even a traumatic medical event. Exposure alone to a traumatic event is not sufficient to trigger PTSD. An individual does not need to personally experience the event; observing one can be equally traumatic. The exposed individual must respond to the event with feelings of extreme fear and helplessness. Studies of survivors of motor vehicle accidents and their loved ones demonstrate that a person does not need to be injured to develop PTSD; simply experiencing the fear of death or injury is sufficient (Jeavons, Greenwood, & deHorne, 2000). As many as 50 percent of survivors of motor vehicle accidents develop PTSD, and half still manifest symptoms 1 year after the accident.

The incidence of the disorder is variable, with estimates of its frequency ranging from 7 to 9 percent, with women being diagnosed with the disorder twice as often as men. Further, women who live in poverty or in an urban neighborhood are more likely to develop PTSD. Minority women are twice as likely to have PTSD as nonminority women, and minority women living in poverty in urban areas may have rates as high as 23 percent (Gill et al., 2009). This may represent cumulative risk from multiple risk factors. Individuals who have been abused or traumatized as children are more likely to develop this disorder after a traumatic event they experience as an adult. PTSD is most prevalent in areas where there is war and political upheaval. Among individuals who have been exposed to violence, as many as 51 percent may develop the disorder (Sampson, Benson, Beck, Price, & Nimmer, 1999). Although between 50 and 60 percent of the population is exposed to a traumatic stressor, only 8 percent of men and 20 percent of women will develop PTSD (Bobo, Warner, & Warner, 2007).

For a diagnosis of PTSD to be made, symptoms must last for at least 1 month. Many would argue that the symptoms of PTSD are a normal response to an overwhelming situation. However, it becomes pathological when the stimulus (danger) has passed, yet the response continues. A range of symptoms are associated with PTSD and other anxiety disorders that are significant for health care providers. Evidence suggests that the stressful event triggers an overactivity of the sympathetic nervous system and the chronic release of cortisol and other stress hormones. This can lead to dysfunction of the cardiopulmonary system that is manifested in hyperventilation, shortness of breath, and increased blood pressure and heart rate. Lowered immune system function can also occur. Increased muscle tension may result in back and neck problems or other joint pain, as well as fatigue and an increased susceptibility to injury. Clients may also experience gastrointestinal distress, dizziness, and headaches. Proper diagnosis of the cause of these complaints is necessary for appropriate and effective treatment. Women with PTSD are likely to have chronic pain, coronary artery disease, hypertension, and thyroid disorders (Gill et al., 2009), as well as at least one co-occurring additional psychiatric disorder (DeJonghe, Bogat, Levendosky, & von Eye, 2008).

Medical procedures, prolonged illness and disability, and sudden onset of medical crises may also trigger PTSD (Alonzo, 2000). This may be especially challenging for clients with human immunodeficiency virus (HIV) and cardiac conditions that require extensive invasive procedures and involve the threat of dying (Rourke, Stuber, Hobbie, & Kazak, 1999). Some feel that the treatment of cancer can also trigger PTSD (Bush, 2009). When the triggering event is a medical procedure or setting, clients may be unable to adhere to medical treatment plans or prescribed medication and may miss appointments (Alonzo, 2000). In fact, they may be unable to enter the medical setting at all. PTSD can have a significant impact on the client's symptoms and response to medical care. Consider Marie, a woman in her early 40s. She was diagnosed with lung cancer and had an entire lung removed, followed by a long, difficult stay in the pulmonary intensive care unit (ICU). Five years later her husband developed significant respiratory distress and was admitted to the same ICU with pulmonary fibrosis. The first time Marie entered the ICU, she "melted down" and had to leave immediately. She has been unable to return, and her husband is being supported by other members of the family and their friends. Some of the nursing staff do not understand how she can be so insensitive. Many mental health practitioners feel PTSD is underdiagnosed due to medical practitioners' failure to question their clients about prior exposure to abuse or trauma. Perhaps that is because many clients with this disorder will see their primary care provider with symptoms of PTSD, but will have complaints about symptoms in other areas. It is important to be ready to screen for these disorders and ask each patient with suspicious symptoms if they or a loved one has been exposed to trauma or violence.

Three clusters of symptoms must be present for a diagnosis of PTSD to be made (refer to Table 13–4 for a summary of key aspects of PTSD). One cluster of symptoms involves persistent reexperiencing of the traumatic event. This can happen in a number of ways. Some clients have intrusive, disturbing thoughts of the event, perhaps in dreams or flashbacks. Seemingly innocuous cues or events may trigger these thoughts; for example, the smell of the cologne that an attacker wore when he raped his victim, a loud or sudden noise, a crowded space, or even driving under a bridge (this last trigger is particularly common in recent combat veterans). The health care professional may unknowingly trigger these reactions by being in an environment where medical equipment is present and procedures occur. People who have experienced torture may have flashbacks triggered by the presence of medical equipment and procedures or by having a body part restrained or being confined to a small space. Having traumatized body parts examined

| **Table 13–4** | Post-Traumatic Stress Disorder (PTSD) |
| --- | --- |
| *Cognitive* | Painful reexperiencing of traumatic event(s)<br>Flashbacks<br>Intrusive thoughts or memories<br>May have amnesia for the event |
| *Physiological* | Hypervigilance<br>Hyperresponsiveness to stimuli<br>Increased levels of sympathetic nervous system arousal<br>Increased startle reactions<br>Insomnia |
| *Mood/emotion* | Emotional numbing<br>Flat affect<br>Feeling disconnected from reality—dissociation |
| *Behavioral* | Persistent avoidance of emotionally charged people, places, and events<br>Persistent avoidance of triggers for memories of traumatic event(s)<br>Irritability<br>Self-injurious behavior<br>Poor impulse control |
| *Appraisal problems* | Faulty judgment of current environment for safety, based on memories of past traumatic event(s)<br>Hypersensitivity to danger cues |

(i.e., a gynecological examination for a woman who has been sexually abused) and undergoing uncomfortable procedures may be unbearable to clients with this disorder. Even gentle physical contact may not be tolerated, which can pose challenges to rehabilitation professionals.

A second cluster of symptoms is avoidance behaviors. These are intended to limit exposure to triggering events, such as avoiding physical or emotional stimuli associated with the traumatic event. Clients may refuse to talk about the event or discuss related situations. Survivors typically avoid activities, places, or people that can trigger memories of the event. For example, a student who has been sexually assaulted at school may be unable to return to school. These avoidance behaviors can severely limit the client's ability to function and enjoy life.

Another form of avoidance behavior is to become emotionally detached with a flattened affect (APA, 2000). This interferes with the client's ability to develop trusting relationships with others. The client may dissociate or experience an altered mental state. In a popular series of children's books, the main character, Harry Potter, dissociates while he experiences flashbacks of watching the murder of his parents. Consider this vignette:

> An intense cold swept over them all. Harry felt his own breath catch in his chest. The cold went deeper than his skin. It was inside his chest; it was inside his very heart. Harry's eyes rolled up into his head. He couldn't see. He was drowning in cold. There was a rushing in his ears as though of water. He was being dragged downward, the roaring growing louder. And then, from far away, he heard screaming, terrible, terrified, pleading screams. He wanted to help whoever it was, to move his arms, but couldn't—a thick white fog was swirling around him, inside him. (Rowling, 1999, pp. 83–84)

The third cluster of symptoms arises from a persistent state of hypervigilance (APA, 2000). This is a consequence of the sympathetic nervous system being chronically overaroused. The client constantly monitors the environment for danger and triggers the alarm at the earliest sign of threat. There is a hyperactive startle response and difficulty focusing, paying attention, sleeping, and eating. There also may be irritability and outbursts of anger.

## Conversion Disorder

Whereas clients who malinger intentionally feign illness or disability for personal gain, clients with conversion disorder develop symptoms of physical illness that have no obvious physiological cause. It is one of the somatoform disorders, a group of psychiatric disorders in which clients manifest physical symptoms that cannot be otherwise explained (APA, 2000). The client believes the symptoms (i.e., weakness/paralysis, numbness/other sensory disturbances, pseudo-seizures, tremors) and the illness are real. The term *conversion* dates back to the 19th-century psychiatrist Sigmund Freud (Breuer & Freud, 1895/1957), who believed that anxiety becomes "converted" into physical symptoms, to keep it out of conscious awareness. The process of converting underlying psychological conflict, stress, or need into "pseudo-neurological" symptoms is presumed to be unconscious.

An important diagnostic feature of conversion disorder is *la belle indifference,* that is, the client seems not to be concerned about the symptoms. In conversion disorder, symptoms do not match known physical conditions. For example, loss of sensation may follow a "gloved hand" pattern rather than the normal dermatomal distribution. Paralysis may only be seen during certain movements or in certain positions. The onset of conversion disorder is usually acute but may be progressive. Clients who are hospitalized with conversion disorder typically recover within 2 weeks (APA, 2000).

Frank is a 23-year-old Marine who presents with apparent paraplegia. He was referred to physical therapy with a diagnosis of conversion disorder, and we're supposed to rehabilitate him. When I took his history, he told me that his legs were completely paralyzed and that he could not move them at all. However, when I transferred him from the wheelchair to the examination table, he supported his weight on his legs. He could not extend his knee or do a straight leg raise, but he tightened his thigh in the strongest quadriceps setting exercise I have ever seen. He doesn't seem to have a clue that this makes no sense.

—*From the journal of Dan Wu, physical therapist student*

Significant diagnostic challenges accompany conversion disorder, and a thorough neurological and medical examination must be conducted to rule out physical disorders, such as multiple sclerosis. To further complicate establishing a diagnosis, certain symptoms of conversion disorder may reflect cultural mores about socially acceptable ways to express illness. The clinician must, therefore, assess whether symptoms can be explained in a cultural/social context (APA, 2000). It is difficult to accurately determine the prevalence of conversion disorder, but it is believed to occur in about 3 percent of clients seen in outpatient mental health clinics (APA, 2000). This disorder is more common in women than men and is generally seen in clients who are young adults through middle age (Iverson & Binder, 2000).

In addition to psychiatric intervention, physical rehabilitation is often beneficial. For example, three women (ages 18, 20, and 34) treated in a hospital-based inpatient rehabilitation setting had resolved symptoms and resumed their previous level of independence, mobility, school, and work following a course of physical therapy that incorporated behavioral modification and shaping techniques with neurological treatment (Ness, 2007). An example of a younger client is that of a 12-year-old-boy who entered an emergency department with paralysis of both legs and an inability to walk. After treatment that included relaxation exercises, guided imagery, and antidepressants, he walked independently (Gallizzi, Kaly, & Takagishi, 2008).

## IMPLICATIONS FOR HEALTH CARE PROFESSIONALS

Each health care discipline has its own role to play in providing care for clients who have physical and psychiatric disorders. It is beyond the scope of this text to address each individually, but some strategies are useful to all disciplines. It is common for new psychiatric residents to be told "When interviewing clients, you should listen to the music, not the song." The implication is that while the clients may appear to be speaking coherently, their actions and demeanor may not "make sense."

Impaired judgment, slovenly appearance, risky behavior, off-putting comments, and general social incompetence carry a powerful message. When evaluating and treating clients with medical symptoms, it is important to be constantly aware of the possibility that mental illness may also be present. Having a low threshold of suspicion for psychiatric disorders may help health care professionals identify these conditions. Recognizing symptoms that suggest mental health problems will enable health care providers to make referrals to appropriate practitioners, improve the outcome of all interventions, and, perhaps, prevent a suicide. Remember that clients with mental health disorders usually present with neurovegetative symptoms, such as changes in eating or sleeping patterns, altered states of arousal, hyperventilation, cardiovascular changes, and changes in muscle tone. When we perform our assessments, we need to ask about these functions. We must focus our evaluations and interventions on determining the scope of the client's problems and treating the symptoms for which we are responsible. We need to develop mechanisms to refer clients to the appropriate professionals when necessary. If we feel comfortable asking follow-up questions and making referrals, the client may also feel comfortable.

Confidentiality is an ethic that we are obligated to observe with all our clients. There is, however, an exception to this rule. If you believe that clients present a risk to themselves or to the safety of others, confidentiality must be broken and appropriate authorities informed. The ethics of nonmaleficence (to do no harm) and beneficence (to provide the best possible care) (see Chapter 1) supercede the client's right to confidentiality. Of course, this information is given only on a "need-to-know" basis and is not shared with others.

Clients with psychiatric disorders may present with altered levels of sensory perception (Everett, Dennis, & Ricketts, 1995). It is our responsibility to assess how the client responds to us and to the environment. Then we must individualize our approach. This may mean lowering the level of sensory stimulation by providing a calm, quiet treatment environment with a structured, unhurried approach. Other clients may respond better to increasing the level of stimulation or making the activities more exciting. It is imperative that we always ask the client's permission before initiating physical contact and continue to seek approval as we proceed.

We must establish a therapeutic relationship built on trust and create an environment in which the client feels safe. This may take longer to do than you or your administration would like, but it is time well spent. Any client who comes for a health care visit may have a mental health problem that he or she may not disclose. Therefore, it is crucial to proceed cautiously with all clients. Respect clients' responses to your questions, and during interventions, work within their tolerance to stress, demands, and levels of stimuli.

Finally, we must not forget to take care of our own mental health needs. Working with clients who are physically or mentally ill can be stressful, and the behavior of clients with mental illness can be challenging. To provide the best quality care, we must be calm, focused, and able to cope with unexpected and difficult events. Practicing what we preach in terms of taking care of ourselves will set a healthy example for our clients and help us be more competent and effective care providers.

## EXERCISE AS AN INTERVENTION FOR MENTAL ILLNESS

Although significant evidence exists that antidepressants are efficacious in treating MDD, there is less evidence that they are effective in less severe forms of depression. A 2010 meta-analysis published in the *Journal of the American Medical Association* (Fournier et al., 2010) demonstrated that, for people with mild to moderate depression, these medications are no more effective than a placebo. This is congruent with other research data that indicate that 30 to 35 percent of people who take antidepressants do not have a positive response (Blumenthal et al., 1999). Although mild to moderate depression may not cause as many functional impairments or present as great a burden of illness, they do present pain and suffering for those who are affected. Fortunately, very good treatment options are available that are effective for these milder forms of depression and other mental illnesses.

Due to symptoms of mental illness, symptoms of other comorbid illnesses, and the side effects of medication, people with mental illness tend to lead very sedentary lifestyles, with limited amounts of physical activity (McDevitt & Wilbur, 2006). Multiple studies support the efficacy of exercise for depression, anxiety, and schizophrenia (Beebe et al., 2005; Blumenthal et al., 1999; McDevitt & Wilbur, 2006; Schmitz, Kruse, & Kugler, 2004). Evidence suggests that exercise improves cognitive function, mood, and a sense of well-being. A significant positive factor in the use of exercise as an alternative to medication is that there are no unpleasant side effects, and the activity can improve many co-occurring medical conditions, such as diabetes, obesity, hypertension, and cardiovascular disease. This research has also shown that exercise is associated with health-related quality of life for people with mood disorders, anxiety, and substance abuse disorders.

Blumenthal and colleagues (1999) performed a study comparing the results of an exercise program to those achieved through the use of antidepressant medication. The subjects were 50 years of age or older and were randomly assigned to an exercise program, a medication regime, or a combination of the two for 16 weeks. At the end of the study, all clients had significant improvements in mood symptoms, and there were no differences between groups. This indicates that in this population of older adults, with moderate depression, exercise is as effective as medication. Further, the two groups that included exercise demonstrated improvements in aerobic capacity.

A walking program is another effective way to provide mild exercise to improve mood symptoms. People with mental illness benefit more from group exercise than individual programs. Groups provide support and motivation, significant factors for people whose symptoms include loss of interest and initiative. For example, McDevitt and Wilbur (2006) designed a successful group walking program for clients with Serious and Persistent Mental Illness. An additional contributing factor that proved important to the group's achievement was the use of positive feedback measures, such as weight loss, activity logs, pedometer scores, and group reinforcement.

## Summary

This chapter explored several common psychiatric diagnoses: depression, bipolar spectrum disorder, and anxiety disorders, including post-traumatic stress disorder. Diagnostic features of these disorders were described, as well as the effects of these symptoms on coexisting physical disorders.

In addition, strategies for health care professionals to use when treating clients with psychiatric disorders were presented. We need to recognize and address every presenting symptom and provide treatment or referral as appropriate.

## Reflective Questions

1. a. What symptoms of mental illness have you observed in family or friends?
   b. How did these symptoms affect the person's ability to function? How did they affect interpersonal relationships?
   c. What are your feelings about these experiences (positive or negative)? Did you feel confused, angry, helpless, scared, embarrassed?
2. a. What have been your experiences with clients who have a diagnosis of mental health?
   b. What symptoms have you observed?
3. a. Do you suspect you had some clients who were undiagnosed for mental health issues?
   b. How did these symptoms affect the client's ability to function?
   c. How did these symptoms affect the client's ability to participate in medical interventions/therapy?
   d. How did these symptoms affect the client's ability to participate in goal achievement?
4. a. How do you think that people with a mental illness should be integrated into the community?
   b. What kinds of supports should be available?
   c. What techniques or strategies can you use to provide the best possible care to meet all of the client's needs?
5. a. Will your profession be involved in caring for people with psychiatric problems? Why or why not?
   b. What professional supports or information might you need? Where can you find them?

## Case Study

Mr. Richards is a 68-year-old man with a history of cardiac disease. Recently discharged from the hospital following coronary artery bypass graft surgery, he now comes to your facility as an outpatient. He is having increasing difficulty following directions, staying focused and concentrating, and remembering what to do. His progress has been very slow. Mr. Richards lives alone since his wife died 2 years ago, but his sister comes to his home every day to help. Although he says that he is very lonely, he has given up going to church and playing cards with friends. He also says that he does not see the point of working hard with his postsurgical exercise regime because he will not be using the skills the health professionals are trying to help him learn. Mr. Richards' social withdrawal, isolating behaviors, and loss of interest in activities that were previously enjoyable raise warning flags of a depressed mood, among other possibilities.

1. a. What questions need to be asked to clarify the situation?
   b. How can these questions be phrased to avoid offending or embarrassing Mr. Richards?
2. What impact might these symptoms have on his progress in cardiac rehabilitation and on other health conditions?
3. a. What is the most appropriate plan of action to address Mr. Richards' symptoms?
   b. What referrals might be helpful?
   c. How can this plan be discussed with Mr. Richards to ensure his collaboration?
   d. Who else might you need to get involved to support his recovery?
4. How can the cardiac rehabilitation plan of care be adjusted to accommodate these challenges?

## References

Abram, K. M., Teplin, L. A., McClelland, G. M., & Dulcan, M. K. (2003). Co-morbid psychiatric disorders in youth in juvenile detention. *Archives of General Psychiatry, 60*(11), 1097–1108.

Akiskal, H. (1996). The prevalent clinical spectrum of bipolar disorders: Beyond DSM-IV. *Journal of Clinical Psychopharmacology, 16*(2, Suppl.), 4s–14s.

Alexopoulos, G. S., Raue, P. J., Sirey, J. A., & Arean, P. A. (2007). Developing an intervention for depressed, chronically medically ill elders: A model from COPD. *International Journal of Geriatric Psychiatry, 23*, 447–453.

Alonzo, A. (2000). The experience of chronic illness and post-traumatic stress disorder: The consequences of cumulative adversity. *Social Science and Medicine, 50,* 1475–1484.

Alpers, G. W. (2009). Ambulatory assessment of panic disorder and specific phobias. *Psychological Assessment, 21*(4), 476–485.

American Academy of Child and Adolescent Psychiatry (AACAP) Official Action. (1997). Practice parameters for the assessment and treatment of children and adolescents with bipolar disorders. *Journal of the American Academy of Child and Adolescent Psychiatry, 36*(10, Suppl.), 157s–176s.

American Psychiatric Association. (2000). *Diagnostic and statistical manual of mental disorders* (4th ed., text rev.). Washington, DC: Author.

Beebe, L. H., Tian, L., Morris, N., Goodwin, A., Allen, S. S., & Kuldae, J. (2005). Effects of exercise on mental and physical health parameters of persons with schizophrenia. *Issues of Mental Health Nursing 26,* 661–667.

Blumenthal, J. A., Babyak, M. A., Moore, K. A., Craighead, W. E., Herman, S., Khatri, P., . . . Krishman, K. R. (1999). Effects of exercise training on older patients with major depression. *Archives of Internal Medicine, 159,* 2349–2356.

Bobo, W. V., Warner, C. H., & Warner, M. (2007). The management of post-traumatic stress disorder (PTSD) in the primary care setting. *Southern Medical Journal, 100*(8), 797–802.

Breuer, J., & Freud, S. (1957). *Studies in hysteria* (J. Strachey, Trans.). New York, NY: Basic Books. (Original work published 1895)

Bush, N. J. (2009). Post-traumatic stress disorder related to the cancer experience. *Oncology Nursing Forum, 36*(40), 395–400.

Butcher, H. K., & McGonigal-Kenney, M. (2005). Depression and dispiritedness in later life: A "gray drizzle of horror" isn't inevitable. *American Journal of Nursing, 105*(12), 52–61.

Caspi, A., Sugden, K., Moffitt, T. E., Taylor, A., Craig, I. W., Harrington, H., . . . Poulton, R. (2003). Influence of life stress on depression: Moderation by a polymorphism in the 5-HTT gene. *Science, 301*(5631), 386–389.

Chapman, D. P., Perry, G. S., & Strine, T. W. (2005). The vital link between chronic disease and depressive disorders. *Preventing Chronic Disease, 2*(1). Retrieved from http://www.cdc.gov/pcd/issues/2005/jan/04_0066.htm

Cheung, A., Ewigman, B., Zuckerbrot, R. A., & Jensen, P. S. (2009). Adolescent depression: Is your young patient suffering in silence? *Journal of Family Practice, 58*(4), 187–192.

DeJonghe, E. S., Bogat, G. A., Levendosky, A. A., & von Eye, A. (2008). Women survivors of intimate partner violence and post-traumatic stress disorder: Prediction and prevention. *Journal of Postgraduate Medicine, 54*(4), 294–300.

DiMatteo, M. R., Lepper, H. S., & Groghan, T. W. (2000). Depression is a risk factor for noncompliance with medical treatment: Meta-analysis of the effects of anxiety and depression on patient adherence. *Archives of Internal Medicine, 160*(14), 2101–2106.

Dowbiggin, I. R. (2009). High anxieties: The social construction of anxiety disorders. *Canadian Journal of Psychiatry, 54*(7), 429–436.

Everett, T., Dennis, M., & Ricketts, E. (1995). *Physiotherapy in mental health.* London, England: Butterworth-Heinemann.

Fournier, J. C., DeRubeis, R. J., Hollon, S. D., Dimidjian, S., Amsterdam, J. D., Shelton, R. C., & Fawcett, J. (2010). Antidepressant drug effect and depression severity. *Journal of the American Medical Association, 303*(1), 47–53.

Gallizzi, G., Kaly, P., & Takagishi, J. (2008). Lower extremity paralysis in a male preadolescent. *Clinical Pediatrics, 47*(1), 86–88.

Gill, J. M., Szanton, S., Taylor, T. J., Page, G. G., & Campbell, J. C. (2009). Medical conditions and symptoms associated with post-traumatic stress disorder in low-income urban women. *Journal of Women's Health, 18*(2), 261–267.

Glod, C. (1998). *Contemporary psychiatric-mental health nursing.* Philadelphia, PA: F. A. Davis.

Haggman, S., Maher, C. G., & Refshauge, K. M. (2004). Screening for symptoms of depression by physical therapists managing low back pain. *Physical Therapy, 84*(12), 1157–1166.

Hariri, A. R., Mattay, V. S., Tessitore, A., Kolachana, B., Fera, F., Goldman, D., . . . Weinberger, D. R. (2002). Serotonin transporter genetic variation and the response of the human amygdala. *Science, 297*(5580), 400–403.

Harris, Y., & Cooper, J. K. (2006). Depressive symptoms in older people predict nursing home admission. *Journal of the American Geriatric Society, 54,* 593–597.

Insel, T. R., & Charney, D. S. (2003). Research on major depression: Strategies and priorities. *Journal of the American Medical Association, 289*(23), 3167–3168.

Iverson, G. L., & Binder, L. M. (2000). Detecting exaggeration and malingering in neuropsychological assessment. *Journal of Head Trauma and Rehabilitation, 15*(2), 829–858.

Jeavons, S., Greenwood, K., & deHorne, D. (2000). Accident cognitions and subsequent psychological trauma. *Journal of Traumatic Stress, 13*(23), 359–365.

Karp, D. A., & Sisson, G. E. (2010). *Voices from the inside: Readings on the experience of mental illness.* New York, NY: Oxford University Press.

Kessler, R. C., Berglund, P., Demler, O., Jin, R., Koretz, D., Merikangas, K. R., . . . Wang, P. S. (2003). The epidemiology of major depressive disorder: Results from the National Co-morbidity Survey Replication. *Journal of the American Medical Association, 289*(23), 3095–3105.

Kinnier, R. T., Hofsess, C., Pongratz, R., & Lambert, C. (2009). Attributions and affirmations for overcoming anxiety and depression. *Psychology and Psychotherapy, Theory, Research and Practice, 82,* 153–169.

Kiraly, D., Gunning, K., & Leiser, J. (2008). Primary care issues in patients with mental illness. *American Family Physician, 78*(3), 355–362.

Korczak, D. J., & Goldstein, B. I. (2009). Childhood onset major depressive disorder: Course of illness and psychiatric comorbidity in a community sample. *Journal of Pediatrics, 155*(1), 118–123.

Kuehn, B. M. (2005). Mental illness takes heavy toll on youth. *Journal of the American Medical Association, 294*(3), 293–295.

Mahan, V. (2006). Challenges in the treatment of depression. *Journal of the American Psychiatric Nurses Association, 11*(6), 336–370.

McDevitt, J., & Wilbur, J. (2006). Exercise and people with serious, persistent mental illness: A group walking program may be an effective way to lower the risk of co-morbidities. *American Journal of Nursing, 106*(4), 50–54.

Murphy, F. D., & Sahakian, B. J. (2001). The neurobiology of bipolar disorder. *British Journal of Psychiatry* (Suppl. 41), s120–s127.

Mynatt, S. L. (2004, Winter). Depression in the older adult: Recognition and nursing intervention. *Tennessee Nurse,* pp. 8–10.

Ness, D. (2007). Physical therapy management for conversion disorder: Case series. *Journal of Neurologic Physical Therapy, 31*(1), 30–39.

Reeves, R. R., Parker, J. D., & Konkle-Parker, D. J. (2005). War-related mental health problems of today's veterans: New clinical awareness. *Journal of Psychosocial Nursing and Mental Health Services, 43*(7), 18–28.

Rourke, M. T., Stuber, M. L., Hobbie, W. L., & Kazak, A. (1999). Post-traumatic stress disorder: Understanding the psychological impact of surviving childhood cancer into young adulthood. *Journal of Oncology Nursing, 16*(3), 126–135.

Rowling, J. K. (1999). *Harry Potter and the prisoner of Azkaban.* New York, NY: Scholastic.

Sampson, A., Benson, S., Beck, A., Price, D., & Nimmer, C. (1999). Post-traumatic stress disorder in primary care. *Journal of Family Practice, 48*(3) 222–227.

Schmitz, N., Kruse, J., & Kugler, J. (2004). The association between physical exercise and health-related quality of life in subjects with mental disorders: Results from a cross-sectional survey. *Preventive Medicine, 39,* 1200–1207.

Steer, R., Cavalieri, T., Leonard, D., & Beck, A. (1999). Use of the Beck inventory for primary care to screen for major depression disorders. *General Hospital Psychiatry, 21,* 106–111.

Stern, T., Herman, J., & Slavin, J. (1998). *The Massachusetts General Hospital (MGH) guide to psychiatry in primary care.* New York, NY: McGraw-Hill.

Stewart, W. F., Ricci, J. A., Chee, E., Hahn, S., & Morganstein, D. (2003). Cost of lost productive work time among US workers with depression. *Journal of the American Medical Association, 289*(23), 3135–3144.

Weisman, A. (1998). The patient with acute grief. In T. Stern, J. Herman, & J. Slavin (Eds.), *The Massachusetts General Hospital (MGH) guide to psychiatry in primary care* (pp. 25–31). New York, NY: McGraw-Hill.

Wells, K. B., & Miranda, J. (2007). Reducing the burden of depression. *Journal of the American Medical Association, 298,* 1451–1452.

Whitley, R. (2009). The implications of race and ethnicity for shared decision-making. *Psychiatric Rehabilitation Journal, 32*(3), 227–230.

Williams, S. M., Chapman, D., & Lando, J. (2005). The role of public health in mental health promotion. *Journal of the American Medical Association, 294*(18), 2293–2294.

CHAPTER

# Self-Destructive Behaviors

Heather Pomeroy came into the infant follow-up clinic again today with Paul, who is now 4 months old. When he was born, he was small for his gestational age, which is why we are monitoring him. He's not developing as quickly as expected, and his head is still floppy. The doctor says he has low muscle tone. Despite our help, his weight is not catching up, and neither are his milestones. The pediatrician referred him to a specialist, who looked at his face and asked if his mother drank during her pregnancy. Heather does have a long history of alcohol abuse, and during her prenatal visits, she was counseled about not drinking. She swore she had stopped and would do nothing that might hurt her baby.

*—From the journal of Larissa Montgomery, nursing student*

One of the motivators to enter a health profession is a desire to want to help people. Health care providers often assume that clients are both motivated and able to follow their advice and work toward improvement. Therefore, it can be puzzling and frustrating when clients fail to follow treatment plans and continue engaging in behaviors that are unhealthy or harmful. Self-destructive behaviors, especially those that cause severe negative consequences, may be puzzling to health professionals. It is easy to assume an attitude of judgment and wonder "Why don't they just stop doing those things?"

In this chapter, we describe several types of self-destructive behaviors, including substance use disorders, eating disorders, self-injurious behaviors, and suicide. These disorders frequently co-occur and may also coexist with psychiatric disorders, as discussed in Chapter 13. Our goals in this chapter are for readers to recognize the signs and consequences of these behaviors and to develop strategies to support clients and refer them to other health professionals who can provide them with appropriate care.

# SUBSTANCE USE DISORDERS

Anthropological data tell us that alcohol has been used for 8,000 years. In addition, marijuana, peyote, cocoa leaves, and tobacco have been used for over 1,000 years, most commonly in religious rituals and ceremonies (Betz, Mihalic, Pinto, & Raffa, 2000). Currently, alcohol-related advertising and its catchy slogans seem to be everywhere, and there are several movements afoot to legalize marijuana. For most people, occasional recreational or ceremonial use of psychoactive substances or use of medications to alleviate pain does not result in harm. However, some individuals are predisposed to developing addictions, and even occasional use may place them at high risk. Others will use substances at a frequency or intensity that cause significant negative consequences. These individuals will have substance use disorders, which include the categories of abuse or addiction, depending on the severity of the involvement. Table 14–1 notes key elements of substance use, abuse, and dependence or addiction.

All substances that have the capacity to alter thinking or consciousness are considered psychoactive substances. They can be taken through many routes, including drinking, eating/swallowing, inhaling, or injecting. Although each drug causes unique physical and psychological effects, intoxication occurs when the substance changes mood, behavior, perception, or judgment (Schuckit, 2000). In the discussion of substance use disorders, we use the term *substance* to refer to alcohol and all other psychoactive substances, such as marijuana, cocaine, opioids, and hallucinogens. These disorders constitute the most commonly reported psychiatric diagnosis, with men more likely to be affected than women (American Psychiatric Association [APA], 2000a). Fifteen to 20 percent of the population has a lifetime risk for a substance use disorder (Baldisseri, 2007).

## Substance Use

Two out of every three Americans report using alcohol, and 35.6 percent admit using illicit drugs (Schuckit, 2000). Although substance users' thinking or motor skills are impaired during intoxication, they may still be able to fulfill major life roles and function competently when not under the influence of these substances. A person whose substance use is under control does not risk job, family, reputation, or financial security for the short-term pleasure of being intoxicated.

| Table 14–1 Key Elements of Substance Use, Abuse, and Dependence or Addiction | | |
|---|---|---|
| **Use** | **Abuse** | **Dependence or Addiction** |
| • Occasional recreational use | • Intoxication accompanied by dangerous or reckless activities | • Includes all problems of substance abuse, *plus:* |
| • Creates no problems for the user | • Drug use causes significant problems at home, work, or school | • Daily activities revolve around acquiring, using, and recovering from drug use |
| | • Personal, financial, and/or legal difficulties occur | • Person is unable to control or curtail use due to cravings |
| | • Substance use continues despite significant and persistent negative consequences | • Tolerance and withdrawal impact use |

## Substance Abuse

The *Diagnostic and Statistical Manual of Mental Disorders, fourth edition, text revision,* lists several categories of substances of abuse, including alcohol, cocaine and amphetamines (speed), caffeine, cannabis (marijuana), opiates (e.g., morphine, heroin, and prescription pain medications), hallucinogens (e.g., LSD), inhalants, nicotine, sedatives, hypnotics, and antianxiety drugs (APA, 2000a). Alcohol is the most frequently abused substance, and marijuana is the most frequently abused illicit drug. Many individuals abuse more than one drug, a situation known as polysubstance abuse. However, most people have a drug that they use most often, and this is referred to as the "drug of choice."

Substance abuse is a maladaptive pattern of drug use that causes significant impairment and distress (APA, 2000a). It leads to difficulty performing major life role expectations at home, work, or school. Someone with a substance abuse disorder continues to use the drug(s) of choice, despite persistent personal, social, or legal difficulties. The individual may lose a job, due to repeated mistakes and absences, have conflicts with family members or friends, or get arrested by police for driving under the influence or for disorderly conduct. In addition, the abuser often partakes in potentially dangerous activities while intoxicated, such as driving a car or boat, skiing, flying a plane, fighting, unsafe sexual practices, or stunts and pranks. Symptoms of substance abuse problems in the workplace include frequent absences, especially on Mondays when the user is hung over; arriving late or taking long lunches; producing substandard work; and interacting inappropriately with coworkers or supervisors (Baldisseri, 2007).

## Substance Dependence or Addiction

To be considered a dependence or addiction, drug use must be compulsive, even when it results in serious negative consequences (Betz et al., 2000). For the person who is addicted, life revolves around drug use, which becomes increasingly more difficult to control. An individual who is addicted spends considerable time obtaining, using, and recovering from using the substance, as well as spending considerable sums of money purchasing it. Social, recreational, or occupational activities are sacrificed, with devastating consequences for the individual and his or her family. Although the person knows that persistent physical or psychological problems are caused by the substance abuse, he or she is unable to curtail use (APA, 2000a). Drug dependence results in expensive social problems, such as lost time from work, accidents and injuries, crimes, and destroyed families, which may result in the need for foster care for children (McLellan, Lewis, O'Brien, & Kleber, 2000).

Two other criteria that determine dependence or addiction involve the issues of tolerance and withdrawal. Tolerance for a substance develops with habitual use. It is evident when a person must ingest larger quantities of the substance to achieve the same level of intoxication or to feel "high." After prolonged use, when the substance leaves the body, withdrawal symptoms develop. However, the inclusion of tolerance and withdrawal as criteria for addiction is controversial. Some people who abuse substances, but are not addicted, need increasing quantities of their drug(s) of choice to provide the desired results, whereas some substances, such as cocaine, cause few withdrawal symptoms (Schuckit, 2000).

Although substance use can become abuse, there is no simple progression to addiction. The addicted brain is neurobiologically different from the nonaddicted brain (Ketchum & Asbury, 2000). Researchers believe that different drugs use multiple neurochemical pathways in the central nervous system (CNS). All addictive substances affect dopamine receptors that regulate pleasure responses. Stimulating these pleasure responses positively reinforces a pattern of drug-seeking behavior and causes withdrawal symptoms when the drug is no longer present in the body (Betz et al., 2000). These CNS effects can cause permanent changes in synaptic function that make abstinence and treatment difficult.

The effects of substance abuse and addiction can be devastating. People cause injury to themselves and others while under the influence of a drug, or they may even die. Employees, including stockbrokers, lawyers, construction workers, and even health care professionals, may come to work with impaired judgment, secondary to drug use, and be unable to perform their jobs competently or safely. Others, such as medical professionals, put their clients at risk (Baldisseri, 2007).

Substance abuse and dependence also have significant effects on both physical and mental health. An individual with a substance use disorder may become dizzy, with frequent losses of balance or falls, have cognitive impairments that affect judgment and impulse control, have changes in physical appearance or hygiene, and become impotent. Substance use disorder causes serious and life-threatening conditions and, therefore, significantly more emergency department, inpatient, and intensive care unit admissions. Those who used drugs other than alcohol have longer lengths of hospital stays (French, McGeary, Chitwood, & McCoy, 2000). Emotional changes also occur that affect behavior and relationships, such as mood swings, manipulative behavior, withdrawal from family and social activities, defensiveness, lying or denial about substance use, and belligerent or confrontational interactions.

## Alcoholism

I have been working with Tom for the last three months trying to find an appropriate wheelchair and seating system for him. He's 26 years old and has a spinal cord injury at the sixth cervical level, as a result of an automobile accident he caused while driving drunk. When he was referred to us, he had a deep pressure sore in the area of his left buttock that kept him from getting out of bed and into his old wheelchair. He had been in bed for months and was very depressed.

My supervisor and I identified a seating system that allowed him to be out of bed for up to 6 hours a day without any signs of redness. Since he's been home, he's having problems again. He swears he's using the equipment the right way and limiting his use to 6 hours a day. Last night, I saw him steering his wheelchair into a local tavern. I wonder if this has anything to do with his current problem.

*—From the journal of Zack McIntyre, physical therapist student*

Alcohol is the most frequently used and abused substance in the United States. Although many individuals use it without harm, its negative consequences are significant and far reaching. Three criteria are necessary to establish a diagnosis of alcoholism (Ketchum & Asbury, 2000): (1) A large quantity of alcohol is consumed over a number of years; (2) there is a chronic loss of control over alcohol use, with an inability to curtail or stop alcohol use; and (3) there are significant negative effects on physical health and social functioning.

Alcoholism affects every organ and system of the body. Chronic alcohol use affects the cardiovascular system, causing hypertension, arrhythmia, and increased risk of stroke. The digestive system, the liver, kidneys, stomach, and pancreas may also be affected. Risk is significantly increased for pancreatitis, gastritis, ulcers, diabetes, cirrhosis, and cancer. The nervous system is affected by loss of nutrients, leading to brain damage, with memory loss and poor judgment. Chronic alcohol abuse can also cause peripheral neuropathies (Ketchum & Asbury, 2000).

It is no surprise that people with alcohol-related problems use more health care resources than others, utilizing from 10 to 50 percent of available hospital beds (Epperly & Moore, 2000). In Canada, 10 percent of deaths each year are caused by hazardous drinking, as are 50 percent of fatal car accidents (Ogborne, 2000). Unfortunately, when clients are ill or hospitalized for an alcohol-related disorder, many health care providers fail to recognize or address the antecedent problem and do not question them about substance use and abuse. This omission results in a missed opportunity for intervention. Health-related effects of alcohol are not limited to the poor health of the person who uses the substances. There is a clear link between alcohol and all forms of trauma. Further, even in moderate amounts, alcohol can have profound effects on a developing fetus, causing low birth weight, social and learning problems, and fetal alcohol syndrome (Olson et al., 1997). Alcohol abuse affects spouses, children, and friends, leading to depression, family violence, and behavioral problems. The personal and social costs are enormous and may last a lifetime.

Accidents and violent crimes are also frequently associated with alcohol use. Alcohol-impaired drivers cause thousands of deaths and millions of injuries annually in motor vehicle accidents (Schuckit, 2000). For example, between 25 and 49 percent of clients with spinal cord injuries were intoxicated at the time of their injury. These clients are also more likely to have difficulty adhering to rehabilitation plans (McKinley, Kolakowsky, & Kreutzer, 1999).

Health care professionals need to know the signs and medical consequences of alcohol abuse, so it can be diagnosed and the appropriate treatment recommendations made. The simple, cost-effective CAGE questionnaire can be used to screen for alcohol abuse. This acronym gets to the heart of the problems and involves asking the client four questions (Epperly & Moore, 2000), as shown in Box 14–1. This questionnaire is easy to administer and takes only a minute or two. One "yes" answer is a red flag for alcohol problems. Two or more "yes" answers are a signal for the care provider to open a dialogue with the goal of encouraging treatment.

The relationship between substance use disorders and psychiatric disorders is a complex one. Studies note that "dual diagnosis" of substance abuse and mental illness is highly prevalent (de Lima, Lorea, & Carpena, 2002). In a study of clients seeking psychiatric care for personal difficulties, 60 percent were found to have both a substance abuse disorder and a personality disorder (Skodol, Oldham, & Gallagher, 1999). In the psychiatric population, polydrug use is common, and psychoactive substances frequently exacerbate the psychiatric disorder (de Lima et al., 2002). Because substance use and withdrawal produce symptoms that mimic psychiatric diagnoses, a differential diagnosis may be difficult to establish when a client presents with behavior that is "out of control."

---

### BOX 14–1    CAGE Questionnaire Used to Screen for Alcohol Abuse

- Have you ever tried unsuccessfully to Cut down your drinking?
- Does it make you Angry when people suggest that you stop drinking?
- Do you feel Guilty when you drink?
- Do you need an Eye-opener to get started in the morning?

## Treatment Interventions for Substance Use Disorders

Many health professionals consider substance use a social rather than a physical or medical disorder (McLellan et al., 2000). This is unfortunate because most physicians do not screen for alcohol or drug use during routine visits. Substance use disorders are often missed, even when a client is ill or in the hospital with an alcohol-related sickness. Many allied health professionals can assess and treat clients who have not been seen by a physician first. Therefore, as part of routine care, all medical professionals should screen clients for substance use during initial examinations. It might be uncomfortable to ask the CAGE questions (see Box 14–1) or to inquire about other substance use, but a straightforward, nonjudgmental attitude can put clients at ease. Many people with a substance abuse problem will not be truthful when questioned, and not everyone with a substance use problem will admit it. However, each time a client is asked, a seed is planted, and the probability of change is increased.

When interviewing the client, the health professional should assess his or her motivation for change. Possible treatment options can be explained, and the client should be encouraged to select the choices that feel right for him or her. If possible, the client should leave the office with information about drug or alcohol treatment programs, the employee assistance programs offered by many companies, or locations of Alcoholics Anonymous meetings.

Unfortunately, there are no proven medications or other interventions that "cure" substance abuse disorders and restore the client to a permanently sober state. However, several treatment options are available, although they have varying levels of efficacy. If a client is in an acute state of toxicity or withdrawal, inpatient treatment may be needed. Some individuals may stay for prolonged periods of time at drug and alcohol rehabilitation facilities to change unhealthy behaviors and learn to live substance free. Others may choose to attend outpatient or day treatment programs.

At this time, there are many promising medications that can alleviate drug withdrawal symptoms or cravings. However, these alone will not lead to prolonged sobriety, so other forms of intervention are also needed. Various forms of psychotherapy, such as relaxation and stress management, marital and family therapy, cognitive behavioral therapy, and motivational interviewing have proven efficacious (Carroll & Onken, 2005; Ogborne, 2000). Another source of intervention might be attendance at a peer support group meeting, such as Alcoholics Anonymous. Al-Anon helps families and friends who have been affected by someone else's drinking, by providing understanding, hope, and strength. Alateen, a part of Al-Anon, is available for young people who have been affected by the problem drinking of a friend or relative.

Alcoholics Anonymous (AA) and Narcotics Anonymous (NA) are self-help groups that support users to become abstinent by attending meetings, finding support from other members, and calling on a higher power to provide guidance. It is difficult to perform research on outcomes with people who attend NA and AA, in part because of the importance of anonymity; therefore, there are few controlled studies. However, there is convincing evidence that AA is an effective intervention with good outcomes. In fact, we do know that in the first year of treatment, AA is as effective as motivational interviewing or cognitive behavioral therapy (Vaillant, 2005). The evidence shows that the more meetings a client attends, the better the outcome. AA and NA are free, and meetings are held in multiple locations at different times of day and night. These groups provide literature that explains these disorders and outlines meeting schedules. This is helpful information that you could have available in your facility.

## EATING DISORDERS

> Jayme is so thin! She came in for a nutritional assessment today because her family and her pediatrician are worried about all the weight she has lost. When she was 13, she was a little chubby and was unhappy about it. Now that she is 15, it is just the opposite. She has lost too much weight and is so frail, you can see all her bones and count her ribs. She still thinks that she's too heavy and worries about the little bit of fat that she carries on her hips. It makes her sick to think about food. To look at her, you'd think she's 12 instead of 15. Our measurements indicate she has only 4 percent body fat, and her Body Mass Index (BMI) is only 15, which is *way* below normal. I've heard about eating disorders, but I've never actually seen someone with one before.
>
> — *From the journal of Christy Marks, nutrition student*

Eating disorders are a heterogeneous group of abnormal eating behaviors with complex and, as yet, unclear causes. Because multiple known factors lead to these disorders, it is likely that each client has unique issues and needs individualized treatment. A category of serious and life-threatening health challenges that include a broad range of problematic eating behaviors, psychological states, and weights, eating disorders include anorexia nervosa (AN), bulimia nervosa (BN), binge-eating disorder (BED), and purging disorder (PD). It is generally believed that these patterns of eating are utilized as a way to manage feelings and emotions, moderate emotional stress, and provide the experience of rewards and punishments. Most people with eating disorders lose the capacity to monitor true hunger and differentiate it from emotional needs. "Eating or not eating often becomes the person's main way of coping with frightening, painful, intense or unacceptable emotions" (Phillips & Pratt, 2005, p. 90). A significant concern is that abnormal eating behaviors and the inability to normally regulate food intake interfere with biological processes, psychological integrity, and sociocultural norms (Tyler, 2003). Thus, disordered eating can cause considerable emotional instability and affect interpersonal behaviors, as well as cause physical harm and even death.

Many authorities consider eating disorders to be spectrum disorders, with some individuals meeting full diagnostic criteria. Others have sub-threshold or partial eating disorders because they have an insufficient number or intensity of symptoms to meet the criteria for diagnosis. The APA estimates that between 0.5 and 1 percent of women will develop full criteria for anorexia nervosa, and 1 to 3 percent will develop full criteria for bulimia nervosa. However, as many as 12 percent of adolescent girls demonstrate some degree of disordered eating (Stice, Marti, Shaw, & Jaconis, 2009), as do 7.7 to 19 percent of college women (Phillips & Pratt, 2005). This is significant because many clients with sub-threshold symptoms and partial symptoms may progress to fully diagnosed conditions. Further, people with sub-threshold disorders, as well as those with fully diagnosed conditions, demonstrate significant functional impairment, emotional distress, psychiatric comorbidity, risk of medical complications, and increased mortality. Although some variations are reported in the literature, most eating disorders first appear in midadolescence to the early 30s. The duration of these disorders may become chronic (Cyr, 2008).

Approximately 90 percent of those diagnosed with eating disorders are women, with the overwhelming majority residing in Western, developed countries. These disorders occur across all socioeconomic groups and in all cultures, although differences exist among various ethnic groups (Franko & George, 2008). There is little literature on the incidence or prevalence in minority women, and some variability in reported data. For example, some studies report that Latina women have approximately the same incidence as Caucasian women (Tyler, 2003), whereas others show Latina women having an increased risk for developing eating disorders (Franko & George, 2008). Native American women have a higher incidence, and African American women are less likely to have an eating disorder (Tyler, 2003). The incidence among men is extremely low. There is concern that lower numbers of Latina women with disordered eating are referred for treatment (Franko & George, 2008). Some speculate that the lower number of African American women having anorexia nervosa or bulimia nervosa is a result of cultural factors that focus on food as a source of comfort and an opportunity for family socialization. Further, African American culture places less emphasis on thinness and is more accepting of a range of body types and shapes (Tyler, 2003).

It is extremely rare for a client to present with only an eating disorder. The majority of affected individuals will have other comorbid psychiatric disorders, substance use/abuse disorders, personality disorders, or post-traumatic stress disorder. A particularly strong correlation exists between sexual abuse and eating disorders, especially bulimia nervosa (Brewerton, 2007). Like other psychological and behavioral problems, the causes are complex and not entirely clear. However, multiple factors have been identified that can affect the onset of the disordered eating or weight-maintenance behaviors. These include genetics, neuroendocrine effects, neurotransmitter function, behavioral reinforcers, and activity/exercise level, as well as psychological issues, family factors, abuse, and traumatic life events (APA, 2000b; Cyr, 2008; Halmi, 2009; Phillips & Pratt, 2005). The brain, in particular the limbic system, is responsible for hunger, thirst, and feeling satisfied with the amount of food ingested. Research related to brain mechanisms that control eating behaviors is ongoing. Studies suggest that genetic sensitivities within the limbic system make certain individuals vulnerable to eating disorders as a mechanism to manage stress. This may explain the common comorbidity with substance abuse (Halmi, 2009).

Most clients with eating disorders will seek medical care for medical or psychological symptoms rather than their eating disorders. They may have low energy, difficulty concentrating, anxiety, depression, blood in the stool, and heart palpitations (Phillips & Pratt, 2005). Unfortunately, many health care providers are unaware of the symptoms of disordered eating and often do not adequately diagnose or provide follow-up treatments.

At one end of the eating disorders spectrum are individuals who are obese, being at least 20 percent overweight and having a body mass index (BMI) of 30 or above. At the other end of the spectrum are individuals with anorexia nervosa. These individuals are at least 15 percent below ideal weight, with a BMI of less than 18. The latter may be literally starving to death (APA, 2000b). Clients with bulimia nervosa are between the two ends of the spectrum concerning their weight. However, they also have very disordered eating and weight control behaviors that are both physically and emotionally unhealthy. Binge-eating disorder occurs when an individual has periods of binge eating without purging.

Currently, anorexia nervosa and bulimia nervosa are receiving a great deal of coverage in the press and popular literature. It is important to put these problems in perspective. Anorexia and bulimia occur in 1 to 4 percent of the population (APA, 2000b). There is a significant overlap between symptoms of anorexia and bulimia. "Weight preoccupation and excessive self-evaluation of size and shape are primary symptoms of anorexia and bulimia" (APA, 2000b, p. 3). Fifty percent of clients with anorexia also exhibit symptoms of bulimia, and some clients may switch or alternate between different types of weight-restricting behaviors. Obesity is a much more significant problem, occurring in approximately one third of Americans. All clients with disordered eating face health and quality-of-life problems that are a result of being over- or underweight or using unhealthy weight-management behaviors.

## Anorexia Nervosa

The hallmark symptom of anorexia nervosa is a refusal to maintain an appropriate body weight for age and height. Weight must be at least 15 percent below ideal with a BMI at or below 18. Clients with anorexia nervosa have a distorted perception of body size, weight, and appearance and an extreme fear of getting fat (Phillips & Pratt, 2005) rather than a loss of appetite. Some clients with anorexia control weight by stringently restricting the amount of food eaten. Others combine severe caloric restriction with binge eating, followed by purging through vomiting or use of laxatives or diuretics. Excessive exercising, to the point where it becomes obsessive, may also be used to burn "extra" calories that have been consumed (APA, 2000b).

Anorexia typically begins in adolescence, when a young person, most often female, decides to diet to become more attractive. This is also a time of increased psychosocial angst that may trigger the desire to control emotional distress through food. Many of today's role models, such as actresses, female rock stars, and models in fashion magazines, are shockingly thin. They send a message that in order to be popular and successful, you need to be very thin. Furthermore, many popular activities encourage, or even require, young people to have unrealistically thin bodies. Wrestlers, dancers, gymnasts, ice skaters, and aspiring actors/actresses are all encouraged to keep their weight low, often without regard to health needs or risks.

Depression, anxiety, obsessions, perfectionism, and a rigid cognitive style, with lack of sexual interest, are frequently seen in clients who have anorexia. In addition, many individuals tend to isolate themselves (APA, 2000b). Numerous medical complications are also associated with anorexia, including hypotension, cardiac abnormalities and arrhythmia, dehydration, and anemia. Dysmenorrhea (infrequent periods) and the loss of the menstrual cycle (amenorrhea) are common in post-pubescent women with anorexia. This decreases circulating estrogens and can lead to osteoporosis and serious risk of fractures. One estimate states that 20 percent of those who meet the full criteria for AN will die within 20 years (Cyr, 2008).

## Bulimia Nervosa

Unlike the client with anorexia, a person with bulimia nervosa may have a normal or near-normal body weight or even be overweight. However, eating behaviors are "chaotic," with extremely abnormal patterns of caloric intake and control. People with bulimia nervosa will engage in episodes of uncontrolled, compulsive eating and ingest large quantities of food in a very short time (Cyr, 2008). Clients with bulimia nervosa may consume over 1,000 calories of food in less than 30 minutes (binging). Afterwards, they may feel so distressed by this that they induce purging by vomiting or the use of diuretics or laxatives. Between binges, clients with bulimia nervosa may restrict food or eat "normal" amounts. Excessive exercising, which can interfere with performing other life activities, is also common. Unlike clients with anorexia nervosa, those with bulimia nervosa are aware that their eating patterns are abnormal. They are very ashamed of their disordered eating patterns and hide this behavior from others (APA, 2000a).

Clients with bulimia nervosa often manifest symptoms of depression, anxiety, poor impulse control, sexual conflicts, personality disorders, and addictions. As many as 50 percent of clients with bulimia nervosa have reported being sexually abused (Wolfe, 1998). This comorbidity with addictions suggests a shared genetic vulnerability (Halmi, 2009). Bulimia nervosa carries health risks that are less severe than those of anorexia and are usually not life threatening. Because weight tends to be near normal, severe weight fluctuations and starvation do not occur. However, bradycardia, hypotension, dehydration, hypoglycemia, and anemia can occur. Stomach acids from recurrent vomiting may affect the esophagus and oral area, including the teeth (Wolfe, 1998).

It may not be difficult to recognize an individual with anorexia, especially if the health provider asks the client to undress or checks the client's weight. Additional indicators of anorexia can include electrolyte imbalances, skin changes, cardiac abnormalities, or fatigue. In contrast, bulimia nervosa can be more difficult to identify, with the most visible signs on the hands or oral area, as a result of self-induced vomiting. A careful health history, including questions about activity and exercise levels, may reveal unhealthy eating or weight-maintenance behavior. "Psychiatric management forms the foundation of treatment for patients/clients with eating disorders and should be instituted for all patients/clients in combination with other specific treatment modalities" (APA, 2000b, p. 1). Other treatments may include nutritional counseling to educate the client to eat a range of healthy foods, correct abnormal eating behaviors, and engage in appropriate levels of exercise. Individual or family psychotherapy, behavioral therapy, and 12-step programs may also be useful. Psychiatric interventions can take many forms, and no particular form of counseling has proven more effective than another for eating disorders. However, unlike with anorexia nervosa, medication use, particularly antidepressants, has proven efficacious and should be started as an initial intervention. Nutritional rehabilitation to restore normal nutritional intake is essential (APA, 2000b).

## Obesity

Currently, in the United States, there are strong public health concerns about the "epidemic" of obesity. One third of adults are considered overweight, with a BMI between 25 and 29.9, and another third are obese, with a BMI of over 30. Thus, only one third of adults have normal weight. The incidence of overweight is not evenly distributed among racial groups, and African Americans have the highest rates of overweight, followed by Hispanics (Flegal, Carrol, & Ogden, 2010). Poverty is another factor that increases the prevalence of overweight. The health consequences of obesity impact both morbidity and mortality. Multiple medical problems are caused or exacerbated by significant weight, including cardiovascular disease, hypertension, diabetes, gallbladder disease, metabolic and endocrine diseases, cancer, and strokes. Excess weight also puts added stress on joints and increases the effects of arthritis and other joint dysfunctions.

There are multiple causes for overweight. Although genetics is certainly a factor, culture, lifestyle, health behaviors, and socioeconomic and environmental issues also contribute. A direct correlation exists between calories-in (eating) and calories-out (activity). Simple arithmetic informs us that an abundance of calories-in versus the number of calories-out leads to people gaining extra pounds. It is not unusual for people to gain weight as they age because metabolic rate slows, and muscle mass is lost. Endocrine imbalances and other diseases may play a role in achieving and maintaining ideal weight. In addition, many medications, especially psychotropic drugs, can cause weight gain as a side effect of their therapeutic actions.

A very significant cause of increased weight is living in what has been called a "toxic" food environment. Fast-food outlets are abundantly marketed and located, with inexpensive calorie-dense foods. Healthy foods, such as fresh fruits and vegetables, are more costly, may not be as enticing to many, and may not be as readily available in low-income neighborhoods.

Once weight is gained, it can be extremely difficult to lose. One study compared the results of using Atkins, Ornish, Weight Watchers, and Zone diets (Dansinger, Gleason, Griffith, Selker, &

Schaefer, 2005). The results demonstrated that no diet was better than any other, as long as the dieter adhered to the plan. Unfortunately, this was very difficult for participants, and a 25 percent adherence was considered a good rate. At the end of 1 year, 10 percent of the dieters had lost more than 15 percent of their weight, and 25 percent had lost more than 5 percent of their weight. Although this may sound disappointing, a weight loss of only 5 percent is sufficient to improve the health of people who are obese (Dansinger et al., 2005).

"Weight loss studies are behavioral studies; they require participants to eat less" (Katan, 2009, p. 923). Cognitive, emotional, and cultural issues all impact one's ability to diet. Does the dieter believe that the diet will work? How does he or she feel about food? Does he or she like the taste and texture of the foods expected to be eaten for improved health? How does the food compare to cultural norms and fit into family events and rituals? The most critical factors to ensure adherence include attendance at counseling sessions and availability of support. However, in the studies cited above, even intelligent, educated, well-supported, and highly motivated clients with access to healthy food could not achieve enough weight loss to reverse obesity (Dansinger et al., 2005; Katan, 2009).

Exercise is another factor that contributes to maintaining a healthy weight. As people age, they face increasing career and relationship responsibilities and demands on their time. They may become more sedentary, which can contribute to decreasing metabolism. In addition, people who live in inner cities or who have low incomes may have no safe outdoor recreational spaces and may not be able to afford to join a gym, even if one is available in their neighborhood. Some people who are overweight are unaccustomed to physical activity and may not have good coordination or motor skills. Some consider exercise unpleasant, and they may find it difficult to elicit and maintain adherence to programs. It is especially important for health care professionals who promote exercise and healthy lifestyles to be supportive and sensitive of clients who are overweight. Entering a gym, wearing form-fitting attire amidst trim people who are comfortable exercising, can be difficult for those who are overweight and self-conscious. They may need to exercise in a more private area, receive a modified exercise program, or receive individualized instructions from a personal trainer until initial weight loss goals are achieved. Special bariatric attention and appropriate equipment needs to be provided to ensure the health and safety of clients in exercise programs. Providing extra praise for efforts to exercise and reinforcement for small successes may help sustain motivation and adherence.

Health care professionals need to be alert to the signs, symptoms, and consequences of eating disorders. Many clients will not present with obvious signs of disordered eating but will have medical complications arising from abnormal eating behaviors. Others will seek care for psychiatric symptoms or substance abuse. Many will have emotional distress and functional impairments as a result of their eating habits or their weight. If we are aware of signs and symptoms of eating disorders, we can ask nonjudgmental questions that can help identify potential problems. Making appropriate referrals to mental health professionals, physicians, and nutritionists who specialize in eating disorders and weight management can help clients acquire healthier eating habits that can improve health and reduce morbidity and mortality.

## SELF-INJURIOUS BEHAVIOR

All of the behaviors we have discussed in this chapter can be considered self-injurious. Substance abuse and eating disorders cause harm to the client, but may not cause visible tissue damage or injury. The physical effects of disordered eating behavior and substance abuse may take many years to develop. However, some disturbing behaviors result in immediate, direct, physical harm.

Self-injurious behaviors (SIB) may also be called self-mutilation, deliberate self-harm (DSH), or nonsuicidal self-injury (NSSI).

"Self-injury is defined as the intentional destruction of body tissue without suicidal intent and for purposes not socially sanctioned" (Klonsky, 2007, p. 1039). Seen more often in women, self-harm typically begins in adolescence or young adulthood. Prevalence figures vary, but Klonsky (2007) reported that 14 to 17 percent of adolescents and young adults have self-injured at least once. A random sample of college students found that 7 percent had injured themselves in the previous 4 weeks, with Black women less likely to self-harm than White women (Gollust, Eisenberg, & Golberstein, 2008). The range of behaviors is both lengthy and disturbing. Cutting, burning, biting, head banging, eye gouging, skin picking or scratching, and hair pulling are classic behaviors. It has been suggested that excessive body piercing and tattooing may also be forms of self-mutilation in mainstream culture in the United States, but this idea remains controversial. Many clients who harm themselves also have other self-destructive behaviors, such as eating disorders and substance abuse disorders. Self-injurious behavior is a symptom, not a diagnosis, and is seen in heterogeneous groups of clients and settings. It can be classified into three distinct types of behaviors: major self-mutilation, superficial or moderate self-mutilation, and stereotypical self-injurious behavior (Favazza, 1998).

Major self-mutilation is a particularly horrifying form of self-harm. It consists of extremely bloody acts that cause permanent or severe damage, such as removing one or both eyes or other body parts. These acts are rare, and are most commonly committed by clients who are in a psychotic state and may be "hearing" commands or experiencing hallucinations. People who are extremely intoxicated may also cause severe self-harm. When the clients' minds clear, they are aghast at what they have done (Favazza, 1998).

Superficial or moderate self-harm describes behaviors that cause pain but do not inflict permanent injury, such as nail biting, hair pulling, scratching, cutting, or burning. These types of behaviors, particularly burning and cutting, are the most common. Many clients who exhibit moderate self-harm have been sexually abused and may have post-traumatic stress syndrome. Self-injurious behavior is most often seen in people with borderline personality disorder and may also be seen with affective disorders or anxiety. It may also be evident in clients with eating and substance use disorders (Gollust et al., 2008). These individuals are vulnerable and emotionally fragile. Surprisingly, it can also occur in people who are high functioning, without obvious pathology (Klonsky, 2007).

Stereotypical self-injurious behavior refers to behaviors that are repetitive, rhythmic, and monotonous, as is sometimes seen in individuals with certain types of autism and intellectual impairments. Many of these actions are "mild" or benign, such as rocking, spinning, or twirling. However, head banging, eye poking, self-biting, and repetitive hitting are also common (Favazza, 1998). Because autism and intellectual impairments are notable for producing abnormal sensory control and processing functions, clients respond atypically to normal levels of stimuli. They may be easily overwhelmed or feel understimulated, and it is believed that self-stimulation or self-harm may help to manage stress.

Clients who cause intentional self-harm often feel either significant emotional pain or numbing. Some clients report feelings of agitation or distress, and the physical act of self-injurious behavior calms them. Other clients describe being in a dissociative state prior to cutting themselves, and seeing blood or feeling pain reconnects them to reality. Inflicting self-harm causes pain that triggers the release of endorphins, the body's internal pain-reducing drugs, modulating the emotional pain. It provides a mechanism to regulate emotions or release tension (Jacobson, Muehlenkamp, Miller, & Turner, 2008). Others have suggested that self-injurious behavior is a maladaptive coping strategy, like disordered eating or substance abuse, that can relieve stress, decrease tension, and provide relief from distressing emotions (Gollust et al., 2008). However, these other behaviors do not cause tissue damage, and self-injury may be a red flag for a later suicide attempt (Nafisi & Stanley, 2007).

Because multiple emotional and biological mechanisms cause self-injurious behavior, a variety of approaches to treatment is needed. Behavioral therapy, especially applied behavior analysis, has been shown to be most effective with clients who have intellectual impairments or autism. For clients who cause severe self-harm while in an altered mental state due to psychosis, antipsychotic drugs are prescribed and can prevent further self-harm by stabilizing the underlying psychiatric disorder. For the majority of clients who self-injure using moderate or superficial means, treatment options are varied and need to be individualized to the client situation. Psychotherapy, various behavioral therapies, support groups, and medication can all be helpful (Favazza, 1998). Two promising therapeutic approaches, with demonstrated efficacy, are cognitive behavioral therapy and dialectical behavioral therapy. Both of these techniques are provided by skilled psychotherapists with extensive training. Allied health professionals can help by identifying clients who need assistance and referring them to the appropriate providers.

Clients who engage in self-injurious behavior are generally ashamed and take great pains to conceal it or provide excuses for how they became injured. Health care providers need to be extremely sensitive and nonjudgmental to encourage open communication about these behaviors. We can provide physical and emotional support after an episode of injury to help clients feel comfortable and assist them in finding competent medical care. Making a referral to a mental health professional is an essential component of that care. Clients can be assisted in finding alternate, healthier means to deal with the tension or stress they may be feeling prior to self-injury. When we work with people who self-injure, we must take care to be present and listen thoroughly and nonjudgmentally. It is likely to be more difficult for people to reveal their behavior than it is for us to hear about it.

In the past, self-injury was frequently erroneously determined to be a suicide attempt. At first glance, all attempts to self-injure may appear to be suicidal gestures or suggest suicidal intent. In fact, most self-injurious behavior is not severe enough to be life threatening and is characteristically a coping mechanism, intended to ameliorate emotional pain and obtain help.

## SUICIDE

The ultimate act of self-injury is suicide, a permanent solution to a temporary problem. Virtually all clients who attempt suicide have a psychiatric and/or substance abuse disorder. Suicide is more likely to occur if psychiatric and substance abuse disorders are both present because impaired judgment may cause the clients to act impulsively, without regard to consequences.

---

I have been taking an abnormal psych. course this semester, and yesterday, the instructor discussed the symptoms of depression. When I was in high school, my best friend committed suicide, and none of us could figure out why. Her life seemed so perfect. She was smart, pretty, and a good athlete. Now, I see that she had all the symptoms of depression. Why didn't some adult notice? Why couldn't anyone have helped her?

—*From the journal of Susan Lockhart, speech-language pathology student*

Unfortunately, many clients send out distress signals that do not get heard. We are often quick to assume that "all teenagers act like this" or "of course, he's acting withdrawn; his wife recently died." Most people are not trained to recognize symptoms of psychiatric disorders, and many who seek care are not appropriately diagnosed. Half of all people who attempt or complete suicide have visited a health care provider in the month prior to their attempt, and the provider failed to recognize the risk or need for supportive treatment (Vannoy, Fancher, Unutwe, Duberstein, & Kravitz, 2010). This may occur because many clients themselves are not able to articulate their emotional distress. Rather, they present to physicians' offices with complaints of pain or other physical discomforts, such as fatigue or general malaise. "Few clients spontaneously disclose suicidal thoughts, however, and few primary care physicians ask about suicide ideation" (Vannoy et al., 2010, p. 34).

The American Foundation for Suicide Prevention (AFSP, 2010) is a current and reliable source of information on suicide. The AFSP reports that each year, more than 30,000 Americans commit suicide, while at least four times that number make an attempt. Suicide is the fourth leading cause of death for people between ages 18 and 65 and the third leading cause of death for adolescents. Surprisingly, the rate of suicide for women drops after 55, whereas the risks for men increase significantly. White men over age 65 who live alone have the highest rate of suicide.

Men are four times more likely to complete a suicide attempt than women, but women are twice as likely to make an attempt. This disparity in consequences can be understood by looking at the methods used for the attempt. Men are likely to use violent means, such as guns or hanging, whereas women are more likely to use pills or cutting. Among Americans of all ages, more than 50 percent of completed suicides are caused by the use of guns (Miller & Hemenway, 2008).

At least 90 percent of people who commit suicide have a diagnosable and treatable mental illness, the most common being depression and other mood disorders. Substance abuse substantially increases the risk of suicide because it leads to poor judgment and impulsive behavior. Surprisingly, 40 to 80 percent of suicide attempts occur impulsively, when a negative event triggers acute distress (Miller & Hemenway, 2008). Individuals who live alone or are socially isolated are at particularly high risk. Elderly Caucasian males have the highest rate of suicide, and it is notable that 60 percent have seen a physician within a few months prior to their deaths (AFSP, 2010). Unfortunately, the suicide rate of active-duty military personnel is rising rapidly. This can be attributed to very high rates of traumatic brain injury and mental disorders, such as posttraumatic stress disorder, depression, and substance abuse among soldiers returning from Iraq and Afghanistan (Kuehn, 2009).

Clients who verbalize feeling helpless, hopeless, and worthless or have excessive guilt are a concern, especially if they are socially withdrawn or isolated. Other examples of critical cues of suicide risk are giving away beloved items, voicing a plan, or becoming suddenly brighter in affect. Some clients state that they wish they were dead or want to die. In this case, health professionals need to ask the clients if they have a suicide plan. If they answer "yes," the professional needs to determine if the clients have the means to carry out the plan. When a client has the intent, the plan, and the means to attempt suicide, the provider must summon immediate mental health intervention and keep the client under observation until help arrives.

This is an area where all health care providers can intervene and, literally, save someone's life. As with substance abuse, all clients can be screened during regular health care visits for symptoms of emotional distress or disorders by asking a few simple questions. We can ask how things are in their personal lives and if anything is bothering them. If problems are identified, we can ask clients if they have the resources to handle the situation and offer assistance finding appropriate supports. Once again, sensitive, nonjudgmental questioning and listening are essential to allow clients to feel sufficiently safe to talk about their feelings and discuss problems that may threaten their health or well-being. It can be difficult knowing what to say or how to recommend mental health care. Letting clients know that you care, are worried about them, and that you want to make sure they are safe is a good place to start.

## Summary

In this chapter, we discussed destructive behaviors that put clients' well-being at risk, including substance abuse, eating disorders, and other self-injurious behaviors. It can be difficult to broach these subjects during a client interview and find ways to effectively discuss them. Sometimes, it seems easier to remain silent or pretend that these situations do not exist. However, the competent health care provider is concerned about all aspects of the client's health and welfare and needs to develop screening and referral strategies.

## Reflective Questions

1. a. What behaviors or problems would indicate that someone has moved from substance use to abuse?
   b. What behaviors or problems would indicate that someone has moved from substance abuse to addiction?
2. As a health care practitioner, you may need to suggest interventions for people with drug or alcohol problems.
   a. How will your personal experiences affect your judgment in making these decisions?
   b. What strategies do you think you could use to offer help?
3. Appearance and weight are important concerns in our culture.
   a. What signs or symptoms would you expect to see in a client who has an inappropriate weight that suggests an eating disorder?
   b. What would you do if you suspected this?
   c. What strategies could you use to offer clients help with their weight or eating patterns?
   d. Think about your own values, beliefs, and behaviors around food. Would you be a good role model for your clients? Why or why not?
4. Clients sometimes intentionally harm themselves or attempt suicide. It can be shocking to discover these situations.
   a. How might you respond to the client?
   b. What resources will you need to have available?
5. All the problem behaviors described in this chapter can trigger powerful emotions for us, particularly if we have had personal experiences with these problems.
   a. Are there any groups of clients with whom you think you might have difficulty working?
   b. How might you be able to manage your emotional responses to your clients and their behaviors in order to develop a therapeutic relationship?

## Case Study

Samantha Davis is a junior in high school who excels academically and athletically. She is being admitted to an ambulatory surgical center for day surgery. While taking the history and recording vital signs prior to the procedure, the nurse notes that Samantha's weight is well below the standard for someone her age and height. Without solicitation, Samantha comments that she needs to lose a few more pounds. After the client disrobes, the nurse notices several scars that appear to be burn marks on the inner thighs. The nurse is concerned and tells Samantha that there are things she will need to discuss with Samantha's parents. Samantha begins to sob and begs the nurse not to tell them anything because they will "kill" her if they find out she has any problems.

1. What could be possible explanations for all of the physical findings?
2. What are the legal and ethical obligations of a licensed health care provider to document and share this information because the client is a minor?
3. What would you do if Samantha revealed that her parents are abusing her?
4. Identify the next steps in treatment that could lead to optimal care for Samantha.

## References

American Foundation for Suicide Prevention. (2010). Retrieved from http://www.afsp.org

American Psychiatric Association. (2000a). *Diagnostic and statistical manual of mental disorders* (4th ed., text rev.). Washington, DC: Author.

American Psychiatric Association (2000b). Practice guidelines for the treatment of patients with eating disorders (rev. ed.). *American Journal of Psychiatry, 157* (Suppl. 1), 1–23.

Baldisseri, M. R. (2007). Impaired health care professional. *Critical Care Medicine, 35*(2), S106–S116.

Betz, C., Mihalic, D., Pinto, M. E., & Raffa, R. B. (2000). Could a common biochemical mechanism underlie addictions? *Journal of Clinical Pharmacy and Therapeutics, 25,* 11–20.

Brewerton, T. D. (2007). Eating disorders, trauma and co-morbidity: Focus on PTSD. *Eating Disorders, 15,* 285–304.

Carroll, K. M., & Onken, L. S. (2005). Behavioral therapies for drug abuse. *American Journal of Psychiatry, 162,* 1452–1460.

Cyr, N. R. (2008). Considerations for patients who have eating disorders. *Association of Operating Room Nurses, 88*(5), 807–815.

Dansinger, M. L., Gleason, J. A., Griffith, J. L., Selker, H. P., & Schaefer, E. J. (2005). Comparison of the Atkins, Ornish, Weight Watchers, and Zone diets for weight loss and heart disease risk reduction: A randomized trial. *Journal of the American Medical Association, 293*(1), 43–53.

de Lima, M. S., Lorea, C. F., & Carpena, M. P. (2002). Dual diagnosis on "substance abuse." *Substance Use and Misuse, 37*(8–10), 1179–1184.

Epperly, T., & Moore, K. (2000). Health issues in men: Part II. *American Family Physician, 62*(1), 117–124.

Favazza, A. R. (1998). The coming of age of self-mutilation. *Journal of Mental and Nervous Disorders, 185*(5), 259–268.

Flegal, K. M., Carrol, M. D., & Ogden, L. R. (2010). Prevalence and trends in obesity among US adults, 1999–2008. *Journal of the American Medical Association, 303*(3), 235–241.

Franko, D. L., & George, J. B. (2008). A pilot intervention to reduce eating disorder risk in Latina women. *European Eating Disorders Review, 16,* 436–441.

French, M. T., McGeary, K. A., Chitwood, D. D., & McCoy, C. B. (2000). Chronic illicit drug use, health services utilization and the cost of medical care. *Social Science & Medicine, 50*(12), 1703–1713.

Gollust, S. E., Eisenberg, D., & Golberstein, E. (2008). Prevalence and correlates of self-injury among university students. *Journal of American College Health, 56*(5), 491–498.

Halmi, K. A. (2009). Perplexities and provocations of eating disorders. *Journal of Child Psychology and Psychiatry, 50*(1–2), 163–169.

Jacobson, C. M., Muehlenkamp, J. J., Miller, A. L., & Turner, J. B. (2008). Psychiatric impairment among adolescents engaging in different types of deliberate self-harm. *Journal of Clinical Child and Adolescent Psychology, 37*(2), 363–375.

Katan, M. B. (2009). Weight-loss diets for the prevention and treatment of obesity. *New England Journal of Medicine, 360*(9), 923–925.

Ketchum, K., & Asbury, W. (2000). *Beyond the influence.* New York: Bantam Books.

Klonsky, E. D. (2007). Non-suicidal self-injury: An introduction. *Journal of Clinical Psychology: In Session, 63*(11), 1039–1043.

Kuehn, B. M. (2009). Soldier suicide rates continue to rise. *Journal of the American Medical Association, 301*(11), 111–113.

McKinley, W. O., Kolakowsky, S. A., & Kreutzer, J. S. (1999). Substance abuse, violence, and outcome after traumatic spinal cord injury. *American Journal of Medical Rehabilitation, 78,* 306–312.

McLellan, A. T., Lewis, D. C., O'Brien, C. P., & Kleber, H. D. (2000). Drug dependence: A chronic medical illness. *Journal of the American Medical Association, 284*(13), 1689–1695.

Miller, M., & Hemenway, D. (2008). Guns and suicide in the United States. *New England Journal of Medicine, 359*(10), 989–991.

Nafisi, N., & Stanley, B. (2007). Developing and maintaining the therapeutic alliance with self-injuring patients. *Journal of Clinical Psychology: In Session, 63,* 1069–1079.

Ogborne, A. C. (2000). Identifying and treating patients with alcohol-related problems. *Canadian Medical Association Journal, 162*(12), 1705–1708.

Olson, H. C., Streissguth, A. P., Sampson, P. D., Barr, H. M., Bookstein, F. L., & Thiede, K. (1997). Association of prenatal alcohol exposure with behavioral and learning problems in early adolescence. *Journal of the American Academy of Child and Adolescent Psychiatry, 36*(9), 1187–1194.

Phillips, E. L., & Pratt, H. D. (2005). Eating disorders in college. *Pediatric Clinics of North America, 52*(1), 85–96.

Schuckit, M. (2000). *Drug and alcohol abuse.* New York: Kluwer Academic/Plenum Press.

Skodol, A. E., Oldham, J. M., & Gallagher, P. E. (1999). Axis II co-morbidity of substance use disorders among patients referred for treatment of personality disorders. *American Journal of Psychiatry, 156,* 734–738.

Stice, E., Marti, N. C., Shaw, H., & Jaconis, M. (2009). An 8-year longitudinal study of the natural history of threshold, subthreshold, and partial eating disorders from a community sample of adolescents. *Journal of Abnormal Psychology, 118*(3), 587–597.

Tyler, I. D. (2003). A true picture of eating disorders among African American women: A review of literature. *Journal of the Association of Black Nursing Faculty, 14*(3), 73–74.

Vaillant, G. E. (2005). Alcoholics Anonymous: Cult or cure? *Australian and New Zealand Journal of Psychiatry, 39,* 431–436.

Vannoy, D., Fancher, T., Unutwe, J., Duberstein, P., & Kravitz, R. L. (2010). Suicide inquiry in primary care: Creating context, inquiring, and following up. *Annals of Family Medicine, 8,* 33–39.

Wolfe, B. (1998). Eating disorders. In C. Glod (Ed.), *Contemporary psychiatric-mental health nursing* (pp. 461–478). New York: F. A. Davis.

# Abuse and Neglect

*I* am completing my final internship in a hospital outpatient clinic, and today, I observed another therapist treating a small somewhat reserved boy. The boy's diagnosis was status/post dislocation of the left shoulder. I watched the therapist examine and evaluate the boy's injuries. He appeared very quiet and was reluctant to answer the therapist's questions, as his mother sat by and observed. Having recently participated in a course that included abuse and neglect, I had to wonder, could this child be a victim of child abuse. I heard his mother state that he fell off the monkey bars in the playground, but I continued to think about him later in the evening. I know children can be quite active and frequently fall down and get hurt; I certainly did myself. Just how does one differentiate between normal childhood injuries and actual abuse or neglect? I think I'll ask my clinical instructor about that in the morning.

*—From the journal of M. J. Rawls, physical therapist student*

Abuse and neglect are interrelated and can take many forms. Neglect is a failure to adequately provide for an individual's physical, medical, financial, or psychological needs and may be intentional or unintentional. Failure to feed a hungry child, give an older person medication, or provide transportation to a scheduled doctor's appointment, for example, can result in minor or extreme physical or emotional harm (Wang & Holton, 2007).

The legal definition of abuse may vary by state; however, in general, abuse refers to physical, psychological, sexual, or material mistreatment or neglect of an individual that causes harm. What turns neglect into abuse is the situation. It occurs when an individual who is at the mercy of someone he or she should be able to trust is hurt or exploited by that caretaker (Andrews, 2008). It can occur at home, in a hospital or skilled nursing facility, or on the playground. Abuse can occur across the life span, affects males and females, and is found among all cultures and socioeconomic groups. It affects individuals in both heterosexual and homosexual relationships, as well as individuals with and without disabilities. Abuse can occur anywhere and can be perpetrated by strangers, but family relatives are the most frequent abusers, and abuse most commonly occurs in the home (Utley, 1999).

## THE FACES OF ABUSE

Abuse and neglect can be physical, psychological, financial, sexual, or any combination of the four. Harmful in many ways, the psychological effects can be devastating at all stages of development (Taylor & Spencer, 2000). Survivors of abuse may show an array of emotional, behavioral, and physical symptoms at the time of the abuse and throughout their life span (Dube et al., 2005; Wekerle et al., 2009).

Psychological abuse may include name-calling, shaming, bullying, embarrassing, or threatening an individual, their pets, or a friend or family member. Although it may seem less damaging than other forms of abuse, it frequently results in a loss of self-esteem and often culminates in depression, anxiety, or even suicide (Centers for Disease Control and Prevention [CDC], 2009).

Physical abuse includes hitting, kicking, shaking, burning, or otherwise exerting force to injure a victim. Symptoms include unexplained physical injuries, burns, cuts, bruises, traumatic brain injury, and excessive stress (CDC, 2009). It may begin in subtle ways and can escalate to include abduction and murder (Paavilainen, Astedt-Kurki, Paunonen-Ilmonen, & Laippala, 2002).

Sexual abuse involves forcing someone to take part in a sexual act without his or her consent. It may include touching, forcing an individual to watch pornographic materials, or actual sexual penetration (CDC, 2009; Doherty, 2009). People who have been abused sexually are more likely to smoke, drink, or use drugs, have low self-esteem, develop eating disorders, consider suicide, and become abusers themselves (CDC, 2009).

Financial abuse includes stealing or misusing an individual's money, property or assets; forging someone's signature; or using a person's property without permission. It may be perpetrated by friends, family, or even strangers through personal contact or via the telephone or Internet. Signs of financial abuse include unpaid bills, missing checkbooks, missing property, and new "best friends." People who have been financially abused may find they are unable to pay their bills, lose their homes, and be unable to pay for adequate care and assistance (Brickner, 2009; MetLife Mature Market Institute, 2009).

Abuse is always about power and control. Typically, a stronger, more powerful individual attempts to control a weaker or more vulnerable person. Infants, children, adolescents, spouses or partners, people who are elderly, and those with disabilities are often easy targets for abuse. Many abusers have been abused themselves and have not learned appropriate nurturing skills. Others may have a psychiatric disorder or abuse alcohol or drugs. Although it is tempting to look for an easy formula to identify potential abusers, there are few clear descriptors because abuse occurs across the spectrum of lifestyles and family situations.

The exact number of individuals abused each year is difficult to estimate because clients may be reluctant to divulge information, deny a problem exists, be embarrassed, or fear retaliation. Children may be afraid or lack the power to report incidents of abuse, and parents may deny it (Kellogg & Committee on Child Abuse and Neglect, 2007; Lazenbatt & Freeman, 2006). Teenagers may believe that abuse is a normal part of a relationship or may be too embarrassed to report abuse to parents or authorities (Betz, 2007). Intimate partners may prefer to remain in a relationship rather than risk the financial loss and potential lack of intimacy, which might be a consequence of reporting abuse (Buel, 2002). Older people, fearing being removed from their homes and relocated to a nursing home or other residential facility, may prefer to remain silent (Utley, 1999). Individuals with cognitive impairments may be unable to define the problem (Gray-Vickrey, 2001; Swagerty, Takahashi, & Evans, 1999).

Accurate statistics on the incidence of domestic violence are difficult to obtain. These events usually occur behind closed doors, and those involved make great efforts to ensure that they remain private, due to shame and fear of social or legal consequences. Furthermore, there is no consensus for an exact description or definition of behaviors that constitute abuse. There is, however, a consensus that abuse is underreported and underidentified (DeHart, Webb, & Cornman, 2009; Doherty, 2009; Flaherty, Jones, & Sege, 2004).

Research shows that the cycle of violence perpetuates future violence. Following an abusive episode, the abuser often expresses feelings of guilt or remorse. He or she then makes excuses for the behavior, and life returns to business as usual. Later, the cycle resumes, and abuse continues. Abuse has an enormous impact on health care resources. Early recognition and treatment might significantly reduce medical costs, as well as personal consequences (Krugman, 2001).

In the late 1990s, in recognition of the problems related to family violence, the government assessed the educational curricula of health care professionals. It is believed that changes in education, research, practice, and recognition of family violence as a health issue, not just a social or legal issue, can break the cycle of violence (Krugman, 2001). Those who are aware and educated about this issue are more likely to detect and report cases of abuse (Andrews, 2008).

## CATEGORIES OF ABUSE

### Child Abuse (Maltreatment)

Child abuse is an important global public health problem that affects children of all ages, genders, ethnicities, and socioeconomic groups (Kellogg & Committee on Child Abuse and Neglect, 2007; Runyon, Deblinger, Ryan, & Thakkar-Kolar, 2004). In the United States during 2007, 1,760 children died from abuse, and Child Protective Services considered 794,000 to be victims of maltreatment (U.S. Department of Health and Human Services, 2009). Children who are abused often have longer hospital stays, more severe injuries, poorer medical outcomes, and higher health care costs than children who are not abused (Rivara et al., 2007; Rovi, Chen, & Johnson, 2004). Although many cases of abuse go unreported, a conservative estimate of costs related to abuse and neglect in 2007 was $103.8 billion. These costs are borne not only by the family but also by society. Additionally, costs for medical care do not include the emotional costs of pain, suffering, reduced quality of life, and long-term affects (Wang & Holton, 2007).

Child maltreatment includes all types of abuse and neglect that occur among children under the age of 18 (CDC, 2009). Two of every 10 girls and one of every 10 boys are sexually abused before they reach the age of 14 (Child Molestation Research & Prevention Institute, 2010). Abuse is twice as high in children with a disability or chronic illness, premature children, and children with low birth weights (American Medical Student Association, 2008). Although the risk of physical abuse increases with age, fatal abuse and more serious injuries are more common among children under the age of 2 (U.S. Department of Health and Human Services, 2006). Estimates regarding the number of childhood injuries resulting from abuse that require an emergency department visit range from as low as 1.3 percent to as high as 15 percent (Kellogg & Committee on Child Abuse and Neglect, 2007).

A child who is vulnerable may place significant stress or demands on a potential abuser that are beyond the abuser's ability to meet. Consider Vanessa, a fussy and demanding baby, the youngest of four children, all living in a small home with their parents. During the day, her father worked two jobs, and her mother cared for the children. In the evenings, her mother went to work. After a long workday, her father was tired and unable to tolerate Vanessa's continual need to be held and comforted. He often yelled and slapped her in an effort to get her to be quiet. One night, he went too far, and Vanessa ended up in the emergency department with multiple fractures. Had her father been better educated about strategies to reduce stress, had a social support system been in place, and had he understood the potential dangerous consequences of his actions, this incident may have been prevented.

Neglect is the most common type of child maltreatment, ahead of physical, sexual, and emotional abuse (Kellogg & Committee on Child Abuse and Neglect, 2007). Indicators of child neglect include hunger, poor hygiene, lack of appropriate supervision, unattended physical problems or medical needs, unexplained injuries, and clothing inappropriate for weather conditions (Doherty, 2009). Physical abuse may include bruises, slashes, fractures, orofacial injuries (Paavilainen et al., 2002), traumatic brain injuries, and death (Kellogg & Committee on Child Abuse and Neglect, 2007) and always includes a component of psychological abuse. Physical abuse may lead to low self-esteem, depression or anxiety, problems at school, and signs of withdrawal or aggression (Doherty, 2009).

Emotional abuse creates a climate of fear in the home and teaches children that relationships include punishment, thus jeopardizing their chances of having healthy future relationships. Although emotional abuse may appear subtle, its effects may be both long lasting and profound (Wekerle et al., 2009).

Childhood sexual abuse occurs among both boys and girls. Psychosocial indicators of sexual abuse may include low self-esteem, depression, anxiety, eating disorders, and difficulty making friends. Abused adolescents may manifest "acting-out" behaviors that can be self-destructive, provocative, and harmful to others. They may become truant from school, abuse alcohol or drugs, run away, become sexually promiscuous, or get into trouble with the law (Dube et al., 2005).

Childhood abuse and neglect have been linked to adult psychiatric disorders. Anxiety, post-traumatic stress disorder, depression, fear, and anger can be sequelae of childhood abuse and sexual molestation, affecting the survivors for a lifetime (Dube et al., 2005). In addition, childhood survivors of abuse often have difficulty developing intimate relationships built on mutual trust, especially if the abuse was sexual (Cyr, McDuff, & Wright, 2006). This may result in the abuser or the abused individual becoming involved in teen dating violence, intimate partner abuse, or elder abuse (Merrill et al., 2005).

Children usually sustain abuse at the hands of a family member who reacts inappropriately to a child's behavior. Parents are more likely to abuse their children if they themselves were abused as children or teenagers. Parents who abuse alcohol and/or drugs and live in an impoverished community with a lower percentage of two-parent families are also more likely to abuse their children. Additional risk factors include high stress levels, depression, anxiety, isolation, interpersonal problems, and a higher number of children living in the household (Black, Heyman, & Smith-Slep, 2001).

## Intimate Partner Violence

Intimate partner violence (IPV), also known as domestic violence, occurs between two people in a close relationship. IPV occurs in both teenage and adult relationships and in both heterosexual and homosexual partnerships. It includes current and former spouses and dating partners. IPV often begins with emotional abuse but can escalate to ongoing battering, resulting in physical or sexual assault and even death. Women who experience intimate partner violence have significantly elevated health care utilization and cost both during and long after the abuse stops. According to the CDC (2009), 4.8 million women and 2.9 million men are victims of IPV annually. In 2005, 1,510 deaths occurred as a result of IPV, 78 percent females and 22 percent males. Costs related to IPV in 2005 were estimated to be $5.8 billion dollars. Because many people do not report abuse, these numbers are likely to be low estimates (Buel, 2002). Many suffer from physical injuries, which can include long-lasting disabilities, broken bones, internal bleeding, and head injuries. They are more likely to smoke, abuse drugs and alcohol, and engage in risky sexual activities (Goodkind & Sarri, 2006).

**TEEN INTIMATE PARTNER VIOLENCE**     Although teenagers who have been abused as children may continue to be abused by family members in their teenage years, intimate partner violence in dating relationships is becoming quite commonplace and has been largely ignored by health practitioners (Barter, 2009; Betz, 2007; Sears, Byers, Whelan, & Saint-Pierre, 2006; Wolitzky-Taylor et al., 2008). Findings suggest that childhood abuse may be one of the most common factors associated with partner abuse, whether during the teen years or later in life. The abused becomes the abuser (Dube et al., 2005; Merrill et al., 2005; Simonelli, Mullis, Elliot, & Pierce, 2002). Teenage boys are prone to engage in more violent acts, including threats, beatings, and the use of weapons. Teenage girls are more likely to resort to acts of self-protection, including kicking, slapping, shoving, pushing, and emotionally abusing their partners (Banyard, Cross, & Modecki, 2006). Teenagers are less likely to seek help in cases of dating violence, and if they do seek help, they are more likely to talk with peers rather than parents, other adults, or authority figures (Black, Tolman, Callahan, Saunders, & Weisz, 2009).

Dating violence occurs in teen heterosexual and same-sex relationships and cuts across ethnic/racial and socioeconomic strata. Research findings vary as to whether the incidence of abuse in gay or lesbian relationships is higher or lower than that in heterosexual teen relationships (Barter, 2009). Lesbian women or gay men may be less likely to report partner abuse fearing authorities will question the validity of their relationships (Freedner, Freed, Yang, & Austin, 2002; Lamberg, 2000; Rivara et al., 2007). Teens may be particularly vulnerable due to their inexperience in dating, susceptibility to peer pressure, and reluctance to tell adults about what is happening. They may also have difficulty defining abuse and may think that they are in love (Betz, 2007).

Adolescents may really want advice from parents and adults on how to make good choices; however, they rarely receive such advice (Wolfe, 2006). In effect, teens primarily receive warnings and threats of possible punitive consequences from parents, thus making teens less likely to communicate with them (Wolfe, 2006). Because dating violence is a significant problem among adolescents, it needs to be addressed by early detection, prevention, and intervention. School-based programs may assist in alleviating this problem (Wolitzky-Taylor et al., 2008). Health care providers who treat adolescents and teens need to be aware of the incidence of teenage dating violence and be vigilant in screening clients for signs of abuse, providing them with educational information, and referring them to appropriate resources.

**ADULT INTIMATE PARTNER VIOLENCE**     Although men are abused, the incidence of women being abused is much more frequent (Lamberg, 2000). Women with a history of abuse have significantly higher utilization of health care services, and costs continue to rise, even if the woman leaves the abusive situation. Increased utilization of services includes inpatient hospitalizations, outpatient and emergency visits, and mental health services. IPV has a major impact on health care resources, and efforts to identify its occurrence, its resulting consequences, and ways of addressing the problem are clearly needed (Rivara et al., 2007; Wong et al., 2008).

IPV may involve isolation, threats, intimidation, blaming, or using children to control a spouse. Those who experience it and those who witness it both suffer. Domestic violence damages family and social relationships, from early childhood throughout one's adult life.

Abusers may cancel their partners' medical appointments, change medications, or threaten to carry out violent acts while the partner sleeps, thus resulting in sleep deprivation. For gay men and women, there may be an added threat that the abuser will reveal the partner's sexual orientation to friends and colleagues who are unaware of the living arrangements. Same-sex partners may also be afraid to report abuse for fear of repercussions from prejudiced health care providers (Lamberg, 2000; Rivara et al., 2007).

Individuals in abusive relationships may have frequent injuries that they claim were accidental. Emergency department or primary care physicians may miss or dismiss cases of abuse, not wanting to ask or know how an injury occurred (Lamberg, 2000; Sugg, Thompson, Thompson, Maiuro, & Rivara, 1999). Clients may also have decreased self-esteem, be depressed or anxious, have headaches and chronic pain, and gastrointestinal and gynecological symptoms (Coker, Smith, Bethea, King, & McKeown, 2000).

When domestic violence begins or increases during pregnancy, both the mother and the unborn child are at risk. Studies show that women abused before or during pregnancy often continue to experience abuse after delivery, putting the health of both the mother and child in jeopardy (Martin, Mackie, Kupper, Buescher, & Moracco, 2001; Reichenheim, Patricio, & Moraes, 2008). Children who grow up in abusive homes are more likely to have behavioral problems than other children and are also more likely to become abusers themselves (Mayo Clinic, 2009). The issue of domestic violence is a public issue, as well as a criminal matter. Early identification and development of prevention strategies are key to reducing and eventually eradicating domestic abuse (Klevens & Whitaker, 2007).

## Elder Abuse

Elder abuse, a growing problem, includes any intended or careless action that results in harm or serious risk of harm to an older person, usually identified as anyone over the age of 60 (Hildreth, 2009). Although evidence suggests that many thousands of older Americans have been abused, there are no official national statistics. Conservative estimates indicate 1 to 2 million older Americans have been injured, abused, exploited, or otherwise mistreated. This number may be grossly underestimated, because only 1 in 14 elder abuse incidents are brought to the attention of the authorities (National Center on Elder Abuse, 2006). It is imperative that we develop and implement prevention and management strategies (Ploeg, Fear, Hutchinson, MacMillan, & Bolan, 2009).

When we think of abuse, we tend to think of physical abuse, yet this is the least common form of elder abuse. When physical abuse does occur, it can be difficult to distinguish from the normal changes that occur during aging. Depression, weight loss, bruising, and poor wound healing may all be attributed to normal aging, yet they can also be signs of abuse or neglect. Conversely, bruises and fractures may be attributed to abuse but be the result of poor balance and falls in the home or in a nursing facility (Utley, 1999). Common age-related changes, including use of blood thinners, may increase normal or accidental bruising, and frequent trips to the doctor are not uncommon with elderly people.

Signs of abuse may include slap marks, burns, withdrawal of the individual from normal activities, bruises around the breasts or genital areas, sudden changes in finances, untreated bedsores, lack of medical or dental care, poor hygiene, and unclean clothing (National Center on Elder Abuse, 2006). Bruises 5 cm or greater and bruises on the head, neck, lateral arm, or posterior torso should alert a health care provider that the client may be being abused (Wiglesworth et al., 2009).

The majority of abusers are family members, most frequently a spouse or adult child who is caring for and living with the individual. Most often, the abuse takes place in the home; however, abuse can also occur in a long-term care facility, a nursing home, or an assisted living facility (DeHart et al., 2009; Ploeg et al., 2009). Underreporting of elder abuse may be the result of lack of knowledge, fear of making the wrong decision, or a tendency to deny the behavior. Abused older people may also be ashamed of their child's or partner's behavior and thus not want to admit there is a problem. Fear of retaliation, being sent to a nursing home, or being abandoned are other reasons why they may choose not to report abuse. Should a competent individual refuse assistance, those wishes must be honored. Educational pamphlets, providing helpful resources, should be left with the older person for future reference, if desired (Utley, 1999).

The United States has nearly 17,000 nursing homes with a total of 1.6 million residents, and numbers are expected to climb to 6.6 million by 2050 (National Center on Elder Abuse, 2006; U.S. Census Bureau, 2002). Forms of mistreatment in nursing homes are similar to those found in home settings and include physical and sexual assault, neglect, inappropriate restraints, financial abuse, isolation, threats, and denial of personal choice. Residents may be irritable, disoriented, or uncooperative, and busy health providers may lose patience with them.

## Abuse of Individuals with Disabilities

People with disabilities are at greater risk for experiencing neglect and abuse than those without disabilities (Curry, Hassouneh-Phillips, Johnston-Silverberg, 2001; Hassouneh-Phillips & Curry, 2002; Powers et al., 2002; Powers, McNeff, Curry, Saxton, & Elliott, 2004). Types of abuse experienced by individuals with disabilities are similar to those experienced by other groups and include physical, sexual, emotional, and financial abuse, as well as neglect and manipulation of medications. One additional form of abuse experienced by these individuals includes destroying or disabling medical equipment or refusing to provide necessary personal assistance (Hassouneh-Phillips, 2005).

Individuals with disabilities may rely on social support services, face inaccessible buildings, be unable to drive, and live in situations where they are isolated. These environmental factors have been shown to increase risk of abuse (Hassouneh-Phillips, 2005). Many people fail to report abuse because of fear of the abuser, who may be someone with whom they live and depend on for assistance. In addition, shelters are rarely equipped to meet the needs of individuals with disabilities so they have few, if any, options. In addition, they may not have access to tools and resources to protect themselves (Powers et al., 2002).

Women with physical disabilities are frequently abused by more than one individual, and they experience abuse for longer periods of time than women who do not have disabilities (Curry et al., 2001; Hassouneh-Phillips & Curry, 2002; Young, Nosek, Howland, Chanpong, & Rintala, 1997). When a woman with a disability is abused, her chances of maintaining her health and living independently in the community decrease (Powers et al., 2002). Previous studies have suggested that women with disabilities are abused more than men, but those statistics may be skewed because men may be less likely than women to be asked about abuse and more reluctant to report abuse and admit their lack of control (Cohen, Forte, DuMont, Hyman, & Ronans, 2006).

Consequences of abuse can be severe for people with disabilities because they may not be able to get out of bed independently, be unable to leave the house, lack access to a telephone, or be totally reliant on the abuser for many of their needs. Abuse by personal care attendants (PCAs) has been well documented. PCAs may arrive for work late or leave early, steal from their employers, verbally abuse the client, or refuse to provide medication or other medically necessary services. Clients may endure abuse because of how difficult it is to find replacements (Hassouneh-Phillips, 2005).

As discussed, all victims of abuse and neglect may experience ramifications, including depression, anxiety, physical injury, stress-related illness, migraine headaches, drug or alcohol abuse, and even suicide. Those with disabilities face even more problems, such as health deterioration and inability to provide self-care, resulting in difficulty maintaining a job or living independently (Powers et al., 2002). In a study of abused women with disabilities, Hassouneh-Phillips (2005) documented disturbing scenarios. Several women said caregivers taunted them. One pretended to give a woman her telephone, then laughed and pulled it away at the last moment. Another PCA threatened to leave and never come back from break. Still another PCA would put the client's cushion backwards in the chair and put her pants on twisted, laughing at her and leaving her quite uncomfortable. One woman spoke of how the PCA's boyfriend pulled her hair and kicked her chair. Another said she remained in an abusive relationship because she could not go to a shelter with her male caregiver; the facility was for women only.

Strategies to reduce or eliminate abuse and violence include increasing education programs for individuals with disabilities and for their health care providers; modifying regulations so that clients who rely on public assistance are able to select their own PCAs and pay them competitive wages and benefits; establishing wheelchair-accessible emergency transportation systems and shelters; and ensuring that all individuals with disabilities have an accessible telephone or alert system (National Research Council, 1996).

## STRATEGIES FOR HEALTH PROFESSIONALS

Health professionals work closely with clients and families, often in home settings, and are in a unique position to identify abuse and neglect. As noted earlier in this chapter, though, many health care professionals find it difficult to identify and report suspected cases of abuse, even though they are mandated reporters of certain forms of abuse.

Barriers may include cultural customs, fear of offending or erring in judgment, unclear policies, limited resources, legal complications, clinician or victim detachment, personal history of abuse, gender bias, or failure to recognize abuse (Andrews, 2008; Flaherty et al., 2004; Pinn & Chunko, 1997; Sugg & Inui, 1992; Sugg & Maiuro, 1999). Providers may have difficulty defining abuse and feel that asking probing questions may negatively affect their relationship with clients or family members (Lamberg, 2000; Lazenbatt & Freeman, 2006; Rosenberg, Fenley, Johnson, & Short, 1997; Wong et al., 2008). They may not think there is time to adequately question family members and make reports to appropriate authorities (Kellogg & Committee on Child Abuse and Neglect, 2007; Sugg & Inui, 1992; Sugg & Maiuro, 1999). Sufficient training, knowledge, and resources may be lacking (Flaherty et al., 2004; Lazenbatt & Freeman, 2006).

One study of nurses, doctors, and dentists working in primary care settings found that 60 percent (251) said they had seen a case of suspicious child physical abuse; however, only 47 percent (201) had reported it to the authorities (Lazenbatt & Freeman, 2006). In a *Nursing Standard* survey conducted in 2007, 50 percent of the nurses reported they would not report abuse for fear of misinterpreting the situation; 16 percent did not know what to do if they suspected abuse, and 34 percent reported they would have benefited from greater support and additional education (Andrews, 2008).

Emergency department or primary care physicians may miss or dismiss cases of abuse, not wanting to ask or know how an injury occurred (Lamberg, 2000; Sugg et al., 1999). Consider the case of the pregnant woman who went to her doctor with bruises on her abdomen and face. She told the doctor she was clumsy and fell into a bookcase. The physician noted in the medical record that the injuries were inconsistent with the claimed injury but said nothing to the client, and the woman remained with her abusive husband for several years. If the doctor had questioned her about the injuries and mentioned suspected abuse, she might have felt more comfortable disclosing the abuse and sought help earlier (Buel, 2002).

Health providers need to be vigilant about observing bruises, burns, and other unexplained or atypical injuries suggestive of abuse. Other indicators include the appearance of malnutrition, dehydration, and poor hygiene, especially among people who are dependent on others for care. Failure to administer medication, provide wound care, or frequently change a client's position is medical neglect, whether or not a personal or professional caregiver is responsible.

In all 50 states, health care providers are mandated to report child abuse. Practitioners have statutory protection against professional liability suits for reports made in good faith (Kellogg & Committee on Child Abuse and Neglect, 2007). Although there are currently no nationally mandated requirements for reporting elder abuse, some states may protect older adults. It is important for health care providers to know state regulations regarding mandatory reporting (National Center on Elder Abuse, 2006) and to make referrals to appropriate professionals. Student interns suspecting abuse should notify their immediate supervisors so proper action can be taken. In most instances, failure to report suspected abuse or neglect where mandated can result in legal penalties or fines, loss of license, and imprisonment, as well as further abuse to the victim (Barnett, Miller-Perrin, & Perrin, 1997; Bird et al., 1998; Buel, 2002; Swagerty et al., 1999).

The Joint Commission (formerly the Joint Commission on Accreditation of Healthcare Organizations) requires that all hospitals institute written policies to improve documentation of abuse (Commission on Accreditation of Healthcare Operations, 1997; Hyman, 1996). Although health care professionals practicing outside of the hospital setting may not be held to this standard, it is imperative that all providers develop screening policies, safety planning, and referral systems to meet the needs of individuals who may be experiencing neglect or abuse (Doherty, 2009). Too often medical records lack sufficient details about injuries or other signs of abuse. If a client later becomes involved in criminal or civil actions, a health care provider's testimony or records may be critical.

Care must be taken, however, when making assumptions about possible neglect and abuse. If health professionals are concerned, it is essential to establish a safe environment where one can open a dialogue with the client by saying, for example, "I'm concerned that some of your medical problems may be the result of someone hurting you" or "I am aware that abuse and neglect are commonplace, so I ask all of my clients these questions" (see Box 15–1).

Listen carefully to client responses and document conversations (Cole, 2000). Studies have shown that women will disclose abuse in response to screening (Ramsay, Richardson, Carter, Davidson, & Feder, 2002; Wathen & MacMillan, 2003). An approach that includes empathy and empowerment is important to assist people who have been abused to disclose their situations to health providers (Wong et al., 2008).

An attempt should be made to interview clients and caregivers separately, take notes, and compare information. Discrepancies must be documented, using the exact words used by each. If the client says the name of an abuser, that should be included in the documentation. Furthermore, a body map or photographs may be useful in documenting injuries (Buel, 2002). Should a competent adult refuse assistance, those wishes must be honored.

## BOX 15–1   Sample Questions

- Do you feel safe?
- Is anyone hurting you at home or anywhere else?
- Does your partner humiliate you?
- Has your partner ever made you engage in sex when you didn't want to?
- Are you receiving adequate care?
- Is there anything I can do to help you?
- Has anyone touched you without your consent?
- Has anyone made you do things you didn't want to do?
- Has anyone taken anything that was yours without asking permission?
- Has anyone scolded or threatened you?
- Have you signed any documents you did not understand?
- Are you afraid of anyone at home?
- Has anyone failed to help you take care of yourself when you needed help?

(American Medical Association guidelines, 1996)

Informational brochures can be important tools in providing information to clients (Utley, 1999). The American Medical Association provides manuals on the topics of child, intimate partner, and elder abuse (American Medical Association, 2000). Providers may want to obtain and place informational brochures in their offices, where they are readily available to clients. Home care providers may consider having brochures with them to distribute to clients in their homes. Additional information is available on the Internet from the CDC. Providers should be available to assist clients in reading and interpreting information.

The high rates of childhood sexual abuse suggest that health providers may unknowingly be working with adult survivors. Physical and emotional trauma resulting from abuse may result in chronic headaches, low back pain, depression, fear, anxiety, gastrointestinal disorders, posttraumatic stress disorder, and other medical conditions (Schachter, Stalker, & Teram, 1999). Clients presenting with those symptoms should be screened for potential abuse and neglect.

Maintaining a client's sense of safety in the clinic is of utmost importance for everyone, especially for people who have been neglected and abused. In a study of female clients who had been sexually abused as children and received physical therapy as adults, Schachter, Stalker, and Teram (1999) found that many of the women experienced fear of being hurt or abused during treatments. Some stated that being in an enclosed room with a male therapist led to a state of panic. Others indicated that being undressed behind a curtain made them feel vulnerable, knowing that someone could open the curtain and walk in at any time. Some women were unable to do exercises in which they had to spread their legs. This would trigger the emotions they experienced during childhood abuse. Some were unable to return to therapy following the first treatment session.

Good communication skills are of the utmost importance to develop rapport and a sense of trust. Appropriate positioning that makes clients feel comfortable is also beneficial. A person's sense of control over his or her own body is of paramount concern. Health care providers should ask permission to progress through each step of treatment, be sensitive to client concerns, and validate their needs. If any touch becomes uncomfortable, stop. Recognize, too, that what might be comfortable for a client one day may not be well tolerated the next.

Research to determine optimal methods for screening clients suspected of being abused is ongoing (MacMillan et al., 2006). Most training for health care providers focuses on detection and mandatory reporting. More training needs to be focused on specific client needs. Understanding the problem, recognizing the signs and symptoms, and developing open lines of communication with clients may assist health professionals in better meeting client needs.

## Summary

In this chapter, we investigated abuse and neglect across the life span. Abuse and neglect can affect anyone, regardless of age, socioeconomic status, gender, sexual orientation, or other factors. Abuse can occur at home and in medical facilities. Although neglect may be intentional or unintentional, abuse is always about power and control and can be physical, psychological, sexual, financial, or a combination of all four. Abuse can lead to long-term psychological and physical impairments. Both abusers and those who are abused may attempt to hide the abuse.

To adequately address this public health issue, health providers need to be educated to screen for signs of abuse or neglect on a regular basis with all clients. Providers may inadvertently be treating victims of abuse and not understand how previous or ongoing abusive relationships may affect interactions. Information regarding abuse and neglect should be included in all health care providers' educational curricula. Evidence suggests that health professionals may be reluctant to report suspected abuse, but this must change. The only way to ensure the safety of those who are vulnerable is to reinforce appropriate methods of screening and encourage providers to take responsibility for reporting abuse to the appropriate authorities, especially where it is mandated by law. However, if a competent adult prefers not to report a case of abuse, those wishes must be respected. Nonetheless, it is important to educate the client about available resources that can provide assistance should the client wish to seek help in the future.

## Reflective Questions

1. Best health care practices require that all health care providers screen clients for abuse and neglect.
   a. How do you feel about screening clients for abuse and neglect?
   b. What barriers do you anticipate?
   c. What would you do/say if a client revealed an ongoing case of abuse to you?
2. Have you ever personally experienced abuse and neglect or do you know someone who has? If so, did you or the individual seek help?
   a. If yes, how did you seek help, and what was the response?
   b. If no, why not?
   c. What might have made it easier to seek help?
3. The most common form of abuse occurs at the hands of men abusing women and children, but men can also be victims of violence. If a male client revealed to you that his wife or teenage son or daughter was abusing him,
   a. how would that make you feel?
   b. how would you respond?
4. a. What might you do to educate clients and members of the community about the prevalence of abuse and neglect across the life span?
   b. How could you make them aware of possible interventions to prevent further abuse?
5. M. J. Rawls, the student introduced at the beginning of this chapter, did not know how to distinguish normal childhood injuries from a case of childhood abuse. What signs and symptoms would you look for to assist in making this determination?

## Case Study

Mrs. Putnam lived independently until 6 months ago when she sustained a cerebral vascular accident (stroke). She was hospitalized for a brief period of time, and then, unable to return home, was discharged to a skilled nursing facility located approximately 12 miles from her son's house. Her speech is currently impaired, and she has difficulty communicating. Unhappy in the facility, she has asked her family to take her home. She complains that staff members often leave her cold and in a state of undress when they are called away to assist others—sometimes right in the middle of her sponge bath. She reports that staff members are stealing her money and candy, that the call bell is frequently left out of her reach, and she cannot signal the staff when she needs to use the bathroom. As a result, she frequently wets the bed and reports that staff members treat her roughly when they change her and the bed linens. Staff members deny these allegations and indicate that Mrs. Putnam is confused. Her son and daughter-in-law love Mrs. Putnam, but both work full time and are unavailable during the day. In addition, they have five children and do not have room in the house to accommodate Mrs. Putnam and her special needs.

1. What types of abuse or neglect may be occurring in the nursing home?
2. Might Mrs. Putnam be exaggerating conditions in the facility in order to return home? What might you do to assess the situation?
3. What might family members do to intervene?
4. a. What obstacles might prevent the family from taking her home?
   b. What accommodations might families make to allow her to come home?

## References

American Medical Association. (2000). *Diagnostic and treatment guidelines.* Retrieved from http://ama-assn.org/pub/releases/assault/orderfrm.html

American Medical Association guidelines for doctors on detecting elder abuse and neglect (1996). *Aging.* Retrieved from http://findarticles.com/p/articles/mi_m1000/is_n367/ai_18200024

American Medical Student Association. (2008). *Child abuse and neglect.* Retrieved from http://www.amsa.org/programs/gpit/child.cfm

Andrews, J. (2008). Travesty of trust. *Nursing Standard, 23*(1), 20–21.

Banyard, V. L., Cross, C., & Modecki, K. L. (2006). Interpersonal violence in adolescence: Ecological correlates of self-reported perpetration. *Journal of Interpersonal Violence, 21,* 1314–1332.

Barnett, O. W., Miller-Perrin, C. L., & Perrin, R. D. (1997). *Family violence across the lifespan: An introduction.* Newbury Park, CA: Sage.

Barter, C. (2009). In the name of love: Partner abuse and violence in teenage relationships. *British Journal of Social Work, 39,* 211–233.

Betz, C. L. (2007). Teen dating violence: An unrecognized health care need. *Journal of Pediatric Nursing: Nursing Care of Children and Families, 22*(6), 427–429.

Bird, P. E., Harrington, D. T., Barillo, D. J., McSweeney, A., Shirani, K. Z., & Goodwin, C. W. (1998). Elder abuse: A call to action. *Journal of Burn Care and Rehabilitation, 19,* 522–527.

Black, A., Heyman, R. D., & Smith-Slep, A. M. (2001). Risk factors for child physical abuse. *Aggression and Violent Behavior, 6,* 121–188.

Black, B. M., Tolman, R. M., Callahan, M., Saunders, D. G., & Weisz, A. N. (2009). When will adolescents tell someone about dating violence victimization? *Violence Against Women, 14*(7), 741–758.

Brickner, P. W. (2009). Elder abuse prevention: Emerging trends and promising strategies. *Care Management Journals, 10*(2), 77–78.

Buel, S. M. (2002). Treatment guidelines for healthcare providers' interventions with domestic violence victims: Experience from the USA. *International Journal of Gynecology and Obstetrics, 78*(1), S49–S54.

Centers for Disease Control and Prevention (2009). *Understanding intimate partner violence.* Retrieved from http://www.cdc.gov/violenceprevention

Child Molestation Research and Prevention Institute, Inc. (2010). *Early diagnosis and effective treatment.* Retrieved from http://childmolestationprevention.org

Cohen, M. M., Forte, T., DuMont, J., Hyman, I., & Ronans, S. (2006). Adding insult to injury: Intimate partner violence among women and men reporting activity limitations. *Annals of Epidemiology, 16*(8), 644–651.

Coker, A. L., Smith, P. H., Bethea, L., King, M. R., & McKeown, R. E. (2000). Physical health consequences of physical and psychological intimate partner violence. *Archives of Family Medicine, 9,* 451–457.

Cole, T. B. (2000). Is domestic screening helpful? *Journal of the American Medical Association, 294*(5), 551–553.

Commission on Accreditation of Healthcare Operations. (1997). *Comprehensive accreditation manual for hospitals* (update 3, pp. PE-10–PE-34). Oakbrook Terrace, IL: Author.

Curry, M. A., Hassouneh-Phillips, D., & Johnston-Silverberg, A. (2001). Abuse of women with disabilities: An ecological model and review. *Violence Against Women International Interdisciplinary Journal, 7*(1), 60–79.

Cyr, M., McDuff, P., & Wright, J. (2006). Prevalence and predictors of dating violence among adolescent female victims of child sexual abuse. *Journal of Interpersonal Violence, 21*(8), 1000–1017.

DeHart, D., Webb, J., & Cornman, C. (2009). Prevention of elder mistreatment in nursing homes: Competencies for direct-care staff. *Journal of Elder Abuse, 21,* 360–378.

Doherty, L. (2009). Recognizing signs of abuse. *Pediatric Nursing, 21*(7), 6–7.

Dube, S. R., Anda, R. F., Whitfield, C. L., Brown, D. W., Felitti, V. J., Dong, M., & Giles, W. H. (2005). Long-term consequences of childhood sexual abuse by gender of victim. *American Journal of Preventative Medicine, 28*(5), 430–438.

Flaherty, E. F., Jones, R., & Sege, R. (2004). Telling their stories: Primary care practitioners' experience evaluating and reporting injuries caused by child abuse. *Child Abuse and Neglect, 28,* 939–945.

Freedner, N., Freed, L. H., Yang, Y. W., & Austin, S. B. (2002). Dating violence among gay, lesbian, and bisexual adolescents: Results from a community survey. *Journal of Adolescent Health, 21,* 469–474.

Goodkind, S., & Sarri, R. C. (2006). The impact of sexual abuse in the lives of young women involved or at risk of involvement with the juvenile justice system. *Violence Against Women, 12*(5), 456–477.

Gray-Vickrey, P. (2001). Protecting the older adult. *Nursing Management, 32*(10), 36–40.

Hassouneh-Phillips, D. (2005). Understanding abuse of women with physical disabilities. An overview of the abuse pathways model. *Advances in Nursing Science, 28*(1), 70–80.

Hassouneh-Phillips, D., & Curry, M. A. (2002). Abuse of women with disabilities: State of the sciences. *Rehabilitation Counseling Bulletin, 45*(2), 96–104.

Hildreth, C. J. (2009). Elder abuse. *Journal of the American Medical Association, 302*(5), 588.

Hyman, A. (1996). Domestic violence: Legal issues for healthcare practitioners and institutions. *Journal of Joint American Medical Associations, 51*(3), 1001–1005.

Kellogg, N. D., & Committee on Child Abuse and Neglect. (2007). Evaluation of suspected child physical abuse. *Pediatrics, 119*1, 1232–1241.

Klevens, J., & Whitaker, D. J. (2007). Primary prevention of child physical abuse and neglect: Gaps and promising directions. *Child Maltreatment, 12*(4), 364–377.

Krugman, R. D. (2001). Time to end health professional neglect of cycle of violence. *The Lancet, 352,* 434.

Lamberg, L. (2000). Domestic violence: What to ask, what to do. *Journal of the American Medical Association, 284*(5), 554–556.

Lazenbatt, A., & Freeman, R. (2006). Recognizing and reporting child physical abuse: A survey of primary healthcare professionals. *Issues in Nursing Practice, 56*(3), 227–236.

MacMillan, H. L., Wathen, C. N., Jamieson, E., Boyle, M., McNutt, L., Worster, A., . . . Webb, M. (2006). Approaches to screening for intimate partner violence in health care settings. *Journal of the American Medical Association, 296*(5), 530–536.

Martin, S. L., Mackie, L., Kupper, L. L., Buescher, P. A., & Moracco, K. E. (2001). Physical abuse of women before, during, and after pregnancy. *Journal of American Medical Association, 285*(12), 1581–1584.

Mayo Clinic. (2009). *Domestic violence against women: Recognizing patterns, seek help.* Retrieved from http://www.mayoclinic.com/health/domestic-violence/WO000444.

Merrill, L. L., Thomsen, C. J., Crouch, J. J., May, P., Gold, S. R., & Milner, J. S. (2005). Predicting adult risk of child physical abuse from childhood exposure to violence: Can interpersonal schemata explain the association? *Journal of Social and Clinical Psychology, 24*(7), 981–1002.

MetLife Mature Market Institute, National Committee for the Prevention of Elder Abuse, & Center for Gerontology at Virginia Polytechnic Institute and State University. (2009, March). *Broken trust: Elders, family and finances.* Westport, CT: MetLife Mature Market Institute. Retrieved from http://www.metlife.com/assets/cao/mmi/publications/studies/mmi-study-broken-trust-elders-family-finances.pdf

National Center on Elder Abuse. (2006). *Nursing home abuse.* Washington, DC: Author. Retrieved from http://www.ncea.aoa.gov.

National Research Council. (1996). *Understanding violence against women.* Washington, DC: National Academy Press.

Paavilainen, E., Astedt-Kurki, P., Paunonen-Ilmonen, M., & Laippala, P. (2002). Caring for maltreated children: A challenge for health care education. *Journal of Advanced Nursing, 37*(6), 551–557.

Pinn, V. W., & Chunko, M. T. (1997). The diverse faces of violence: Minority women and domestic abuse. *Academy of Medicine, 72,* 565–571.

Ploeg, J., Fear, J., Hutchinson, B., MacMillan, H., & Bolan, G. (2009). A systematic review of interventions for elder abuse. *Journal of Elder Abuse, 21,* 167–210.

Powers, L. E., Curry, M. A., Oschwald, M., Maley, S., Saxton, M., & Eckels, K. (2002). Barriers and strategies in addressing abuse. A survey of disabled women's experiences. *Journal of Rehabilitation, 68*(1), 4–13.

Powers, L. E., McNeff, E., Curry, M., Saxton, M., & Elliott, D. (2004). *Preliminary findings on the abuse experiences of men with disabilities.* Portland, OR: Oregon Health & Science University Center on Self-Determination.

Ramsay, J., Richardson, J., Carter, Y. H., Davidson, L. L., & Feder, G. (2002). Should health professionals screen women for domestic violence? Systematic review. *British Medical Journal, 325,* 314.

Reichenheim, M. E., Patricio, T. F., & Moraes, C. L. (2008). Detecting intimate partner violence during pregnancy: Awareness-raising indicators for use by primary healthcare professionals. *Public Health, 122,* 716–724.

Rivara, F. P., Anderson, M. L., Fishman, P., Bonomi, A. E., Reid, R. J., Carrell, D., & Thompson, R. S. (2007). Healthcare utilization and costs for women with a history of intimate partner violence. *American Journal of Preventative Medicine, 32*(2), 89–96.

Rosenberg, M., Fenley, M. A., Johnson, D., & Short, L. (1997). Bridging prevention and practice and family violence. *Academy of Medicine, 72,* 513–518.

Rovi, S., Chen, P. H., & Johnson M. S. (2004). The economic burden of hospitalizations associated with child abuse and neglect. *American Journal of Public Health, 94,* 586–590.

Runyon, M., Deblinger, E., Ryan, E., & Thakkar-Kolar, R. (2004). An overview of child physical abuse: Developing an integrated child treatment programme. *Trauma, Violence and Abuse, 5*(1), 65–85.

Schachter, C. L., Stalker, C. A., & Teram, E. (1999). Toward sensitive practice: Issues for physical therapists working with survivors of childhood sexual abuse. *Physical Therapy, 79*(3), 248–261.

Sears, H. A., Byers, E. S., Whelan, J. J., & Saint-Pierre, M. (2006). "If it hurts you, then it is not a joke." *Journal of Interpersonal Violence, 21*(9), 1191–1207.

Simonelli, F. J., Mullis, T., Elliot, A. N., & Pierce, T. H. (2002). Abuse by siblings and subsequent experiences of violence within the dating relationship. *Journal of Interpersonal Violence, 17,* 103–121.

Sugg, N., & Inui, T. (1992). Opening Pandora's box: Primary care physicians' response to domestic violence. *Journal of the American Medical Association, 267*(3), 3157–3160.

Sugg, N., & Maiuro, R. (1999). Domestic violence and primary care. Attitudes, practices and beliefs. *Archives of Family Medicine, 8,* 301–306.

Sugg, N. K., Thompson, R. S., Thompson, D. C., Maiuro, R., & Rivara, F. P. (1999, July–August). Domestic violence and primary care: Attitudes, practices, and beliefs. *Archives of Family Medicine, 8*(4), 301–306.

Swagerty, D. L., Takahashi, P. Y., & Evans, J. M. (1999). Elder mistreatment. *American Family Physician, 59*(10), 2804–2808.

Taylor, J., & Spencer, N. (2000). Social, economic and political content of parenting. *Advocates of Diseases in Childhood, 82*(2), 113–120.

U.S. Census Bureau. (2002). *Industry statistics sampler: NAICS 62311 nursing care facilities.* Washington, DC: Author.

U.S. Department of Health and Human Services, Administration on Children, Youth, and Families. (2006). *Child maltreatment.* Washington, DC: U.S. Government Printing Office.

U.S. Department of Health and Human Services, Administration on Children, Youth, and Families. (2009). *Child maltreatment.* Washington, DC: Author. Retrieved from http://www.acf.hhs.gov

Utley, R. (1999). Screening and intervention in elder abuse. *Home Care Provider, 4*(5), 198–201.

Wang, C. T., & Holton, J. (2007). *Total estimated cost of child abuse and neglect in the United States. Economic impact study.* Retrieved from https://secure.goozm.com/userfiles/3595 9537961.pdf

Wathen, C., & MacMillan, H. L. (2003). Interventions for violence against women: Systematic review. *Journal of the American Medical Association 289,* 589–600.

Wekerle, C., Leung, E., Wall, A., MacMillan, H., Boyle, M., Trocme, N., & Waechter, R. (2009). The contribution of childhood emotional abuse to teen dating violence among child protective-services-involved youth. *Child Abuse & Neglect, 33,* 45–58.

Wiglesworth, A., Austin, R., Corona, M., Schneider, D., Liao, S., Gibbs, L., & Mosqueda, L. (2009). Bruising as a marker of physical elder abuse. *Journal of American Geriatric Society, 57,* 1191–1196.

Wolfe, D. A. (2006). Preventing violence in relationships: Psychosocial science addressing complex social issues. *Canadian Psychology, 47*(1), 44–50.

Wolitzky-Taylor, K. B., Ruggiero, K. J., Danieldson, C. K., Resnick, H. S., Hanson, R. F., Smith, D. W., . . . Kilpatrick, D. G. (2008). Prevalence and correlates of

dating violence in a national sample of adolescents. *Journal of the American Academy of Child and Adolescent Psychiatry, 47*(7), 755–762.

Wong, S. L. F., Wester, F., Mol, S., Romkens, R., Hezemans, D., & Lagro-Janssen, T. (2008). Talking matters: Abused women's views on disclosure of partner abuse to the family doctor and its role in handling abuse situations. *Patient Education and Counseling, 70,* 386–394.

Young, M. E., Nosek, M. A., Howland, C., Chanpong, G., & Rintala, D. H. (1997). Prevalence of abuse of women with physical disabilities. *Archives of Physical Medicine and Rehabilitation, 78*(12, Suppl. 5), S34–S38.

## Additional Resources

### Domestic Abuse References

National Domestic Violence Hotline
www.ndvh.org
1-800-799-7233

U.S. Department of Justice, Office on Violence Against Women
www.ovw.usdoj.gov

Domestic Abuse Helpline for Men and Women
www.dahmw.org
1-888-7HELPLINE
1-888-743-5754

Office for Victims of Crime
www.ojp.usdoj.gov
1-800-851-3420

National Teen Dating Abuse Hotline
www.loveisrespect.org
1-866-331-9474

Abuse Victim Hotline
www.avhotline.org
1-877-4-IT-TO-STOP

U.S. Department of Justice Federal Abuse Hotline
1-800-799-SAFE

### Child Abuse References

Childhelp
www.childhelp.org
1-800-4-A-CHILD

U.S. Department of Health and Human Services, Administration for Children and Families
www.acf.hhs.gov

Office for Victims of Crime
www.ojp.usdoj.gov
1-800-851-3420

Abuse Victim Hotline
www.avhotline.org
1-877-4-IT-TO-STOP

U.S. Department of Justice Federal Abuse Hotline
1-800-799-SAFE

### Elder Abuse References

National Center on Elder Abuse
www.ncea.aoa.gov
1-800-677-1116

Administration on Aging Elder Abuse Prevention and Treatment Resource Page
www.aoa.dhhs.gov/abuse

U.S. Department of Justice Federal Abuse Hotline
1-800-799-SAFE

Senior Justice League
www.seniorjustice.com

Office for Victims of Crime
www.ojp.usdoj.gov
1-800-851-3420

Abuse Victim Hotline
www.avhotline.org
1-877-4-IT-TO-STOP

# INDEX